Deep Brain Stimulation for Neurological Disorders

Toru Itakura
Editor

Deep Brain Stimulation for Neurological Disorders

Theoretical Background and Clinical Application

Springer

Editor
Toru Itakura, MD, PhD
Department of Neurological Surgery
Koyo Hospital, Wakayama
Japan

ISBN 978-3-319-08475-6 ISBN 978-3-319-08476-3 (eBook)
DOI 10.1007/978-3-319-08476-3
Springer Cham Heidelberg Dordrecht London New York

Library of Congress Control Number: 2014949146

Printed on acid-free paper

Springer is part of Springer Science+Business Media (www.springer.com)

Preface

Chronic electrical stimulation of the brain has become standard surgical therapy for Parkinson's disease and other neurological disorders. Numerous scientific papers have demonstrated that patients with Parkinson's disease who receive deep brain stimulation show excellent outcomes without serious complications. Recently, this surgical intervention has been applied to many other neurological diseases such as involuntary movements, intractable pain and psychiatric disorders, including depression and obsessive-compulsive disorder.

The number of neurosurgeons embarking on this new surgery has recently increased owing to the outstanding development of surgical techniques in the electrical stimulation of the brain. For young neurosurgeons, an introductory textbook is essential for good progress in skills and for safe and accurate surgery in this area. The aim of this book, therefore, is to show the complete range of knowledge requisite to the scientific background of the diseases as well as to explain the detailed surgical techniques necessary. The target audience for this endeavor is young neurosurgeons, neurologists, psychiatrists and other medical staff interested in this operation.

In editing this volume, I have listed outstanding scientists and international experts in the field. The book is divided into two main parts: the basic background of brain stimulation, and clinical studies on deep brain stimulation. The first part will discuss the anatomical and functional scientific background concerning the basal ganglia, thalamus and other related brain structures of movement disorders, pain, epilepsy and psychiatric diseases. The second part describes clinical studies of brain stimulation on symptoms, and surgical techniques in movement disorders and psychiatric diseases.

It is a great honor to publish this updated book on electrical brain stimulation. It is sincerely hoped that it will contribute to the development of this type of surgery for various neurological disorders. I also hope that the book will contribute to the rescue of the lives of sufferers and to the development in the quality of life of patients with various neurological disorders.

Wakayama, Japan　　　Toru Itakura, MD, PhD

Contents

Contributors

Takashi Agari, MD, PhD Department of Neurological Surgery, Okayama University Graduate School of Medicine, Dentistry and Pharmaceutical Sciences, Okayama, Japan

Gordon Baltuch, MD, PhD Department of Neurosurgery, University of Pennsylvania, Philadelphia, PA, USA

Satomi Chiken, PhD Division of System Neurophysiology, National Institute for Physiological Sciences, Okazaki, Japan

Isao Date, MD, PhD Department of Neurological Surgery, Okayama University Graduate School of Medicine, Dentistry and Pharmaceutical Sciences, Okayama, Japan

Chikashi Fukaya, MD, PhD Division of Applied System Neuroscience, Department of Neurological Surgery, Nihon University School of Medicine, Tokyo, Japan

Satoshi Goto, MD, PhD Department of Motor Neuroscience and Neurotherapeutics, Institute of Health Bioscience, Graduate School of Medical Science, University of Tokushima, Tokushima City, Tokushima Prefecture, Japan

Toru Itakura, MD, PhD Department of Neurological Surgery, Koyo Hospital, Wakayama, Japan

Hidefumi Ito, MD, PhD Department of Neurology, Wakayama Medical University, Wakayama, Japan

Yoichi Katayama, MD, PhD Division of Neurosurgery, Department of Neurological Surgery, Nihon University School of Medicine, Tokyo, Japan

Kazutaka Kobayashi, MD, PhD Division of Neurosurgery, Department of Neurological Surgery, Nihon University School of Medicine, Tokyo, Japan

Paul Koch, MD Department of Neurosurgery, University of Pennsylvania, Philadelphia, PA, USA

Nir Lipsman, MD, PhD Department of Neurosurgery, Toronto Western Hospital, Toronto, ON, Canada

Andres M. Lozano, MD, PhD Department of Neurosurgery, Toronto Western Hospital, Toronto, ON, Canada

Patrick Mertens, MD, PhD Neurological Hospital Lyon, Lyon, France

Yasushi Miyagi, MD, PhD Department of Stereotactic and Functional Neurosurgery, Kaizuka Hospital, Fukuoka, Japan

Ryoma Morigaki, MD Department of Motor Neuroscience and Neurotherapeutics, Institute of Health Bioscience, Graduate School of Medical Science, University of Tokushima, Tokushima City, Tokushima Prefecture, Japan

Atsushi Nambu, MD, PhD Division of System Neurophysiology, National Institute for Physiological Sciences, Okazaki, Japan

Hiroki Nishibayashi, PhD, MD Department of Neurological Surgery, Wakayama Medical University Hospital, Wakayama, Japan

Mitsuhiro Ogura, MD, PhD Department of Neurological Surgery, Wakayama Medical University, Wakayama, Japan

Gustavo Polo, MD, MSc Department of Neurosurgery, Neurological Hospital Lyon, Lyon, France

Marc Sindou, MD, PhD Neurological Hospital Lyon, Lyon, France

Kenji Sugiyama, MD, PhD Department of Neurosurgery, Hamamatsu University School of Medicine, Hamamatsu, Shizuoka, Japan

Takaomi Taira, MD, PhD Department of Neurosurgery, Tokyo Women's Medical University, Tokyo, Japan

Takamitsu Yamamoto, MD, PhD Division of Applied System Neuroscience, Department of Neurological Surgery, Nihon University School of Medicine, Tokyo, Japan

Atsuo Yoshino, MD, PhD Division of Neurosurgery, Department of Neurological Surgery, Nihon University School of Medicine, Tokyo, Japan

Functional Circuitry of the Basal Ganglia

1

Atsushi Nambu

1.1 Introduction

The basal ganglia are a group of nuclei lying at the base of the forebrain. They control cortical activity through the thalamus together with the cerebellum, and control voluntary movements and other higher cortical functions. Lesions in the basal ganglia result in severe disturbances in the execution of voluntary movements as typically observed in movement disorders such as Parkinson's disease and dystonia. On the other hand, stereotactic surgery by making a small lesion or applying electrical stimulation (i.e., deep brain stimulation, DBS) in the basal ganglia ameliorates the symptom of movement disorders. In order to understand the pathophysiology of these movement disorders and the mechanism of stereotactic surgery, it is essential to understand the circuitry of the basal ganglia. Knowledge on the electrophysiological properties, such as firing rates and patterns, and the somatotopic organization of the individual nucleus of the basal ganglia also helps us to identify the right target during stereotactic surgery.

A. Nambu, MD, PhD
Division of System Neurophysiology, National Institute for Physiological Sciences, Okazaki, Japan

Department of Physiological Sciences, Graduate University for Advanced Studies, Okazaki, Japan
e-mail: nambu@nips.ac.jp

1.2 Composition of the Basal Ganglia

The basal ganglia are composed of the following four nuclei (Fig. 1.1).

1. The striatum, which comprises the caudate nucleus, putamen, and ventral striatum (including the nucleus accumbens and olfactory tubercle).
2. The globus pallidus, which consists of the external (GPe) and internal (GPi) segments.
3. The subthalamic nucleus (STN).
4. The substantia nigra, which is divided into the pars reticulata (SNr) and pars compacta (SNc).

The above nuclei can be grouped functionally into four categories.

1. Input nuclei: striatum and STN, which receive cortical inputs.
2. Output nuclei: GPi and SNr, which project outside the basal ganglia to the thalamus and the brain stem.
3. Connecting nucleus: GPe, which connects the input nuclei to the output nuclei.
4. Modulatory nucleus: SNc, which modulates the activity of the basal ganglia.

The caudate nucleus and putamen can be considered as a continuum, as they share similar morphological and electrophysiological properties. Actually, they form a single entity in rodents. The striatum of primates and carnivores is separated by dense fiber bundles of the internal

T. Itakura (ed.), *Deep Brain Stimulation for Neurological Disorders: Theoretical Background and Clinical Application*, DOI 10.1007/978-3-319-08476-3_1,

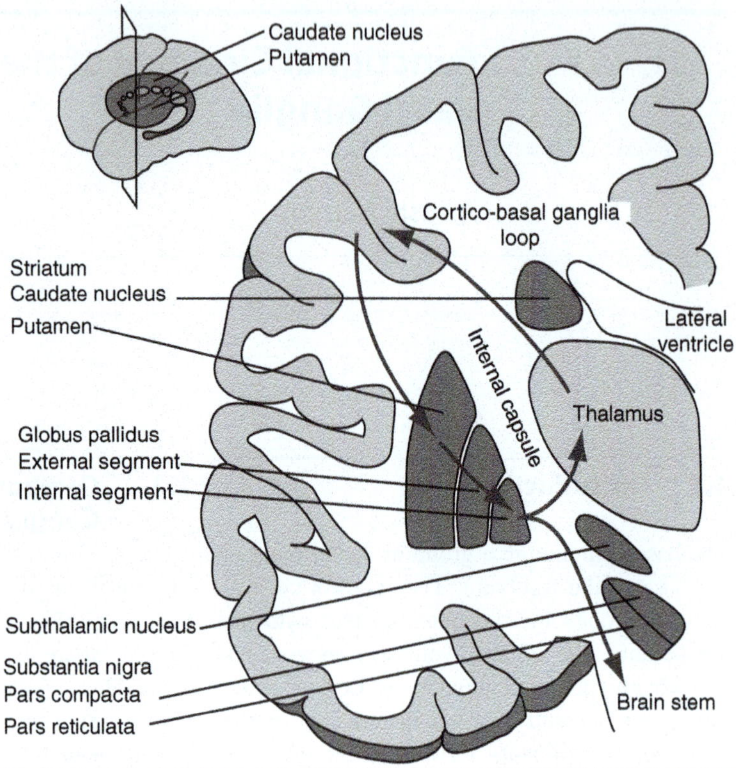

Fig. 1.1 Basal ganglia. Human basal ganglia shown in a frontal section and in a lateral view (*inset*). The basal ganglia receive cortical inputs and return processed information to the cerebral cortex through the thalamus (cortico-basal ganglia loop) and to the brain stem (Modified from Nambu (2009) with permission)

capsule into the caudate nucleus and putamen. The caudate nucleus receives inputs mainly from the prefrontal cortex and the putamen from the motor cortices. The GPi and SNr can also be considered as a continuum separated by the internal capsule. In rodents and carnivores, the GPi is small and buried in the fibers of the internal capsule, thus classically named the entopeduncular nucleus, and the GPe is called simply as the globus pallidus.

The basal ganglia receive inputs from wide areas of the cerebral cortex. Information processed in the basal ganglia returns mainly to the cerebral cortex, especially to the frontal lobe, via the thalamus (Fig. 1.1). Thus, the basal ganglia and the cerebral cortex form a loop circuitry (cortico-basal ganglia loop) (Alexander et al. 1986; Albin et al. 1989; Alexander and Crutcher 1990; Middleton and Strick 2000). Through this loop, the basal ganglia control cortical activity. Minor output of the basal ganglia descends to the brain stem.

1.3 Circuitry of the Basal Ganglia

The striatum as the input nucleus receives excitatory glutamatergic inputs from the wide areas of the cerebral cortex. Striatal projection neurons can be classified into two groups based on projection sites and neurotransmitters. Information in the striatum is transferred to the output nuclei, GPi/SNr, via following two different pathways (Fig. 1.2) (Albin et al. 1989; Alexander and Crutcher 1990).

1. *Direct* pathway: striatal neurons containing gamma-aminobutyric acid (GABA), substance P, and dopamine D1 receptors project monosynaptically to the GPi/SNr.
2. *Indirect* pathway: striatal neurons containing GABA, enkephalin, and dopamine D2 receptors project polysynaptically to the GPi/SNr by way of sequential connections with the GPe (composed of GABAergic neurons) and STN (composed of glutamatergic neurons).

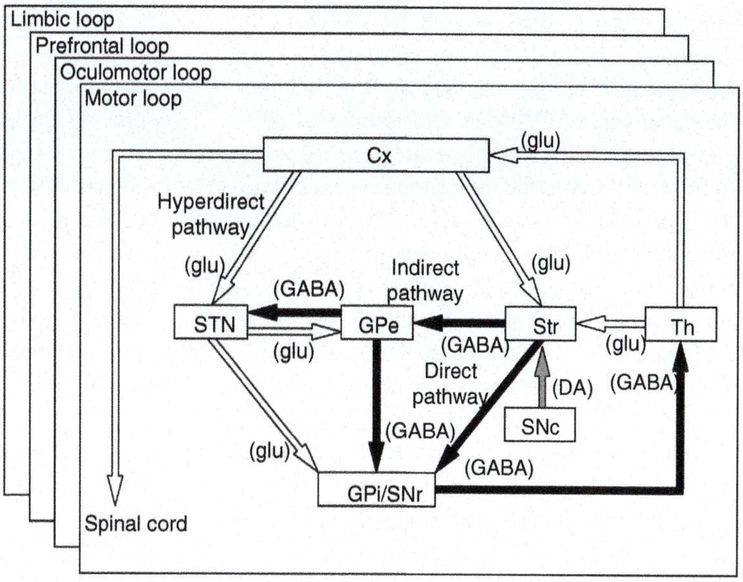

Fig. 1.2 Basic circuitry of the basal ganglia. *Open and filled arrows* indicate excitatory and inhibitory projections, respectively. *Cx* cerebral cortex, *DA* dopamine, *GABA* gamma-aminobutyric acid, *glu* glutamate, *GPe and GPi* external and internal segments of the globus pallidus, *SNc* substantia nigra pars compacta, *SNr* substantia nigra pars reticulata, *STN* subthalamic nucleus, *Str* striatum, *Th* thalamus (Modified from Nambu et al. (2002a) with permission)

Signals through the *direct* pathway have inhibitory effects on GPi/SNr neurons. On the other hand, signals through the *indirect* pathway have net excitatory effects on GPi/SNr neurons, because both striato-GPe and GPe-STN projections are inhibitory and STN-GPi/SNr projections are excitatory.

The STN, the other input nucleus, also receives direct cortical inputs mainly from the frontal cortex in a topographically organized manner and sends information to the output nuclei through the following pathway (Fig. 1.2) (Nambu et al. 2002a).

3. *Hyperdirect* pathway: STN neurons receiving cortical inputs project monosynaptically to the GPi/SNr. The *hyperdirect* pathway conveys strong excitatory signals from the cortex to the GPi/SNr with shorter conduction time than the *direct* and *indirect* pathways.

The output nuclei of the basal ganglia, GPi/SNr, are composed of inhibitory GABAergic neurons and project to the ventral anterior and ventral lateral nuclei (VA/VL) of the thalamus and brain stem nuclei, such as the pedunculopontine tegmental nucleus (PPN) and superior colliculus. VA/VL thalamic neurons project to the frontal cortex. Ascending projections from the basal ganglia to the cerebral cortex through the thalamus control the learned movements of hands and the higher brain functions. On the other hand, descending projections to the motor centers in the brain stem control the innate motor functions, such as eye movements, trunk movements, locomotion, mastication, and vocalization.

Dopaminergic neurons in the SNc project to the striatum and modulate differentially the activity of striatal projection neurons in the *direct* and *indirect* pathways (Fig. 1.2) (Albin et al. 1989; Alexander and Crutcher 1990; DeLong 1990; Gerfen and Surmeier 2011). Dopamine excites the *direct* pathway striatal neurons through the dopamine D1 receptors, while it inhibits the *indirect* pathway striatal neurons through dopamine D2 receptors.

The cortico-basal ganglia loops are composed of the following several loops (Alexander et al. 1986; Albin et al. 1989; Alexander and Crutcher 1990; Middleton and Strick 2000). The motor loop controlling movements of forelimbs, hindlimbs, and trunk, starts from the motor cortices, such as the primary motor cortex (MI), supplementary motor area (SMA), and premotor cortex (PM), and goes through the somatomotor territories of the basal ganglia, and finally returns to the original cortices through the VA/VL of the thalamus. The somatomotor territories of the basal ganglia include the caudoventral putamen, the caudoventral GPe/GPi, and the dorsal STN, and each territory shows somatotopic organization. In addition to the motor loop, the oculomotor, prefrontal (composed of dorsolateral prefrontal and lateral orbitofrontal loops), and limbic loops connect the cerebral cortical areas (the frontal eye field/supplementary eye field, prefrontal cortex, and limbic cortex, respectively) with corresponding parts of the basal ganglia and thalamic nuclei, and form multiple, parallel, segregated, and functionally distinct but homologous loops (Fig. 1.2). Through these multiple loops, the basal ganglia control eye movements, higher brain functions and emotions, as well as limb movements.

The above basal ganglia circuitry may be oversimplified. There exist other significant projections, such as the following (Nambu 2008).

1. It is supposed that striatal neurons projecting to the GPe and GPi belong to different groups. However, tracing studies of a single neuron have shown the existence of neurons projecting to both the GPe and GPi (Levesque and Parent 2005). It has also been reported that some striatal projection neurons express both D1 and D2 receptors. Moreover, electrophysiological experiments have failed to show the expected effect of dopamine on striatal projection neurons.
2. Thalamic neurons, such as those in the VA/VL and centromedian-parafascicular complex (CM/Pf), project also to the striatum, suggesting a short circuit of striato-GPi-thalamo-striatal loop (McFarland and Haber 2000).
3. The cortico-basal ganglia loops are considered to be composed of several segregated and parallel loops. However, there exists partial overlap of projections. Thus, these loops should be viewed more as a continuum rather than subdivisions with strict boundaries.
4. The GPe gives rise to GABAergic projections to the GPi/SNr, striatum and GPe itself through local axon collaterals. Thus, the GPe may be viewed as a center nucleus projecting to multiple sites of the basal ganglia.
5. The STN projects to the GPe, as well as to the GPi, using axon collaterals. The STN and GPe have intimate interconnections, and the interconnected groups of neurons in the GPe and STN innervate the same population of neurons in the GPi (Shink et al. 1996). Thus, the STN and GPe are coupled to each other and may work together.
6. The basal ganglia and cerebellum are classically considered to function independently without interactions. However, recent anatomical studies suggest that the basal ganglia communicate with cerebellum through the cerebello-thalamo-striatal and STN-ponto-cerebellar pathways (Bostan et al. 2013).

1.4 Functions of the Basal Ganglia

Physiological functions of the basal ganglia are not yet fully understood; most probable hypothesis on the basal ganglia functions is the focused selection of intended movements, which may also explain pathophysiology of movement disorders of the basal ganglia origin.

Neurons in the output nuclei of the basal ganglia are inhibitory GABAergic and fire at high frequency (40–100 Hz), and thus, neurons in the target structures, such as the thalamus, are inhibited continuously (Fig. 1.3). When striatal neurons are activated by cortical inputs, the striatal neurons inhibit GPi/SNr activity through the striato-GPi/SNr *direct* pathway. The continuous inhibition from the output nuclei to the target structures is temporally removed (disinhibition), and neurons in the target structures, including thalamic and cortical neurons, are activated, resulting in the release of a selected motor program (Fig. 1.3) (Hikosaka et al. 2000). These mechanisms have been investigated in saccadic eye movements.

On the other hand, signals through the *hyperdirect* and *indirect* pathways have excitatory effects on the GPi/SNr, and thus, have inhibitory effects on thalamic neurons. Considering the

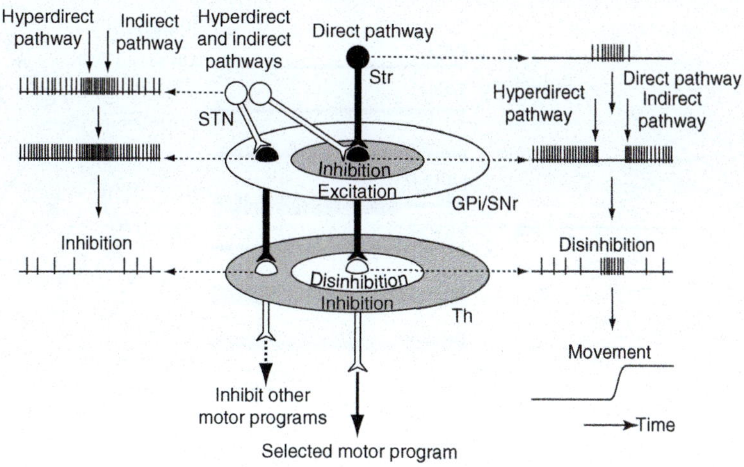

Fig. 1.3 Spatial and temporal distribution of basal ganglia activity during behavior. Signals from the motor cortices through the *direct* pathway inhibit GPi/SNr neurons, activate thalamic neurons by disinhibition, and finally release a selected motor program. On the other hand, signals through the *hyperdirect* and *indirect* pathways have broad excitatory effects on GPi/SNr neurons in temporal and spatial domains, make clear initiation and termination of the selected motor program, and inhibit other unnecessary competing motor programs (Modified from Nambu (2008) with permission)

conduction time, signals through the *hyperdirect* pathway first actively inhibit thalamic neurons, then those through the *direct* pathway disinhibit them, and finally those through the *indirect* pathway inhibit them again. Thus, signals through the *hyperdirect* and *indirect* pathways make clear initiation and termination of the selected motor program (Fig. 1.3) (Nambu et al. 2002a; Nambu 2007).

In addition to such a temporal aspect, the enhancement by differential inputs through the *hyperdirect*, *direct*, and *indirect* pathways may work in spatial domain as well (Mink 1996). Anatomical studies have shown that STN-GPi fibers arborize more widely and terminate on more proximal neuronal elements than striato-GPi fibers. Signals through the *hyperdirect* and *indirect* pathways activate GPi/SNr neurons extensively, thereby inhibiting large areas of the thalamus, whereas signals through the *direct* pathway disinhibit thalamic neurons only in the center area (Fig. 1.3). Thus, signals through the *hyperdirect* and *indirect* pathways inhibit thalamic neurons in the surrounding area, which are related to other unnecessary competing motor programs (Mink 1996; Nambu et al. 2002a; Nambu 2007).

Based on the temporal and spatial inputs to the target structures through the *hyperdirect*, *direct*, and *indirect* pathways, only the selected motor program is executed at the selected timing, and other competing motor programs are canceled. In addition to the motor loop, the oculomotor, prefrontal, and limbic loops control the activity of corresponding cortical areas in a similar manner.

1.5 Firing Properties and Somatotopy of the Basal Ganglia

Neurons in each nucleus of the basal ganglia show characteristic firing rates and patterns reflecting their membrane properties, such as ion channels and receptors, and afferent inputs. Afferent and efferent connections of each nucleus of the basal ganglia maintain functional topography, and thus somatomotor territories of the basal ganglia show somatotopic organization. The following description on the firing properties and somatotopy of the basal ganglia and thalamus is derived mainly from animal experiments, especially using subhuman primates, and is also applicable to humans.

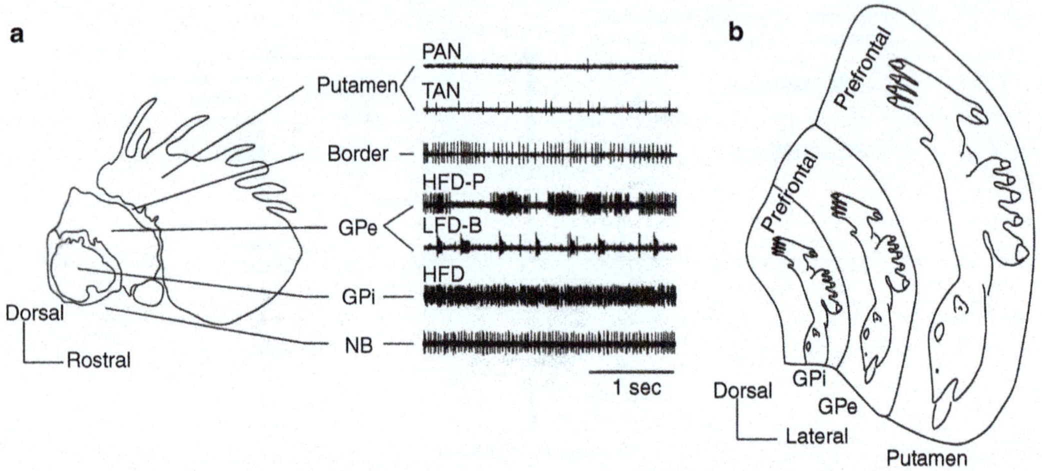

Fig. 1.4 (**a**) Firing properties of the putamen, GPe, and GPi. Each structure of the basal ganglia shows characteristic firing rates and patterns (*right*). *HFD* high frequency discharge, *HFD-P* high frequency discharge with pauses, *LFD-B* low frequency discharge with bursts, *NB* nucleus basalis of Meynert, *PAN* phasically active neuron, *TAN* tonically active neuron (Modified from Vitek et al. (1997) with permission). (**b**) Somatotopic organization of the putamen, GPe and GPi on a frontal map (Modified from Nambu (2011) with permission)

1.5.1 Striatum

The striatum is composed of major (80–95 %) projection neurons and minor interneurons (Alexander and DeLong 1985; Kawaguchi 1997; Wilson 2004). Projection neurons are inhibitory GABAergic, medium-sized neurons, and their dendrites are covered by numerous spines. Medium spiny projection neurons are usually silent and fire when they receive inputs, and thus, are described as phasically active neurons (PAN) in unit recording *in vivo* (Fig. 1.4a) (Vitek et al. 1997). Projection neurons can be divided into two groups, i.e., the *direct* and *indirect* pathway neurons, based on the transmitters and projection sites as described earlier, and both show similar firing properties. Interneurons lack spines and are classified into at least four groups: (1) cholinergic large aspiny neurons, (2) parvalbumin-containing GABAergic aspiny neurons, (3) somatostatin/nitric oxide synthase-containing GABAergic aspiny neurons, and (4) calretinin-containing GABAergic aspiny neurons. Interneurons, as well as projection neurons, receive inputs from the cerebral cortex, thalamus, and SNc, ultimately project to projection neurons and control their activity. Cholinergic large aspiny neurons fire spontaneously with broader spikes than PANs at 2–10 Hz and are described as tonically active neurons (TAN) in unit recording *in vivo*. The activity patterns of other interneuron *in vivo* remain to be elucidated.

The striatum receives excitatory glutamatergic inputs from wide areas of the cerebral cortex. Cortical inputs maintain functional topography, for example, the motor and sensory cortices project to the caudal part of the putamen, which is posterior to the anterior commissure, while the prefrontal cortex projects to the caudate nucleus and the rostral part of the putamen. Hindlimb, forelimb, and orofacial areas of the MI project to the dorsal to ventral part of the lateral putamen in a somatotopically organized manner (Fig. 1.4b) (Takada et al. 1998; Nambu et al. 2002b; Nambu 2011). The somatotopy in the putamen is also confirmed by electrophysiological methods. PANs in the somatomotor territories are activated by active and/or passive movements of the corresponding body parts on the contralateral side (Nambu et al. 2002b; Takara et al. 2011), while TANs respond to novel acoustic and visual stimuli (Aosaki et al. 1995). Microstimulation in the somatomotor territories of the putamen produces movements of the corresponding body parts

(Alexander and DeLong 1985; Nambu et al. 2002b).

The prefrontal cortex projects to the rostral part of the putamen anterior to the anterior commissure and the head of the caudate nucleus (prefrontal territory of the striatum), and the limbic cortex projects to the ventral striatum (limbic territory) (Selemon and Goldman-Rakic 1985; Haber et al. 1990; Parent 1990). Eye movement-related neurons are located in the central part of the caudate nucleus (oculomotor territory) (Hikosaka et al. 1989).

1.5.2 GPe and GPi

The GPe and GPi are composed of inhibitory GABAergic projection neurons, which fire spontaneously and irregularly at high frequency, however their firing properties are different.

The GPe is composed of the following two types of neurons that show different firing patterns (Fig. 1.4a) (DeLong 1971; DeLong et al. 1985; Vitek et al. 1997):

1. High-frequency discharge with pauses (HFD-P) neurons, which fire at high frequency (10–100 Hz) with interruption by pauses and comprise a major portion (85 %).
2. Low-frequency discharge with bursts (LFD-B) neurons, which fire at low frequency (1–30 Hz) with intermittent bursts and comprise the rest (15 %).

On the other hand, the GPi is mainly composed of a single type of neurons (Fig. 1.4a) (DeLong 1971; DeLong et al. 1985; Vitek et al. 1997):

3. High frequency discharge (HFD) neurons, which fire at high frequency (10–110 Hz) without pauses.

In addition, the "border" neurons, which fire regularly at 20–50 Hz, are found along the borders between the putamen and GPe and between the GPe and GPi.

The somatomotor territory of the striatum (i.e., the caudal aspect of the putamen) projects to the ventral two thirds of the caudal GPe and GPi, and thus, these areas are the somatomotor territories (Smith and Parent 1986; Parent 1990) and show somatotopic organization (Fig. 1.4b). The orofacial, forelimb, and hindlimb areas are represented along the ventral-to-dorsal axis in the GPe and GPi (Yoshida et al. 1993). GPe/GPi neurons change their activity in relation to active and/or passive movements of the corresponding body parts on the contralateral side (DeLong 1971; Georgopoulos et al. 1983; DeLong et al. 1985). Border neurons do not respond to somatosensory stimulation. Microstimulation in the GPe/GPi does not induce any movements.

The prefrontal territory of the striatum projects to the rostral GPe and dorsal one third of the caudal GPe/GPi, and thus, these areas are the prefrontal territory (Smith and Parent 1986; Parent 1990). Ventral striatum projects to the ventral pallidum, the most rostral part of the GPe and the most medial part of the GPi, and thus, these areas correspond to the limbic territory (Haber et al. 1990; Parent 1990).

1.5.3 STN

The STN is composed of excitatory glutamatergic projection neurons, which fire irregularly at medium frequency rates (25–45 Hz) (Fig. 1.5a) (DeLong et al. 1985). The STN receives excitatory inputs from the frontal cortex including the motor cortices in a somatotopically organized manner. The dorsal part of the STN belongs to the somatomotor territory and shows somatotopic organization (Fig. 1.5b) (Nambu et al. 1996). The MI projects to the lateral part (MI territory), and the SMA projects to the medial part (SMA territory). The orofacial, forelimb, and hindlimb areas of the MI project to the lateral to medial parts of the lateral STN, while those of the SMA project to the medial to lateral parts of the medial STN. Therefore, two sets of somatotopic body maps, which are mirror-imaged to each other, are represented in the lateral and medial parts of the STN. STN neurons in the MI territory change their activity (mostly excitation) in relation to active and/or passive movements of the corresponding body parts on the contralateral side (DeLong et al. 1985; Wichmann et al. 1994). Neurons in the SMA territory may also show task-related activity. Microstimulation in the STN does not evoke movements.

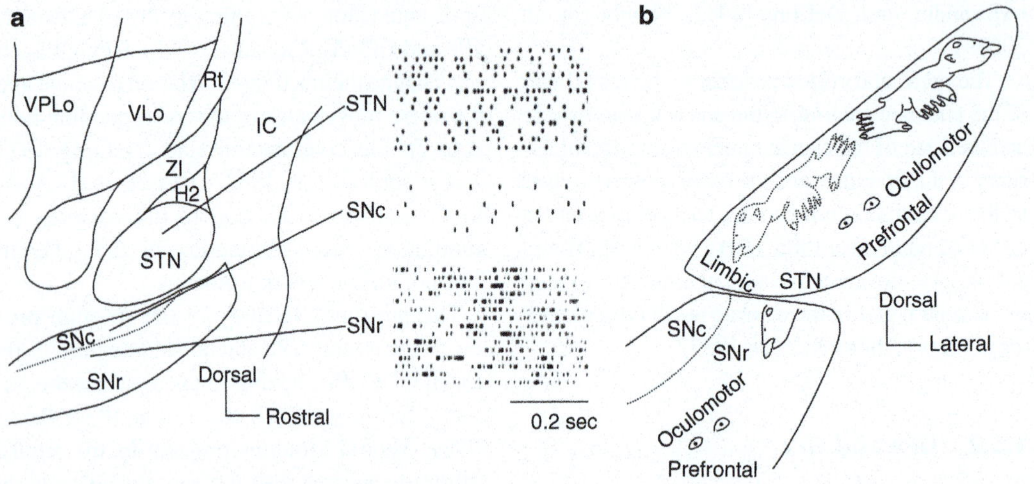

Fig. 1.5 (**a**) Firing properties of the STN, SNc, and SNr. Firing patterns of each structure are shown in a raster display (*right*). Each small vertical bar represents a neuronal firing. *H2* Forel's field H2 (lenticular fasciculus), *IC* internal capsule, *Rt* thalamic reticular nucleus, *VLo* oral part of the ventral lateral nucleus of the thalamus, *VPLo* oral part of the ventral posterolateral nucleus of the thalamus, *ZI* zona incerta (Modified from DeLong et al. (1983, 1985) with permission). (**b**) Somatotopic organization of the STN and SNr on a frontal map (Modified from Nambu (2011) with permission)

The ventral part of the STN to the somatomotor territory belongs to the prefrontal territory (Fig. 1.5b) (Monakow et al. 1978; Parent 1990), including the oculomotor territory (Matsumura et al. 1992). The most ventromedial part of the STN is occupied by limbic territory (Parent 1990).

1.5.4 SNr and SNc

The SNr is mainly composed of inhibitory GABAergic projection neurons, which fire spontaneously and irregularly at high frequency like HFD neurons in the GPi (Fig. 1.5a). The somatomotor territory of the striatum projects to the dorsal one third of the SNr (Smith and Parent 1986; Parent 1990), and thus, this area is considered to be the somatomotor territory of the SNr (Fig. 1.5b). Neurons in this area change their activity in relation to active and/or passive movements of the orofacial region (DeLong et al. 1983; Kitano et al. 1998). The orofacial area of the SNr is considered to be a continuation of the orofacial area of the GPi (Figs. 1.4b and 1.5b). The prefrontal territory of the striatum projects to the rostromedial two thirds of the SNr including the oculomotor territory (Fig. 1.5b) (Hikosaka and Wurtz 1983; Smith and Parent 1986). The limbic territory of the striatum projects to the most medial part of the SNr (Haber et al. 1990).

On the other hand, the SNc is composed of dopaminergic neurons, which are characterized by broad spikes and low firing rates (less than 6 Hz) (DeLong et al. 1983; Schultz and Romo 1990). SNc neurons do not respond to active or passive movements of body parts, but respond to novel sensory stimuli and/or rewards (DeLong et al. 1983; Schultz and Romo 1990). The SNc has no clear somatotopy.

1.5.5 Thalamus

The thalamus is a target structure of the basal ganglia. Subnuclei located in the rostral part of the motor thalamus receive inputs from the basal ganglia. The oral part of the ventral lateral nucleus (VLo) and the parvicellular part of the ventral anterior nucleus (VApc) receive inputs from the GPi, and the medial part of the ventral lateral nucleus (VLm) and the magnocellular part of the ventral anterior nucleus (VAmc) receive inputs from the SNr. On the other hand, subnuclei located in the caudal part, such as the oral part of the ventral posterolateral nucleus (VPLo), the caudal part of the ventral lateral nucleus (VLc), and area X, receive cerebellar inputs (Jones 2007). Thus, projections from the SNr, GPi, and cerebellar nuclei terminate in the rostral to caudal parts of the motor thalamus with minimal overlap of their terminals. The VApc, VLo, VPLo, and VLc project to the motor cortices, and most of them receive inputs from both the basal ganglia and cerebellum through the motor thalamus (Jones 2007). The MI receives basal ganglia inputs through the VLo and cerebellar inputs through the VPLo (Holsapple et al. 1991). Thalamic neurons fire at 10–20 Hz and do not show characteristic firing patterns unlike basal ganglia neurons. Firing rates in the VLo, which receives tonic inhibitory inputs from the GPi, are lower than those in the VPLo, which receives tonic excitatory inputs from the cerebellar nuclei (Vitek et al. 1994).

The VLo and VPLo display clear somatotopic organization (Fig. 1.6). The orofacial, forelimb, and hindlimb areas are represented in the medial to lateral parts (Asanuma et al. 1983; Vitek et al. 1994). VLo neurons change their activity in relation to active movements of the corresponding body parts. However, sensory inputs are not clearly identified, and the microstimulation in the VLo does not induce any movements. On the other hand, VPLo neurons respond clearly to active and passive movements of discrete body parts (one to several joints) on the contralateral side (Anderson and Turner 1991; Nambu et al. 1991; Vitek et al. 1994). Microstimulation in the VPLo induces movements in the corresponding body parts, contralateral to the stimulation side (Buford et al. 1996; Vitek et al. 1996).

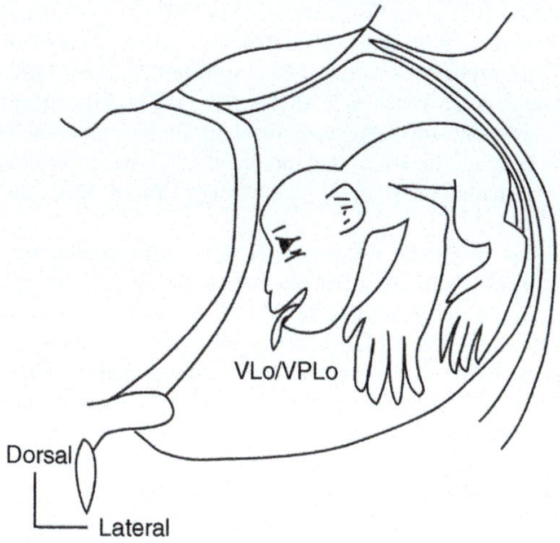

Fig. 1.6 Somatotopic organization of the thalamus on a frontal map. Both the VLo receiving pallidal projections and the VPLo receiving cerebellar projections have their own somatotopic representations. Their somatotopic representations are continuous rostrocaudally (Modified from Asanuma et al. (1983) with permission)

Summary and Conclusions

The basal ganglia circuitry can be summarized as follows:

1. The basal ganglia control not only voluntary movements, but also other higher brain functions through the multiple and parallel cortico-basal ganglia loops.
2. The output of the basal ganglia is controlled differentially by the *hyperdirect*, *direct*, and *indirect* pathways.
3. The function of the basal ganglia is proposed to be the focused selection of intended movements.
4. Each structure of the basal ganglia shows characteristic firing rates and patterns.
5. Connections of the basal ganglia maintain functional topography, and somatomotor territories of the basal ganglia show somatotopic organization.

References

Albin RL, Young AB, Penney JB (1989) The functional anatomy of basal ganglia disorders. Trends Neurosci 12:366–375

Alexander GE, Crutcher MD (1990) Functional architecture of basal ganglia circuits: neural substrates of parallel processing. Trends Neurosci 13:266–271

Alexander GE, DeLong MR (1985) Microstimulation of the primate neostriatum. II. Somatotopic organization of striatal microexcitable zones and their relation to neuronal response properties. J Neurophysiol 53: 1417–1430

Alexander GE, DeLong MR, Strick PL (1986) Parallel organization of functionally segregated circuits linking basal ganglia and cortex. Annu Rev Neurosci 9:357–381

Anderson ME, Turner RS (1991) Activity of neurons in cerebellar-receiving and pallidal-receiving areas of the thalamus of the behaving monkey. J Neurophysiol 66:879–893

Aosaki T, Kimura M, Graybiel AM (1995) Temporal and spatial characteristics of tonically active neurons of the primate's striatum. J Neurophysiol 73:1234–1252
Asanuma C, Thach WR, Jones EG (1983) Anatomical evidence for segregated focal groupings of efferent cells and their terminal ramifications in the cerebellothalamic pathway of the monkey. Brain Res 286: 267–297
Bostan AC, Dum RP, Strick PL (2013) Cerebellar networks with the cerebral cortex and basal ganglia. Trends Cogn Sci 17:241–254
Buford JA, Inase M, Anderson ME (1996) Contrasting locations of pallidal-receiving neurons and microexcitable zones in primate thalamus. J Neurophysiol 75:1105–1116
DeLong MR (1971) Activity of pallidal neurons during movement. J Neurophysiol 34:414–427
DeLong MR (1990) Primate models of movement disorders of basal ganglia origin. Trends Neurosci 13: 281–285
DeLong MR, Crutcher MD, Georgopoulos AP (1983) Relations between movement and single cell discharge in the substantia nigra of the behaving monkey. J Neurosci 3:1599–1606
DeLong MR, Crutcher MD, Georgopoulos AP (1985) Primate globus pallidus and subthalamic nucleus: functional organization. J Neurophysiol 53:530–543
Georgopoulos AP, DeLong MR, Crutcher MD (1983) Relations between parameters of step-tracking movements and single cell discharge in the globus pallidus and subthalamic nucleus of the behaving monkey. J Neurosci 3:1586–1598
Gerfen CR, Surmeier DJ (2011) Modulation of striatal projection systems by dopamine. Annu Rev Neurosci 34:441–466
Haber SN, Lynd E, Klein C, Groenewegen HJ (1990) Topographic organization of the ventral striatal efferent projections in the rhesus monkey: an anterograde tracing study. J Comp Neurol 293:282–298
Hikosaka O, Wurtz RH (1983) Visual and oculomotor functions of monkey substantia nigra pars reticulata. I. Relation of visual and auditory responses to saccades. J Neurophysiol 49:1230–1253
Hikosaka O, Sakamoto M, Usui S (1989) Functional properties of monkey caudate neurons. I. Activities related to saccadic eye movements. J Neurophysiol 61:780–798
Hikosaka O, Takikawa Y, Kawagoe R (2000) Role of the basal ganglia in the control of purposive saccadic eye movements. Physiol Rev 80:953–978
Holsapple JW, Preston JB, Strick PL (1991) The origin of thalamic inputs to the "hand" representation in the primary motor cortex. J Neurosci 11:2644–2654
Jones EG (2007) The thalamus, 2nd edn. Cambridge University Press, New York
Kawaguchi Y (1997) Neostriatal cell subtypes and their functional roles. Neurosci Res 27:1–8
Kitano H, Tanibuchi I, Jinnai K (1998) The distribution of neurons in the substantia nigra pars reticulata with input from the motor, premotor and prefrontal areas of the cerebral cortex in monkeys. Brain Res 784: 228–238
Levesque M, Parent A (2005) The striatofugal fiber system in primates: a reevaluation of its organization based on single-axon tracing studies. Proc Natl Acad Sci U S A 102:11888–11893
Matsumura M, Kojima J, Gardiner TW, Hikosaka O (1992) Visual and oculomotor functions of monkey subthalamic nucleus. J Neurophysiol 67:1615–1632
McFarland NR, Haber SN (2000) Convergent inputs from thalamic motor nuclei and frontal cortical areas to the dorsal striatum in the primate. J Neurosci 20:3798–3813
Middleton FA, Strick PL (2000) Basal ganglia and cerebellar loops: motor and cognitive circuits. Brain Res Brain Res Rev 31:236–250
Mink JW (1996) The basal ganglia: focused selection and inhibition of competing motor programs. Prog Neurobiol 50:381–425
Monakow KH, Akert K, Kunzle H (1978) Projections of the precentral motor cortex and other cortical areas of the frontal lobe to the subthalamic nucleus in the monkey. Exp Brain Res 33:395–403
Nambu A (2007) Globus pallidus internal segment. Prog Brain Res 160:135–150
Nambu A (2008) Seven problems on the basal ganglia. Curr Opin Neurobiol 18:595–604
Nambu A (2009) Basal ganglia: physiological circuits. In: Squire LR (ed) Encyclopedia of neuroscience, vol 2. Academic, Oxford, pp 111–117
Nambu A (2011) Somatotopic organization of the primate basal ganglia. Front Neuroanat 5:26
Nambu A, Yoshida S, Jinnai K (1991) Movement-related activity of thalamic neurons with input from the globus pallidus and projection to the motor cortex in the monkey. Exp Brain Res 84:279–284
Nambu A, Takada M, Inase M, Tokuno H (1996) Dual somatotopical representations in the primate subthalamic nucleus: evidence for ordered but reversed body-map transformations from the primary motor cortex and the supplementary motor area. J Neurosci 16:2671–2683
Nambu A, Tokuno H, Takada M (2002a) Functional significance of the cortico-subthalamo-pallidal 'hyperdirect' pathway. Neurosci Res 43:111–117
Nambu A, Kaneda K, Tokuno H, Takada M (2002b) Organization of corticostriatal motor inputs in monkey putamen. J Neurophysiol 88:1830–1842
Parent A (1990) Extrinsic connections of the basal ganglia. Trends Neurosci 13:254–258
Schultz W, Romo R (1990) Dopamine neurons of the monkey midbrain: contingencies of responses to stimuli eliciting immediate behavioral reactions. J Neurophysiol 63:607–624

Selemon LD, Goldman-Rakic PS (1985) Longitudinal topography and interdigitation of corticostriatal projections in the rhesus monkey. J Neurosci 5:776–794

Shink E, Bevan MD, Bolam JP, Smith Y (1996) The subthalamic nucleus and the external pallidum: two tightly interconnected structures that control the output of the basal ganglia in the monkey. Neuroscience 73:335–357

Smith Y, Parent A (1986) Differential connections of caudate nucleus and putamen in the squirrel monkey (Saimiri sciureus). Neuroscience 18:347–371

Takada M, Tokuno H, Nambu A, Inase M (1998) Corticostriatal projections from the somatic motor areas of the frontal cortex in the macaque monkey: segregation versus overlap of input zones from the primary motor cortex, the supplementary motor area, and the premotor cortex. Exp Brain Res 120:114–128

Takara S, Hatanaka N, Takada M, Nambu A (2011) Differential activity patterns of putaminal neurons with inputs from the primary motor cortex and supplementary motor area in behaving monkeys. J Neurophysiol 106:1203–1217

Vitek JL, Ashe J, DeLong MR, Alexander GE (1994) Physiologic properties and somatotopic organization of the primate motor thalamus. J Neurophysiol 71: 1498–1513

Vitek JL, Ashe J, DeLong MR, Kaneoke Y (1996) Microstimulation of primate motor thalamus: somatotopic organization and differential distribution of evoked motor responses among subnuclei. J Neurophysiol 75:2486–2495

Vitek JL, Bakay RAE, DeLong MR (1997) Microelectrode-guided pallidotomy for medically intractable Parkinson's disease. In: Obeso JA, DeLong MR, Ohye C, Marsden CD (eds) The basal ganglia and new surgical approaches for Parkinson's disease, advances in neurology. Lippincott-Raven, Philadelphia, pp 183–198

Wichmann T, Bergman H, DeLong MR (1994) The primate subthalamic nucleus. I. Functional properties in intact animals. J Neurophysiol 72:494–506

Wilson CJ (2004) The synaptic organization of the brain. In: Shepherd GM (ed) Basal ganglia, 5th edn. Oxford, New York, pp 361–413

Yoshida S, Nambu A, Jinnai K (1993) The distribution of the globus pallidus neurons with input from various cortical areas in the monkeys. Brain Res 611: 170–174

Mechanism of DBS: Inhibition, Excitation, or Disruption?

2

Atsushi Nambu and Satomi Chiken

2.1 Introduction

Deep brain stimulation (DBS) that applies high-frequency electrical stimulation to a specific target in the subcortical structures was introduced in the early 1990s as a surgical treatment for movement disorders (Benabid et al. 1991, 1994; Siegfried and Lippitz 1994a, b; Limousin et al. 1995). DBS has now been widely accepted as an effective and safe alternative to lesion therapy, conventional stereotactic surgery. DBS targeting the motor thalamus dramatically alleviates essential and resting tremor (Benabid et al. 1991, 1996; Siegfried and Lippitz 1994b; Koller et al. 1997; Rehncrona et al. 2003). DBS targeting the subthalamic nucleus (STN) and the internal segment of the globus pallidus (GPi) has been largely used for treatment of advanced Parkinson's disease (PD) and dyskinesia, a major side effect of L-DOPA treatment, and GPi-DBS has marked effects on the improvement of dystonic symptoms (Limousin et al. 1995; Deep-Brain Stimulation for Parkinson's Disease Study Group 2001; Coubes et al. 2004; Wichmann and DeLong 2006; Kringelbach et al. 2007; Ostrem and Starr 2008; Vitek 2008; Vidailhet et al. 2013). However, the exact mechanism underling its effectiveness remains to be elucidated.

Since DBS gives rise to similar beneficial effects to those of lesion therapy, such as pallidotomy and thalamotomy, it was originally considered to inhibit local neuronal elements. In fact, STN- or GPi-DBS inhibited firings of neighboring neurons (Boraud et al. 1996; Dostrovsky et al. 2000; Wu et al. 2001; Filali et al. 2004; Lafreniere-Roula et al. 2010). On the other hand, other studies suggested that DBS excited local neuronal elements: STN-DBS increased activity of GPi neurons through the excitatory STN-GPi projections (Hashimoto et al. 2003; Galati et al. 2006; Reese et al. 2011), and GPi-DBS reduced activity of thalamic neurons through the inhibitory GPi-thalamic projections (Anderson et al. 2003; Pralong et al. 2003; Montgomery 2006). In addition, other studies reported that GPi-DBS induced multiphasic responses consisting of excitation and inhibition in GPi neurons (Bar-Gad et al. 2004; Erez et al. 2009; McCairn and Turner 2009; Leblois et al. 2010). In this chapter, we will critically review recent studies and discuss possible mechanisms for the effectiveness of DBS.

A. Nambu, MD, PhD (✉) • S. Chiken, PhD
Division of System Neurophysiology,
National Institute for Physiological Sciences,
Okazaki, Japan

Department of Physiological Sciences,
Graduate University for Advanced Studies,
Okazaki, Japan
e-mail: nambu@nips.ac.jp

T. Itakura (ed.), *Deep Brain Stimulation for Neurological Disorders: Theoretical Background and Clinical Application*, DOI 10.1007/978-3-319-08476-3_2,

2.2 DBS Inhibits Local Neuronal Elements

Both DBS and lesion therapy are found to produce similar beneficial effects on the alleviation of symptoms. STN-DBS has similar effects on PD motor signs (Benazzouz et al. 1993; Benabid et al. 1994; Limousin et al. 1995) to the STN lesion (Bergman et al. 1990; Aziz et al. 1991; Levy et al. 2001) and to the blockade of the STN (Luo et al. 2002) or STN-GPi neurotransmission (Graham et al. 1991; Brotchie et al. 1991). Thus, DBS is originally assumed to inhibit local neuronal elements.

Actually, one of the most common effects of STN- or GPi-DBS on neighboring neurons is the reduction of the firing rates. In PD patients, distinct suppression of neuronal activity was recorded around the stimulating sites of STN-DBS during stereotactic surgery (Filali et al. 2004; Welter et al. 2004). Similar results were also obtained in animal models, such as PD monkeys (Meissner et al. 2005; Moran et al. 2011) and rats (Tai et al. 2003; Shi et al. 2006). Recent studies using a template subtraction method, which can detect spikes soon after stimulus pulses by removing stimulus artifacts (Wichmann 2000; Hashimoto et al. 2002), confirmed that STN-DBS indeed decreased the firing rate of neighboring neurons (Meissner et al. 2005; Moran et al. 2011). However, complete cessation of STN firings was observed in a limited number of neurons, and other STN neurons exhibited residual neuronal activity (Welter et al. 2004). Similar results were also observed in PD monkeys (Meissner et al. 2005), and PD and normal rats (Tai et al. 2003). The inhibitory effects sometimes outlasted the stimulus period (Tai et al. 2003; Filali et al. 2004; Welter et al. 2004).

Inhibitory effects of GPi-DBS on firings of neighboring neurons were also reported (Boraud et al. 1996; Dostrovsky et al. 2000; Wu et al. 2001; McCairn and Turner 2009). GPi-DBS induced complete inhibition of local neuronal firings more commonly than STN-DBS. GPi-DBS at 100 Hz induced complete inhibition in most of neighboring neurons in normal monkeys, and the inhibition outlasted the stimulus period sometimes over 100 ms (Chiken and Nambu 2013). Similar posttrain inhibition was also observed in PD patients (Lafreniere-Roula et al. 2010).

2.3 Mechanism of Inhibition

Several possible mechanisms can account for the inhibitory responses during DBS: (1) depolarization block, and (2) the inactivation of voltage-gated currents (Beurrier et al. 2001; Do and Bean 2003; Shin et al. 2007). However, they are less probable, because both single-pulse and low-frequency stimulation in the GPi evoked intense short latency inhibition in neighboring neurons (Dostrovsky et al. 2000; Dostrovsky and Lozano 2002; Chiken and Nambu 2013). Another possible mechanism is (3) the inhibition caused by the activation of inhibitory GABAergic afferents in the stimulated nucleus (Boraud et al. 1996; Dostrovsky et al. 2000; Dostrovsky and Lozano 2002; Meissner et al. 2005; Liu et al. 2008; Johnson et al. 2008; Deniau et al. 2010). A recent study confirmed that inhibitory responses induced by GPi-DBS were mediated by $GABA_A$ and $GABA_B$ receptors (Chiken and Nambu 2013). GPi-stimulation induced directly evoked spikes, which are characterized by a short and constant latency, and GPi-DBS also suppressed directly evoked spikes by strong GABAergic inhibition (Chiken and Nambu 2013).

DBS activates afferent axons in the stimulated nucleus, and the effects vary depending on the composition of the inhibitory and excitatory axon terminals. The GPi receives excitatory glutamatergic inputs from the STN, as well as inhibitory GABAergic inputs from the striatum and GPe (Smith et al. 1994; Shink and Smith 1995). Glutamatergic afferents must also be activated by GPi stimulation, but the glutamatergic excitation is probably overwhelmed by predominant GABAergic inhibition (Shink and Smith 1995). In contrast to GPi neurons, GPe neurons exhibited complex responses composed of excitation and inhibition during GPe-DBS (Chiken and Nambu 2013). The balance between GABAergic and glutamatergic inputs may explain the different effects between GPe-DBS and GPi-DBS: The density of GPe terminals on GPi neurons is higher than those on GPe neurons (Shink and Smith 1995). Similarly, STN-DBS generated both excitatory and inhibitory postsynaptic potentials in STN neurons probably through activation of both glutamatergic and GABAergic afferents (Lee et al. 2004).

2.4 DBS Excites Local Neuronal Elements

It is rational to consider that local stimulation excites local neuronal elements. Actually, directly evoked spikes were induced by GPi-DBS in GPi neurons (Johnson and McIntyre 2008; McCairn and Turner 2009). Such excitation may propagate to the target nucleus through efferent projections. Thalamic activity was reduced during GPi-DBS through inhibitory GABAergic GPi-thalamic projections in PD monkeys (Anderson et al. 2003) and dystonia patients (Pralong et al. 2003; Montgomery 2006). GPi activity was increased during STN-DBS through excitatory glutamatergic STN-GPi projections (Hashimoto et al. 2003; Galati et al. 2006; Reese et al. 2011). Both glutamate and GABA levels measured by microdialysis were increased in the substantia nigra pars reticulata (SNr) of normal rats during STN-DBS (Windels et al. 2000; see also Windels et al. 2005). An intraoperative microdialysis study revealed that STN-DBS increased extracellular concentration of cGMP in the GPi (Stefani et al. 2005). Functional MRI and PET studies in humans indicated that DBS excites efferent outputs (Jech et al. 2001; Hershey et al. 2003; Boertien et al. 2011).

According to a modeling study (McIntyre et al. 2004), subthreshold DBS suppresses intrinsic firings in the cell bodies, while suprathreshold DBS induces spikes at the stimulus frequency in the axons without corresponding firings in the cell bodies. Thus, although stimulation may fail to activate the cell bodies due to strong GABAergic inhibition, it can still excite the efferent axons and provide spikes to the target nucleus at the stimulus frequency. Multiphasic responses consisting of excitation and inhibition during GPi-DBS were observed in GPi neurons of PD monkeys (Bar-Gad et al. 2004; Erez et al. 2009; McCairn and Turner 2009) and dystonic hamsters (Leblois et al. 2010).

Abnormal firings, such as bursting and oscillatory activity, are observed in the cortico-basal ganglia (BG) loop of PD and dystonia and are suggested to be a cause of motor and nonmotor symptoms (Wichmann et al. 1994; Bergman et al. 1998; Starr et al. 2005; Brown 2007; Chiken et al. 2008; Nishibayashi et al. 2011; Tachibana et al. 2011). Excitation and/or excitation–inhibition of efferent pathways may reach the target nucleus, change the firing rates and patterns, and normalize such abnormal firings of target nucleus (Anderson et al. 2003: Hashimoto et al. 2003; Hammond et al. 2007; Johnson et al. 2008; Vitek 2008; Deniau et al. 2010).

DBS can also antidromically excite afferent axons. Antidromic activation of GPi neurons induced by STN-DBS in PD monkeys (Moran et al. 2011) and antidromic activation of thalamic (Vop) neurons induced by GPi-DBS in PD patients (Montgomery 2006) were observed. STN-DBS with low intensity induced GABAergic inhibition in the SNr through antidromic activation of GPe neurons projecting to both the STN and SNr (Maurice et al. 2003; see also Moran et al. 2011), whereas stimulation with higher intensity induced glutamatergic excitation in the SNr through activation of STN–SNr projections. STN-DBS also activated neurons in the motor cortex antidromically and suppressed abnormal low-frequency synchronization, including beta-band oscillation in PD rats (Li et al. 2007, 2012; Degos et al. 2013). Recent development of optogenetics has enabled selective stimulation of afferent inputs vs. efferent outputs: Selective stimulation of cortico-STN afferent axons without activation of STN efferent axons robustly ameliorated the symptoms in PD rats (Gradinaru et al. 2009), suggesting that therapeutic effects of STN-DBS may be accounted for exclusively by the activation of cortico-STN afferent axons.

The contradictory results between inhibition and excitation by DBS may be due to differences in stimulus parameters and electrode assembly used in the experiments: Larger axons are easily activated by electrical stimulation than smaller axons (Ranck 1975), and continuous repetitive stimulation might cause the failure of postsynaptic events due to receptor desensitization and/or transmitter depletion (Wang and Kaczmarek 1998; Zucker and Regehr 2002).

2.5 DBS Disrupts Information Flow

Chiken and Nambu (2013) recently examined the responses of GPi neurons evoked by motor cortical stimulation and effects of GPi-DBS on the response in normal monkeys. Cortical stimulation induces a triphasic response composed of early excitation, inhibition, and late excitation in the GPi, which are mediated by the cortico-STN-GPi *hyperdirect*, cortico-striato-GPi *direct,* and cortico-striato-GPe-STN-GPi *indirect* pathways, respectively (Mink 1996; Nambu et al. 2000, 2002). Both cortically evoked responses and spontaneous discharges were completely inhibited during GPi-DBS by strong GABAergic inhibition, suggesting that GPi-DBS blocks information flow through the GPi (Fig. 2.1). In PD and dystonia, abnormal responses to cortical stimulation (Chiken et al. 2008; Nishibayashi et al. 2011; Kita and Kita 2011), and abnormal bursts and oscillatory activity (Wichmann et al. 1994; Bergman et al. 1998; Starr et al. 2005; Brown 2007; Chiken et al. 2008; Nishibayashi et al. 2011; Tachibana et al. 2011) were observed in GPi neurons, and therefore, signal transmission of such abnormal activities in the BG to the thalamus and motor cortex seems to be responsible for motor symptoms. It is reasonable to speculate that the disruption of such abnormal information flow in the GPi could suppress the expression of motor symptoms. This mechanism can explain the paradox that GPi-DBS produces similar therapeutic effects to GPi-lesion: Both GPi-DBS and GPi-lesion block abnormal information flow through the GPi.

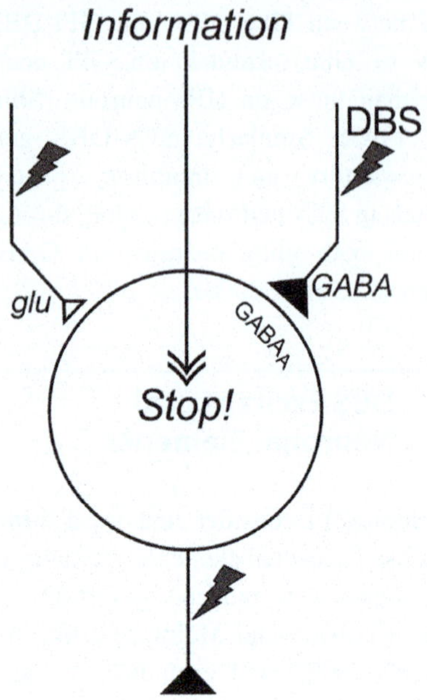

Fig. 2.1 Proposed mechanism underling effectiveness of deep brain stimulation (*DBS*). DBS dissociates input and output signals in the stimulated nucleus, resulting in disruption of abnormal information flow through the cortico-basal ganglia loop in the pathological conditions. *GABA* gamma-aminobutyric acid, *GABA$_A$* GABA$_A$ receptor, *glu* glutamate (Modified from Chiken and Nambu (2014) with permission)

STN-DBS may also block transmission of abnormal signals through the STN. Maurice et al. (2003) examined the effects of STN-DBS on cortically evoked responses in SNr neurons of normal rats. Cortically evoked early and late excitation was abolished or largely reduced during STN-DBS, whereas cortically evoked inhibition was preserved, suggesting that information flow through the *hyperdirect* and *indirect* pathways was blocked by STN-DBS without interrupting the *direct* pathway. The response patterns of SNr neurons during STN-DBS were similar to those of GPi neurons during STN blockade by muscimol injection in normal monkeys (Nambu et al. 2000). Thus, it is rational that STN-DBS has similar effect to the lesion or chemical blockade of the STN. In PD, due to the loss of dopaminergic modulation, the information flow through the striato-GPi *direct* pathway is suppressed, whereas the information flow through the striato-GPe *indirect* pathway is facilitated, resulting in akinesia. Both STN-DBS and STN lesion may block information flow through the STN and normalize the balance between inhibitory inputs through the *direct* pathway and excitatory inputs through the *hyperdirect* and *indirect* pathways to the GPi, leading to the effective alleviation of akinesia. Similar ideas of functional disconnection of the stimulated elements have been proposed by other research groups (Anderson et al. 2006; Deniau et al. 2010; Moran et al. 2011).

2.6 Other Components to Be Considered

It is also probable that STN-DBS induces dopamine release through excitatory glutamatergic STN-SNc projections. STN-DBS induced dopamine release by activation of nigrostriatal dopaminergic neurons in rats (Meissner et al. 2003) and pigs (Shon et al. 2010), although it did not increase the dopamine level in the striatum of human patients (Abosch et al. 2003; Hilker et al. 2003). DBS may also affect neurons whose axons pass close to the stimulating site. A modeling study showed that clinically effective STN-DBS could activate the lenticular fasciculus, a part of GPi-thalamic fibers, by the current spread in addition to STN neurons themselves (Miocinovic et al. 2006).

Nonneuronal glial tissues should also be taken into account as a possible mechanism for the effectiveness of DBS. DBS induced glutamate and ATP release from astrocytes (Fellin et al. 2006; Tawfik et al. 2010). Thalamus-DBS induced an abrupt increase in extracellular ATP and adenosine (Bekar et al. 2008). ATP and glutamate released from astrocytes triggered by DBS may modulate neuronal activity in the stimulated nucleus: A1 receptors activation by adenosine depressed excitatory transmission in the thalamus and alleviated tremor in a mouse model (Vedam-Mai et al. 2012; Jantz and Watanabe 2013).

Conclusion

DBS has a variety of effects on neurons in the stimulated nucleus of the cortico-BG loop, through transmitter release, orthodromic activation of efferent axons, antidromic and orthodromic activation of afferent axons and direct stimulation of passing axons close to the stimulating electrode. The total effects may vary depending on the composition of neural elements in the stimulated nucleus and be more complex than originally expected. However, a common key mechanism should underlie the effectiveness of DBS: DBS dissociates input and output signals in the stimulated nucleus and disrupts abnormal information flow through the cortico-BG loop in the pathological conditions (Fig. 2.1). The proposed mechanism may well explain the paradox that DBS produces similar therapeutic effects to lesion or blockade of the target nucleus. Understanding the exact mechanism of DBS will lead us to better therapeutic options including improvements and upgrading of DBS.

References

Abosch A, Kapur S, Lang AE, Hussey D, Sime E, Miyasaki J, Houle S, Lozano AM (2003) Stimulation of the subthalamic nucleus in Parkinson's disease does not produce striatal dopamine release. Neurosurgery 53:1095–1105

Anderson ME, Postupna N, Ruffo M (2003) Effects of high-frequency stimulation in the internal globus pallidus on the activity of thalamic neurons in the awake monkey. J Neurophysiol 89:1150–1160

Anderson TR, Hu B, Iremonger K, Kiss ZH (2006) Selective attenuation of afferent synaptic transmission as a mechanism of thalamic deep brain stimulation-induced tremor arrest. J Neurosci 26:841–850

Aziz TZ, Peggs D, Sambrook MA, Crossman AR (1991) Lesion of the subthalamic nucleus for the alleviation of 1-methyl-4-phenyl-1,2,3,6-tetrahydropyridine (MPTP)-induced parkinsonism in the primate. Mov Disord 6:288–292

Bar-Gad I, Elias S, Vaadia E, Bergman H (2004) Complex locking rather than complete cessation of neuronal activity in the globus pallidus of a 1-methyl-4-phenyl-1,2,3,6-tetrahydropyridine-treated primate in response to pallidal microstimulation. J Neurosci 24:7410–7419

Bekar L, Libionka W, Tian GF, Xu Q, Torres A, Wang X, Lovatt D, Williams E, Takano T, Schnermann J, Bakos R, Nedergaard M (2008) Adenosine is crucial for deep brain stimulation-mediated attenuation of tremor. Nat Med 14:75–80

Benabid AL, Pollak P, Gervason C, Hoffmann D, Gao DM, Hommel M, Perret JE, de Rougemont J (1991) Long-term suppression of tremor by chronic stimulation of the ventral intermediate thalamic nucleus. Lancet 337:403–406

Benabid AL, Pollak P, Gross C, Hoffmann D, Benazzouz A, Gao DM, Laurent A, Gentil M, Perret J (1994) Acute and long-term effects of subthalamic nucleus stimulation in Parkinson's disease. Stereotact Funct Neurosurg 62:76–84

Benabid AL, Pollak P, Gao D, Hoffmann D, Limousin P, Gay E, Payen I, Benazzouz A (1996) Chronic electrical stimulation of the ventralis intermedius nucleus of the thalamus as a treatment of movement disorders. J Neurosurg 84:203–214

Benazzouz A, Gross C, Féger J, Boraud T, Bioulac B (1993) Reversal of rigidity and improvement in motor performance by subthalamic high-frequency stimulation in MPTP-treated monkeys. Eur J Neurosci 5:382–389

Bergman H, Wichmann T, DeLong MR (1990) Reversal of experimental parkinsonism by lesions of the subthalamic nucleus. Science 249:1436–1438

Bergman H, Feingold A, Nini A, Raz A, Slovin H, Abeles M, Vaadia E (1998) Physiological aspects of information processing in the basal ganglia of normal and parkinsonian primates. Trends Neurosci 21:32–38

Beurrier C, Bioulac B, Audin J, Hammond C (2001) High-frequency stimulation produces a transient blockade of voltage-gated currents in subthalamic neurons. J Neurophysiol 85:1351–1356

Boertien T, Zrinzo L, Kahan J, Jahanshahi M, Hariz M, Mancini L, Limousin P, Foltynie T (2011) Functional imaging of subthalamic nucleus deep brain stimulation in Parkinson's disease. Mov Disord 26:1835–1843

Boraud T, Bezard E, Bioulac B, Gross C (1996) High frequency stimulation of the internal Globus Pallidus (GPi) simultaneously improves parkinsonian symptoms and reduces the firing frequency of GPi neurons in the MPTP-treated monkey. Neurosci Lett 215: 17–20

Brotchie JM, Mitchell IJ, Sambrook MA, Crossman AR (1991) Alleviation of parkinsonism by antagonism of excitatory amino acid transmission in the medial segment of the globus pallidus in rat and primate. Mov Disord 6:133–138

Brown P (2007) Abnormal oscillatory synchronisation in the motor system leads to impaired movement. Curr Opin Neurobiol 17:656–664

Chiken S, Nambu A (2013) High-frequency pallidal stimulation disrupts information flow through the pallidum by GABAergic inhibition. J Neurosci 33: 2268–2280

Chiken S, Nambu A (2014) Disrupting neuronal transmission: mechanism of DBS? Front Syst Neurosci 8:33

Chiken S, Shashidharan P, Nambu A (2008) Cortically-evoked long-lasting inhibition of pallidal neurons in a transgenic mouse model of dystonia. J Neurosci 28: 13967–13977

Coubes P, Cif L, El Fertit H, Hemm S, Vayssiere N, Serrat S, Picot MC, Tuffery S, Claustres M, Echenne B, Frerebeau P (2004) Electrical stimulation of the globus pallidus internus in patients with primary generalized dystonia: long-term results. J Neurosurg 101: 189–194

Deep-Brain Stimulation for Parkinson's Disease Study Group (2001) Deep-brain stimulation of the subthalamic nucleus or the pars interna of the globus pallidus in Parkinson's disease. N Engl J Med 345:956–963

Degos B, Deniau JM, Chavez M, Maurice N (2013) Subthalamic nucleus high-frequency stimulation restores altered electrophysiological properties of cortical neurons in parkinsonian rat. PLoS One 8: e83608

Deniau JM, Degos B, Bosch C, Maurice N (2010) Deep brain stimulation mechanisms: beyond the concept of local functional inhibition. Eur J Neurosci 32:1080–1091

Do MT, Bean BP (2003) Subthreshold sodium currents and pacemaking of subthalamic neurons: modulation by slow inactivation. Neuron 39:109–120

Dostrovsky JO, Lozano AM (2002) Mechanisms of deep brain stimulation. Mov Disord 17:S63–S68

Dostrovsky JO, Levy R, Wu JP, Hutchison WD, Tasker RR, Lozano AM (2000) Microstimulation-induced inhibition of neuronal firing in human globus pallidus. J Neurophysiol 84:570–574

Erez Y, Czitron H, McCairn K, Belelovsky K, Bar-Gad I (2009) Short-term depression of synaptic transmission during stimulation in the globus pallidus of 1-methyl-4-phenyl-1,2,3,6-tetrahydropyridine-treated primates. J Neurosci 29:7797–7802

Fellin T, Pascual O, Haydon PG (2006) Astrocytes coordinate synaptic networks: balanced excitation and inhibition. Physiology 21:208–215

Filali M, Hutchison WD, Palter VN, Lozano AM, Dostrovsky JO (2004) Stimulation-induced inhibition of neuronal firing in human subthalamic nucleus. Exp Brain Res 156:274–281

Galati S, Mazzone P, Fedele E, Pisani A, Peppe A, Pierantozzi M, Brusa L, Tropepi D, Moschella V, Raiteri M, Stanzione P, Bernardi G, Stefani A (2006) Biochemical and electrophysiological changes of substantia nigra pars reticulata driven by subthalamic stimulation in patients with Parkinson's disease. Eur J Neurosci 23:2923–2928

Gradinaru V, Mogri M, Thompson KR, Henderson JM, Deisseroth K (2009) Optical deconstruction of parkinsonian neural circuitry. Science 324:354–359

Graham WC, Robertson RG, Sambrook MA, Crossman AR (1991) Injection of excitatory amino acid antagonists into the medial pallidal segment of a 1-methyl-4-phenyl-1,2,3,6-tetrahydropyridine (MPTP) treated primate reverses motor symptoms of parkinsonism. Life Sci 47:L91–L97

Hammond C, Bergman H, Brown P (2007) Pathological synchronization in Parkinson's disease: networks, models and treatments. Trends Neurosci 30:357–364

Hashimoto T, Elder CM, Vitek JL (2002) A template subtraction method for stimulus artifact removal in high-frequency deep brain stimulation. J Neurosci Methods 113:181–186

Hashimoto T, Elder CM, Okun MS, Patrick SK, Vitek JL (2003) Stimulation of the subthalamic nucleus changes the firing pattern of pallidal neurons. J Neurosci 23: 1916–1923

Hershey T, Revilla FJ, Wernle AR, McGee-Minnich L, Antenor JV, Videen TO, Dowling JL, Mink JW, Perlmutter JS (2003) Cortical and subcortical blood flow effects of subthalamic nucleus stimulation in PD. Neurology 61:816–821

Hilker R, Voges J, Ghaemi M, Lehrke R, Rudolf J, Koulousakis A, Herholz K, Wienhard K, Sturm V, Heiss WD (2003) Deep brain stimulation of the subthalamic nucleus does not increase the striatal dopamine concentration in parkinsonian humans. Mov Disord 18:41–48

Jantz JJ, Watanabe M (2013) Pallidal deep brain stimulation modulates afferent fibers, efferent fibers, and glia. J Neurosci 33:9873–9875

Jech R, Urgosík D, Tintera J, Nebuzelský A, Krásenský J, Liscák R, Roth J, Růzicka E (2001) Functional magnetic resonance imaging during deep brain stimulation: a pilot study in four patients with Parkinson's disease. Mov Disord 16:1126–1132

Johnson MD, McIntyre CC (2008) Quantifying the neural elements activated and inhibited by globus pallidus deep brain stimulation. J Neurophysiol 100: 2549–2563

Johnson MD, Miocinovic S, McIntyre CC, Vitek JL (2008) Mechanisms and targets of deep brain stimulation in movement disorders. Neurotherapeutics 5: 294–308

Kita H, Kita T (2011) Cortical stimulation evokes abnormal responses in the dopamine-depleted rat basal ganglia. J Neurosci 31:10311–10322

Koller W, Pahwa R, Busenbark K, Hubble J, Wilkinson S, Lang A, Tuite P, Sime E, Lazano A, Hauser R, Malapira T, Smith D, Tarsy D, Miyawaki E, Norregaard T, Kormos T, Olanow CW (1997) High-frequency unilateral thalamic stimulation in the treatment of essential and parkinsonian tremor. Ann Neurol 42: 292–299

Kringelbach ML, Jenkinson N, Owen SL, Aziz TZ (2007) Translational principles of deep brain stimulation. Nat Rev Neurosci 8:623–635

Lafreniere-Roula M, Kim E, Hutchison WD, Lozano AM, Hodaie M, Dostrovsky JO (2010) High-frequency microstimulation in human globus pallidus and substantia nigra. Exp Brain Res 205:251–261

Leblois A, Reese R, Labarre D, Hamann M, Richter A, Boraud T, Meissner WG (2010) Deep brain stimulation changes basal ganglia output nuclei firing pattern in the dystonic hamster. Neurobiol Dis 38:288–298

Lee KH, Chang SY, Roberts DW, Kim U (2004) Neurotransmitter release from high-frequency stimulation of the subthalamic nucleus. J Neurosurg 101:511–517

Levy R, Lang AE, Dostrovsky JO, Pahapill P, Romas J, Saint-Cyr J, Hutchison WD, Lozano AM (2001) Lidocaine and muscimol microinjections in subthalamic nucleus reverse Parkinsonian symptoms. Brain 124:2105–2118

Li S, Arbuthnott GW, Jutras MJ, Goldberg JA, Jaeger D (2007) Resonant antidromic cortical circuit activation as a consequence of high-frequency subthalamic deep-brain stimulation. J Neurophysiol 98:3525–3537

Li Q, Ke Y, Chan DC, Qian ZM, Yung KK, Ko H, Arbuthnott GW, Yung WH (2012) Therapeutic deep brain stimulation in Parkinsonian rats directly influences motor cortex. Neuron 76:1030–1041

Limousin P, Pollak P, Benazzouz A, Hoffmann D, Le Bas JF, Broussolle E, Perret JE, Benabid AL (1995) Effect of parkinsonian signs and symptoms of bilateral subthalamic nucleus stimulation. Lancet 345:91–95

Liu Y, Postupna N, Falkenberg J, Anderson ME (2008) High frequency deep brain stimulation: what are the therapeutic mechanisms? Neurosci Biobehav Rev 32:343–351

Luo J, Kaplitt MG, Fitzsimons HL, Zuzga DS, Liu Y, Oshinsky ML, During MJ (2002) Subthalamic GAD gene therapy in a Parkinson's disease rat model. Science 298:425–429

Maurice N, Thierry AM, Glowinski J, Deniau JM (2003) Spontaneous and evoked activity of substantia nigra pars reticulata neurons during high-frequency stimulation of the subthalamic nucleus. J Neurosci 23: 9929–9936

McCairn KW, Turner RS (2009) Deep brain stimulation of the globus pallidus internus in the parkinsonian primate: local entrainment and suppression of low-frequency oscillations. J Neurophysiol 101:1941–1960

McIntyre CC, Savasta M, Walter BL, Vitek JL (2004) How does deep brain stimulation work? Present understanding and future questions. J Clin Neurophysiol 21: 40–50

Meissner W, Harnack D, Reese R, Paul G, Reum T, Ansorge M, Kusserow H, Winter C, Morgenstern R, Kupsch A (2003) High-frequency stimulation of the subthalamic nucleus enhances striatal dopamine release and metabolism in rats. J Neurochem 85:601–609

Meissner W, Leblois A, Hansel D, Bioulac B, Gross CE, Benazzouz A, Boraud T (2005) Subthalamic high frequency stimulation resets subthalamic firing and reduces abnormal oscillations. Brain 128:2372–2382

Mink JW (1996) The basal ganglia: focused selection and inhibition of competing motor programs. Prog Neurobiol 50:381–425

Miocinovic S, Parent M, Butson CR, Hahn PJ, Russo GS, Vitek JL, McIntyre CC (2006) Computational analysis of subthalamic nucleus and lenticular fasciculus activation during therapeutic deep brain stimulation. J Neurophysiol 96:1569–1580

Montgomery EB Jr (2006) Effects of GPi stimulation on human thalamic neuronal activity. Clin Neurophysiol 117:2691–2702

Moran A, Stein E, Tischler H, Belelovsky K, Bar-Gad I (2011) Dynamic stereotypic responses of Basal Ganglia neurons to subthalamic nucleus high-frequency stimulation in the parkinsonian primate. Front Syst Neurosci 5:21

Nambu A, Tokuno H, Hamada I, Kita H, Imanishi M, Akazawa T, Ikeuchi Y, Hasegawa N (2000) Excitatory cortical inputs to pallidal neurons via the subthalamic nucleus in the monkey. J Neurophysiol 84: 289–300

Nambu A, Tokuno H, Takada M (2002) Functional significance of the cortico-subthalamo-pallidal 'hyperdirect' pathway. Neurosci Res 43:111–117

Nishibayashi H, Ogura M, Kakishita K, Tanaka S, Tachibana Y, Nambu A, Kita H, Itakura T (2011) Cortically evoked responses of human pallidal neurons recorded during stereotactic neurosurgery. Mov Disord 26:469–476

Ostrem JL, Starr PA (2008) Treatment of dystonia with deep brain stimulation. Neurotherapeutics 5:320–330

Pralong E, Debatisse D, Maeder M, Vingerhoets F, Ghika J, Villemure JG (2003) Effect of deep brain stimulation of GPI on neuronal activity of the thalamic nucleus ventralis oralis in a dystonic patient. Neurophysiol Clin 33:169–173

Ranck JB Jr (1975) Which elements are excited in electrical stimulation of mammalian central nervous system: a review. Brain Res 98:417–440

Reese R, Leblois A, Steigerwald F, Potter-Nerger M, Herzog J, Mehdorn HM, Deuschl G, Meissner WG, Volkmann J (2011) Subthalamic deep brain stimulation increases pallidal firing rate and regularity. Exp Neurol 229:517–521

Rehncrona S, Johnels B, Widner H, Törnqvist AL, Hariz M, Sydow O (2003) Long-term efficacy of thalamic deep brain stimulation for tremor: double-blind assessments. Mov Disord 18:163–170

Shi LH, Luo F, Woodward DJ, Chang JY (2006) Basal ganglia neural responses during behaviorally effective deep brain stimulation of the subthalamic nucleus in rats performing a treadmill locomotion test. Synapse 59:445–457

Shin DS, Samoilova M, Cotic M, Zhang L, Brotchie JM, Carlen PL (2007) High frequency stimulation or elevated K^+ depresses neuronal activity in the rat entopeduncular nucleus. Neuroscience 149:68–86

Shink E, Smith Y (1995) Differential synaptic innervation of neurons in the internal and external segments of the globus pallidus by the GABA- and glutamate-containing terminals in the squirrel monkey. J Comp Neurol 358:119–141

Shon YM, Lee KH, Goerss SJ, Kim IY, Kimble C, Van Gompel JJ, Bennet K, Blaha CD, Chang SY (2010) High frequency stimulation of the subthalamic nucleus evokes striatal dopamine release in a large animal model of human DBS neurosurgery. Neurosci Lett 475:136–140

Siegfried J, Lippitz B (1994a) Bilateral chronic electrostimulation of ventroposterolateral pallidum: a new therapeutic approach for alleviating all parkinsonian symptoms. Neurosurgery 35:1126–1130

Siegfried J, Lippitz B (1994b) Chronic electrical stimulation of the VL-VPL complex and of the pallidum in the treatment of movement disorders: personal experience since 1982. Stereotact Funct Neurosurg 62:71–75

Smith Y, Wichmann T, DeLong MR (1994) Synaptic innervation of neurones in the internal pallidal segment by the subthalamic nucleus and the external pallidum in monkeys. J Comp Neurol 343:297–318

Starr PA, Rau GM, Davis V, Marks WJ Jr, Ostrem JL, Simmons D, Lindsey N, Turner RS (2005) Spontaneous pallidal neuronal activity in human dystonia:comparison with Parkinson's disease and normal macaque. J Neurophysiol 93:3165–3176

Stefani A, Fedele E, Galati S, Pepicelli O, Frasca S, Pierantozzi M, Peppe A, Brusa L, Orlacchio A, Hainsworth AH, Gattoni G, Stanzione P, Bernardi G, Raiteri M, Mazzone P (2005) Subthalamic stimulation activates internal pallidus: evidence from cGMP microdialysis in PD patients. Ann Neurol 57:448–452

Tachibana Y, Iwamuro H, Kita H, Takada M, Nambu A (2011) Subthalamo-pallidal interactions underlying parkinsonian neuronal oscillations in the primate basal ganglia. Eur J Neurosci 34:1470–1484

Tai CH, Boraud T, Bezard E, Bioulac B, Gross C, Benazzouz A (2003) Electrophysiological and metabolic evidence that high-frequency stimulation of the subthalamic nucleus bridles neuronal activity in the subthalamic nucleus and the substantia nigra reticulata. FASEB J 17:1820–1830

Tawfik VL, Chang SY, Hitti FL, Roberts DW, Leiter JC, Jovanovic S, Lee KH (2010) Deep brain stimulation results in local glutamate and adenosine release: investigation into the role of astrocytes. Neurosurgery 67:367–375

Vedam-Mai V, van Battum EY, Kamphuis W, Feenstra MG, Denys D, Reynolds BA, Okun MS, Hol EM (2012) Deep brain stimulation and the role of astrocytes. Mol Psychiatry 17:124–131

Vidailhet M, Jutras MF, Roze E, Grabli D (2013) Deep brain stimulation for dystonia. Handb Clin Neurol 116:167–187

Vitek JL (2008) Deep brain stimulation: how does it work? Cleve Clin J Med 75(Suppl2):S59–S65

Wang LY, Kaczmarek LK (1998) High-frequency firing helps replenish the readily releasable pool of synaptic vesicles. Nature 394:384–388

Welter ML, Houeto JL, Bonnet AM, Bejjani PB, Mesnage V, Dormont D, Navarro S, Cornu P, Agid Y, Pidoux B (2004) Effects of high-frequency stimulation on subthalamic neuronal activity in parkinsonian patients. Arch Neurol 61:89–96

Wichmann T (2000) A digital averaging method for removal of stimulus artifacts in neurophysiologic experiments. J Neurosci Methods 98:57–62

Wichmann T, Delong MR (2006) Deep brain stimulation for neurologic and neuropsychiatric disorders. Neuron 52:197–204

Wichmann T, Bergman H, DeLong MR (1994) The primate subthalamic nucleus. III. Changes in motor behavior and neuronal activity in the internal pallidum induced by subthalamic inactivation in the MPTP model of parkinsonism. J Neurophysiol 72:521–530

Windels F, Bruet N, Poupard A, Urbain N, Chouvet G, Feuerstein C, Savasta M (2000) Effects of high frequency stimulation of subthalamic nucleus on extracellular glutamate and GABA in substantia nigra and globus pallidus in the normal rat. Eur J Neurosci 12:4141–4146

Windels F, Carcenac C, Poupard A, Savasta M (2005) Pallidal origin of GABA release within the substantia nigra pars reticulata during high-frequency stimulation of the subthalamic nucleus. J Neurosci 25: 5079–5086

Wu YR, Levy R, Ashby P, Tasker RR, Dostrovsky JO (2001) Does stimulation of the GPi control dyskinesia by activating inhibitory axons? Mov Disord 16: 208–216

Zucker RS, Regehr WG (2002) Short-term synaptic plasticity. Annu Rev Physiol 64:355–405

3 Symptoms and Signs of Parkinson's Disease and Other Movement Disorders

Hidefumi Ito

3.1 Parkinson's Disease

3.1.1 General Consideration

Parkinson's disease (PD) has been traditionally regarded as a representative neurodegenerative disorder involving the extrapyramidal system and principally presenting motor symptoms and signs. These motor manifestations are caused by deficiency of dopamine in the striatum. However, recent progress in clinical and basic research on parkinsonism reveals that various nonmotor symptoms frequently manifest in PD patients and that nondopaminergic neurons also degenerate. Therefore, to date PD is considered as a subset of multisystem degenerative disorders.

Nevertheless, the cardinal clinical features of PD are motor symptoms, including tremor, bradykinesia, rigidity, and loss of postural reflex. Flexed posture and freezing may be added to them, collectively designated as six cardinal motor features (Fahn and Przedborski 2010). The onset of PD is so gradual and insidious that patients can rarely indicate the date of beginning. Moreover, not all motor symptoms manifest when they become aware of its presence. Symptoms usually start unilaterally, as the disease progresses slowly, they extend to bilateral involvement. The most common initial motor symptom in PD is tremor, which is first recognized in 70 % of patients. Most of the patients with PD consult a doctor after manifestation of motor symptoms. However, detailed medical history usually reveals the existing nonmotor symptoms, such as constipation, hyposmia, and REM sleep behavior disorder (RBD), at their first visit. The nonmotor symptoms appearing in PD are diverse and troublesome, which considerably impair quality of life of the patients.

3.1.2 Motor Symptoms

3.1.2.1 Tremor

The most prominent feature of parkinsonism is a *rest tremor*. This tremor differs from cerebellar tremor and essential tremor in that it typically occurs when patients sit with their arms supported. The shaking is rhythmic and has a regular rate at a frequency of 4–6 Hz. Rest tremor first manifests in one side of upper or lower extremity distally, but as the disease progresses, it extends to the other ipsilateral limb, then becomes bilateral. It is usually pronounced on the same side of akinesia (see below). Tremor is a simple to-and-fro motion, turning of the forearm, or a back-and-forth motion of the thumb and fingers. The classic rest tremor involves the thumb and index finger and is reminiscent of rolling a pill between them, thus called "*pill-rolling tremor*." At the earliest

H. Ito, MD, PhD
Department of Neurology,
Wakayama Medical University, Wakayama, Japan
e-mail: ito@wakayama-med.ac.jp

T. Itakura (ed.), *Deep Brain Stimulation for Neurological Disorders: Theoretical Background and Clinical Application*, DOI 10.1007/978-3-319-08476-3_3,

stage of the disease, some patients feel a vibrating sensation when no involuntary movements are noticeable by appearance. The tremor may be confined to a very small part, such as the thumb only, or may be present intermittently. It disappears during sleep and when patients are really relaxed. On the contrary, the tremor is induced or enhanced by nervousness or mental task, such as calculating mentally and speaking in public. This is one of the reasons that PD patients avoid social activity. On the other hand, the tremor ameliorates with action, such as writing or holding something in the hand. Therefore, rest tremor is, indeed an embarrassing symptom, not great impairment of the activity of daily living. In certain patients, as the limb maintains a posture for several seconds, the tremor re-emerges; thus, it is called "*re-emergent tremor*" (Jankovic et al. 1999). Rest tremor of the hand is often intensified with walking and could be an important diagnostic sign in early stage of PD. Tremor may involve the tongue, lips, jaw, and sometimes it causes shaking of the neck. However, voice is rarely affected in contrast to being common in patients with essential tremor.

3.1.2.2 Akinesia

A term *akinesia* collectively implies *bradykinesia* and *hypokinesia*. Bradykinesia represents slowness of movement, and hypokinesia signifies reduction in amplitude of movement. Akinesia develops unilaterally, and despite having normal strength and coordination, patients have difficulty moving arms and legs.

For the patient, akinesia is the most debilitating feature, leading to the loss of automatic and spontaneous movement and difficulty of initiating movement. These movements are normally made without being conscious of them. For example, we swallow the saliva and the eyes blink spontaneously several times a minute. While sitting, we shift our weight from one side to the other, rub our face, turn our head, and may tap the chair arm, without significant intention. In PD patients, these automatic motions are much less frequent than normal subjects.

Impairment of minor movements of postural adjustment keeps the patient sitting motionless. Reduction of eye blinking and expressive movements of the face results in the *mask-like face* or *hypomimia*. Speech is devoid of the normal inflection in pitch and cadence; the voice becomes monotonous, hypophonic (low in volume), and tremulous; and the articulation loses clarity. Paucity of trunk and limb movement leads to small and slow handwriting (*micrographia*), and impairment of brushing teeth, combing hair, shaving, dressing, buttoning, bathing, and other "activities of daily living." Drooling saliva is a consequence of decrease of spontaneous swallowing, but not of excessive secretion of saliva. Voluntary swallowing with effort may reduce drooling, however, swallowing function gradually develops impaired in advanced stage, and aspiration and choking become at risk.

Gait is slow, stride length is shortened, and arm swing decreases. When turning, normally the head and eyes turn first, followed by the shoulders, and then the trunk and legs. PD patients fail to lead with the head on turns, the body turns in one piece, called "*en bloc turning*." Rising from a chair and turning over in bed become also difficult due to truncal bradykinesia.

Parkinsonian patients have a difficulty performing two motor acts simultaneously, such as picking up coins from a purse during walking up to a vending machine. Therefore, daily activities such as eating and dressing take much time and appear to be performed in a deliberate manner.

Another peculiar phenomenon is *paradoxical kinesia*, which designates a sudden improvement of akinesia by stimulation of visual or auditory cues.

3.1.2.3 Rigidity

Rigidity is an increase in muscle tone resulted from the failure of reciprocal relaxation of antagonist muscles. Patients sometime feel stiffness, pain, tiredness, or a cramp in rigid muscles, however, they are not usually aware of rigidity. Only physicians can decide the presence or the absence of it by passively moving the patient's limbs, neck, or trunk. In that sense, rigidity is not a symptom, but a sign. To test for it, the physician takes the patient's forearm, hand, lower leg, or foot and bends and straightens it gently repetitively while asking the patient to relax. The presence of persistent and

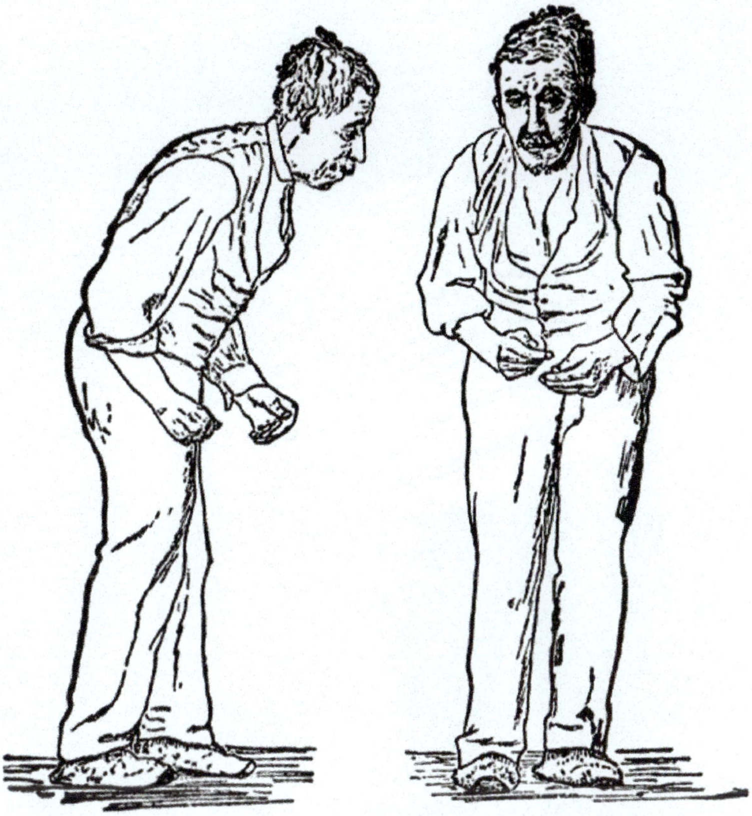

Fig. 3.1 Postural abnormality of a patient with Parkinson's disease. The elbows, hips, and knees are flexed; the trunk is bent forward; and the arms are held in front of the body (Reproduced from the sketch of Sir William Richard Gowers)

constant resistance to passive motion around the elbow, wrist, knee, or ankle joint in all directions throughout the movement implies "*lead-pipe rigidity*." In contrast, a regular and jerky resistance as if there is a ratchet gear in the joint is known as "*cogwheel rigidity*." This cogwheel rigidity is a manifestation of overlapping or underlying tremor. Rigidity is augmented, or only elicited, by another limb being engaged in voluntary movement. To detect rigidity is not only important to diagnose parkinsonism and other extrapyramidal disorders but it is also helpful in distinguishing a parkinsonian tremor from other varieties of tremor.

3.1.2.4 Loss of Postural Reflexes

Loss of postural reflexes is the principal cause of falling. It manifests usually in later stage of PD, and its earlier manifestation in parkinsonian patients suggests the diagnosis of progressive supranuclear palsy (PSP). Postural reflexes can be tested by the *pull test*. The physician stands behind the patient, gives a sudden firm pull on the shoulders after explaining the procedure, and checks for retropulsion. Normal subjects can recover within two steps. Patients who have impairment or loss of postural reflexes, which are the mechanisms that alter muscle tone in response to change in position, could fall without catching the patient by the physician. Loss of postural reflexes, in combination with akinesia and rigidity, leads to gait impairments, called *marche a petit pas* and *festinating gait*, those are characterized by short steps and a tendency to accelerate, respectively.

3.1.2.5 Flexed Posture

Postural abnormality is often found in the arm initially, gradually spreads to the whole body. The elbows, hips, and knees are flexed; the trunk is bent forward; the head is dropped; and the arms are held in front of the body (*stooped posture*) (Fig. 3.1). *Camptocormia* is the extreme anteflexion posture of the trunk, and the sustained lateral bending of the trunk is often referred to as *Pisa syndrome* (Fig. 3.2) (Tassorelli et al. 2012). Deformity of the

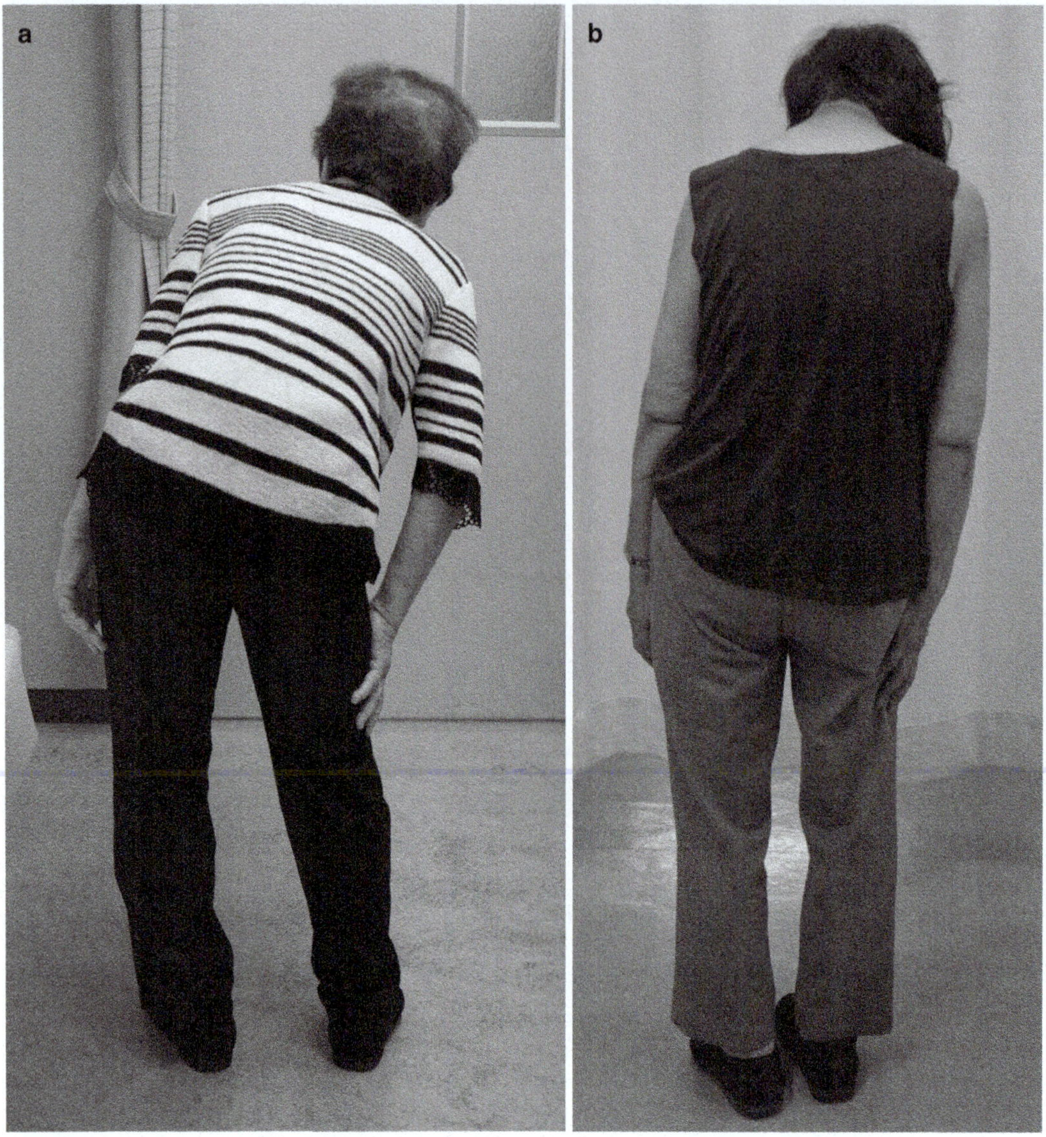

Fig. 3.2 Pisa syndrome. The sustained lateral bending of the trunk is evident (**a**) A 82 year-old woman manifesting Pisa syndrome and camptocormia. (**b**) A 73 year-old woman with Pisa syndrome and a dropped head.

hands includes metacarpophalangeal flexion, proximal interphalangeal extension, distal interphalangeal flexion, and ulnar deviation (*striatal hand*) (Fig. 3.3) (Ashour et al. 2005).

3.1.2.6 Freezing

The freezing phenomenon is sudden, transient inability to perform movements. Freezing occurs in opening the eyelid (*eyelid opening apraxia*), speaking, and writing. However, if walking is affected, it is troublesome for the patient. The feet seem glued to the floor, and starting to walk delays (*start hesitation*). After several seconds, the feet suddenly become unstuck and the patient can start walking with shuffling steps. However, freezing reappears when the patient attempts to turn or approaches a destination (*destination hesitation*), such as a chair in which to sit. Gait freezing is frequently induced when the patient passes through a narrow doorway, especially under hastened situation, such as entering train doors or elevator doors those may close. Interestingly,

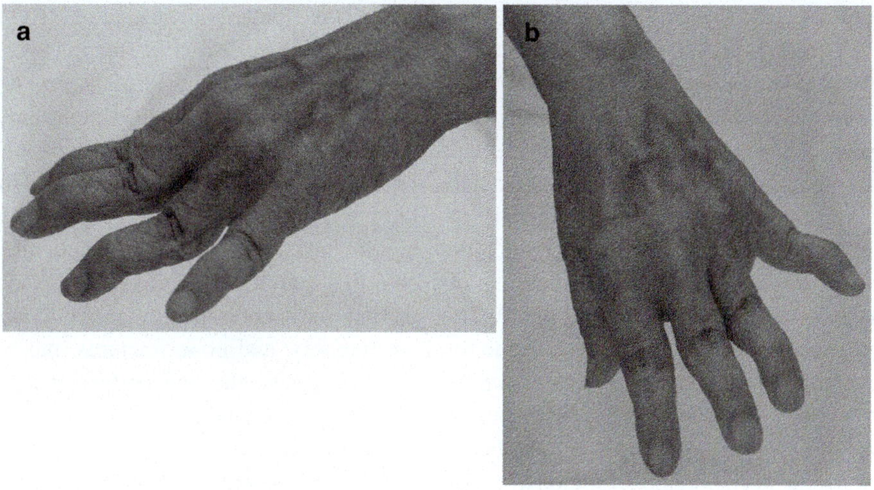

Fig. 3.3 Striatal hand. Note the characteristic deformity of the hands with metacarpophalangeal flexion, proximal interphalangeal extension, and distal interphalangeal flexion, resembling the swan-neck deformities in arthritic disorders (a) viewed sidewise (b) seen from above

entering escalators or stairs causes less trouble because each step acts as visual clues. Freezing accompanied with loss of postural reflexes is a great risk of falling and hip fractures.

3.1.3 Nonmotor Symptoms

3.1.3.1 Autonomic Dysfunction

In PD patients, various autonomic disturbances develop.

Constipation is a representative premotor symptom and a major complaint for many patients. Insufficient movements and drinking little water may contribute its exacerbation. Severe constipation could result in the enlargement of colon and lead to obstructive ileus requiring a surgical procedure.

Bladder dysfunction is a rather later symptom. Difficulty in emptying the urinary bladder leads to *frequent urination*. Nocturnal pollakisuria not only disturbs the patient's sleep, but also increases the risk of fall.

Sexual dysfunction appeared in PD patients includes decreases in libido, sexual intercourse, and orgasm. In men, difficulty in maintaining erection and delayed ejaculation also occur. Dopamine deficiency is presumably related to these problems. Recently, hypersexuality induced by levodopa treatment has drawn attention as a troublesome aspect of impulse control disorder.

Orthostatic hypotension usually becomes apparent in the advanced stage. The patient is aware of the symptoms of faintness, dizziness, or lightheadedness on standing or walking. Orthostatic hypotension is likely aggravated by antiparkinsonian medications. Another disturbance of blood pressure control is *postprandial hypotension*. Symptoms tend to be more severe after eating a large meal or a meal that includes a lot of carbohydrates.

Excessive sweating is a common symptom of PD. It may manifest on a part of the body, but can be generalized. In patients with wearing off phenomenon, it tends to be seen at off period. The excessive sweating appears to be a response to normal stimuli in an exaggerated manner.

Seborrhea is excessive discharge of *sebum*, the oily, waxy substance secreted from the sebaceous gland of the skin. A subsequent infection and inflammation causes seborrheic dermatitis. The skin of the face at the sides of the nose, the forehead, and the scalp is particularly affected.

3.1.3.2 Sensory Symptoms

Hyposmia, a manifestation of olfactory dysfunction, is one of the most important premotor symptoms. It may precede the onset of motor symptom by many years. Furthermore, hyposmia in PD is more severe than that found in patients with other parkinsonian syndromes such as progressive supranuclear palsy, multiple system atrophy, and corticobasal degeneration. Therefore, the recognition of the olfactory deficit in parkinsonian patients helps making a clinical diagnosis of PD. In addition, a recent report suggests that olfactory dysfunction is a prodromal symptom of dementia associated with PD (Baba et al. 2012).

Painful symptoms in PD are quite commonly present, although neurological examinations reveal no objective sensory impairment. Sensory symptoms include numbness, tingling, and burning, those occur in the region of motor involvement. To note, dull pain may be present even before appearance of rigidity or akinesia in the same limb.

Painful symptoms are classified into five categories: (1) musculoskeletal pain, (2) radicular or neuropathic pain, (3) dystonia-related pain, (4) central pain, and (5) akathitic discomfort (Ford and Pfeiffer 2005). Musculoskeletal pain is related to rigidity and akinesia, aggravated at off period, and relieved by levodopa. The postural deformities in PD may predispose to the development of radiculopathy. Dystonia appears not only at off period as the deficit of dopamine, but also at on period as a medication-induced symptom. Central pain is originated from the brain and is resistant to treatment. Akathisia is characterized by subjective inner restlessness. The patient is unable to sit still and bothered especially during off period. Similarly, restless legs syndrome (RLS) is characterized by uncomfortable sensation of legs that disappears with movement. Akathisia is present most of the day, while RLS aggravates during evening and night. However, these two conditions are sometimes difficult to distinguish, because both may respond to dopamine replacement therapy.

3.1.3.3 Sleep and Awakening Disturbances

Sleep problems encompass RBD, RLS, insomnia, and sleep apnea. Awakening problems are encountered with dopaminergic therapy including excessive daytime sleepiness (EDS) and sleep attacks.

RBD is a pathological state of REM in which the normal atonia of REM sleep is lost, enabling motor activity during REM sleep, leading to respond to dreams. Dream content during RBD episodes is often threatened, chased, or attacked ones. Therefore, the patients yell, clap, punch, kick, sit, stand, fall out of bed, and run. These violent behaviors may injure both the patients and bed partners during RBD episodes. The patient may not only suffer from lacerations, ecchymoses, and bone fractures, but also pommel and choke the bed partner. The patient is unable to remember the behavior when awakens in the morning.

The patients with *RLS* feel dysesthesias in the legs at rest, which is aggravated in the evening and at nighttime. The dysesthesias are expressed as tingling, creeping, crawling, burning, itching, aching, or other sensations. It is relieved by moving the legs or walking, thus the patient feels irresistible urge to move the legs. Many patients with RLS also experience periodic limb movements in sleep (PLMS). RLS resembles akathisia, however, RLS can cause sleep fragmentation and EDS.

EDS is defined as an increased propensity to fall asleep at daytime. The causes of EDS in PD patients include antiparkinsonian medications, RBD, PLMS, nightmares, hallucinations, dyskinesias, and symptoms of PD such as tremor, rigidity, nocturia, central pain, sweating, etc.

Sleep attacks is a sudden episode of sleep without warning. Frucht et al. first described PD patients taking nonergot dopamine agonist who had sudden onset of sleep during driving (Frucht et al. 1999). Subsequently, many PD cases with sleep attacks have been reported. The risk factors of sleep attacks include duration of illness, medication of dopamine agonists or levodopa, and EDS. However, it is difficult to precisely predict who is at risk of sleep attacks while driving, and there are no guidelines to determine who is safe to drive.

3.1.3.4 Psychological Disturbance

The most common psychiatric symptom that affects PD patients is *depression*. It is important to discriminate a depressive state as a manifestation of PD from major depression. In PD, a guilty conscience or attempting suicide is not a predominant symptom, instead *apathy* and *anhedonia* could be dominated. Apathy is a state of loss of emotions such as concern, excitement, motivation, and passion. Anhedonia is defined as the inability to experience pleasure from activities usually found enjoyable, such as hobbies, music, sexual activities, or social interactions. The patient becomes dependent, indecisive, passive, and lacks motivations. It is known in PD patients that apathy or anhedonia can manifest independently from depression.

Anxiety is another psychological problem that is frequently seen in PD patients. Anxiety disorder includes panic attack or obsessive–compulsive behavior, manifesting at off state. It can precede motor manifestations.

Fatigue is also common in PD. It may present as one of symptoms of depression, but recently it can manifest by itself in parkinsonian patients. *Mental fatigue* is a subjective tiredness and *physical fatigue* indicates gradual reduction of amplitude or velocity of motion, detectable in finger tapping or rapid alternating movement procedures. Mental fatigue and physical fatigue are known to occur independently in PD.

Impulse control disorder is a behavioral adverse effect associated with dopamine replacement therapy (Voon et al. 2009). Pathological gambling and shopping, compulsive eating, hypersexuality, and compulsive medication use are its representative symptoms. The patient also suffers from punding (abnormal repetitive non-goal oriented behaviors). These symptoms are collectively called as *dopamine dysregulation syndrome*.

3.1.3.5 Cognitive Decline

Dementia is generally not an early feature of PD. In early stage, the patient responds to questions slowly, but when given enough time, correct answers can be obtained (*bradyphrenia*), indicating that memory function itself is not impaired. However, as the disease progresses, higher cognitive dysfunctions become prominent. Dementia in PD is clinically associated with older age and severe motor symptoms. Most of PD patients with dementia have Lewy bodies in cortical neurons (dementia with Lewy bodies: DLB), and the others may develop concurrent Alzheimer pathology, multiple infarctions, or other neurodegenerative disorders. Although it is often difficult to distinguish these disorders in each patient, early features of DLB are executive dysfunction, impaired verbal fluency, and visuospatial disturbances, while memory impairment comes late. The other representative symptoms which characterize DLB include fluctuating attention and concentration, recurrent well-formed visual hallucinations, and severe neuroleptic sensitivity. Mckeith et al. have proposed in the report of the consortium on DLB international workshop that fluctuation in cognitive function, persistent well-formed visual hallucinations, and spontaneous motor features of parkinsonism are core features with diagnostic significance in discriminating DLB from AD and other dementias (McKeith et al. 1996).

3.1.4 Motor Complications

3.1.4.1 Fluctuations

At an early stage of PD, the beneficial effect of levodopa is sustained and motor symptoms are stably controlled throughout the day. This effect is attributed both to a prolonged storage of levodopa-derived dopamine within residual dopaminergic nerve terminals and to a prolonged postsynaptic effect on dopamine receptors. However, with chronic levodopa therapy motor fluctuations gradually appear. *Wearing off phenomenon* or end-of-dose deterioration is, by definition, a return of parkisonian symptoms in less than 4 h after the last intake of medication. Beneficial time of levodopa (*on period*) progressively shortens, and the motor dysfunction in the deteriorated time (*off period*) becomes more profound. Another subset of motor fluctuations is *on–off phenomenon* in that the changes between on and off come abrupt and are not related to the timing of the levodopa dosing. One of the causes of these fluctuations is further reduced dopamine storage in the progressively lost residual dopaminergic nerve terminals. However, the failure of elimination of fluctuations by direct-acting dopamine agonists provokes the possibility that the sensitivity of dopamine receptors is modulated. Large width between the peaks and the bottoms of the striatal dopamine concentrations due to intermittent levodopa administration is hypothesized as a cause of the altered sensitivity of dopamine receptors.

Fluctuations are known to appear not only in motor functions but also in nonmotor symptoms, such as mood, anxiety, and pain. These behavioral and sensory offs can occur in the absence of motor offs. This nonmotor offs may underlie the dopamine dysregulation syndrome.

3.1.4.2 Dyskinesias

Chronic levodopa therapy and altered sensitivity of dopamine receptors affect the dyskinetic effects. Dyskinesias usually take forms of chorea, ballism, dystonia, or their combination. Mild dyskinesias are not troublesome and even unnoticeable. However, severe forms can be disabling.

Dyskinesias are categorized into several forms according to the timing of levodopa intake. The most common is peak-dose dyskinesias, those appear at the peak of levodopa concentration when parkinsonian symptoms are well controlled. Diphasic dyskinesias appear at the beginning and end of the dosing when levodopa concentrations change acutely. In this case the involuntary movements affect mainly the legs.

Off dystonias appear during off periods and is often painful. The patients may experience early morning dystonia, which affects the feet for several minutes. This is ameliorated by levodopa administration.

3.2 Dystonia

3.2.1 General Consideration

Dystonia is defined as a syndrome of sustained muscle contractions, frequently causing twisting and repetitive movements or abnormal postures. To stress its twisting quality of movements and posture, the term torsion is sometimes placed in front of the word dystonia, as *torsion dystonia.* The voluntary muscles in the face, trunk, and limbs can be affected by dystonia. When rhythmic, repetitive muscle spasms of the limbs occur in patients with torsion dystonia, the term *dystonic tremor* is applied.

Dystonia can be elicited by a specific action. This condition is called as *task-specific dystonia,* including writer's cramp and occupational cramp. Dystonia is induced or exacerbated by emotional stresses, fatigue, and also by voluntary movements in parts of the body not affected by dystonia. Exacerbation of truncal dystonia during talking is an example. With progression, dystonic movements can develop while at rest, and finally bizarre dystonic postures become sustained.

A characteristic feature of dystonic movements is that they can be reduced by tactile *sensory tricks.* The patients with cervical dystonia (spasmodic torticollis) can diminish their abnormal muscle contractions by placing a hand on the side of the face. Lying down on the floor can reduce truncal dystonia. The oral dystonia can be suppressed in touching the lips or placing something in the mouth. Dystonia is also relieved with relaxation and sleep.

Some patients with dystonia, especially of young age, may experience a sudden exacerbation of the severity of dystonia, called *status dystonicus.* These patients should be intensely treated by using sedatives such as propofol, because the induced myoglobinuria may cause renal failure.

3.2.2 Classification of Dystonia

Dystonia can be classified by age at onset, by distribution of dystonia, and by etiology (Fahn and Bressman 2010).

Age at onset is in childhood (0–12 years), in adolescence (13–20 years), or in adult (later than 20 years). Patients with the younger age at onset tend to progress severe and generalized symptoms, whereas cases with the older age at onset likely remain focal dystonia. Thus, age at onset is the factor most related to prognosis of dystonia.

Distribution of dystonia may be focal, segmental, multifocal, generalized, or hemidystonia. *Focal dystonias* are those when only a single body part is affected. The most common focal dystonia is spasmodic torticollis, followed by blepharospasm, oromandibular dystonia, or spasmodic dysphonia. Writer's cramp or occupational cramp is less common. When dystonia spreads to involve contiguous body parts, the term *segmental dystonia* is applied. The most common segmental dystonia is Meige syndrome in which blepharospasm is concomitant with oromandibular dystonia. *Generalized dystonia* represents involvements of bilateral legs and some other areas. On the other hand, in multifocal dystonia two or more noncontiguous parts are involved. In patients with *hemidystonia* one-half of the body is affected.

The etiologic classification of dystonia identifies primary, dystonia-plus syndromes, secondary, and heredodegenerative subsets.

3.2.3 Primary Dystonias

Primary dystonia is a pure dystonia, presenting dystonic postures, dystonic movements, and if any, dystonic tremor, but other neurologic abnormalities are not accompanied. Primary dystonias include familial and sporadic cases. Several causative genes have been identified, but in the most of primary dystonias the causes remain to be elucidated.

3.2.3.1 Early Onset Primary Dystonia

DYT1 is the typical early onset primary dystonia, begins in childhood or adolescence. DYT1 was first described by Oppenheim as "dystonia musculorum deformans" in 1911, thus also called as Oppenheim's dystonia. The causative gene is *TOR1A*, being localized to chromosome 9q34, and encoding the protein torsin A (Ozelius et al. 1997). DYT1 is inherited in an autosomal-dominant manner with reduced penetrance of 30–40 %. Moreover, great intrafamilial variability is noted, ranging from severe generalized dystonia to mild writer's cramp or even no dystonia at all. DYT1 is estimated to account for approximately 80–90 % of early onset dystonia in Ashkenazi Jews, and 15–50 % in non-Jews. The increased prevalence in Jews is attributed to a founder effect.

The average age of onset of DYT1 is approximately 12 years. Although onset ranges from 4 to 64 years, rare patients begin after age 26 years.

DYT1 usually starts in a leg or an arm as an action dystonia, being apparent with specific actions. When a leg is first affected, the child walks in a peculiar manner with inversion or eversion of the foot and abnormal flexion of the knee or hip. With arm involvement, writing is interfered by the finger curling, wrist flexion and pronation, and the elbow elevation. Dystonic tremor of the arm is frequently seen. The small minority of individuals have onset in the neck or a cranial muscle, presenting torticollis or blepharospasm.

Dystonic movements usually persist through life. Furthermore, in most patients with onset in a leg, dystonia progresses over several years. The contractions become less action specific and are present at rest, resulting in a fixed twisted posture. Going further, the dystonia spreads to other body parts to "generalized dystonia" involving other limbs and the trunk. In individuals who have onset in an arm, progression is variable and dystonia generalizes in approximately 50 %. Approximately 20 % of DYT1 is restricted to a single limb or the neck, usually as writer's cramp. This occurs in a minority of individuals with adult onset.

Mental activity is generally unaffected. There are no abnormalities in sensory or cerebellar systems, and deep tendon reflexes are preserved. An increased risk for recurrent major depression is reported in individuals with a *TOR1A* mutation with or without dystonia (Heiman et al. 2004). Life span is not supposed to be shortened.

Other early onset non-DYT1 primary dystonias include DYT6 and DYT13. DYT6 is characterized by focal, predominantly cranio-cervical involvements with dysarthria, dysphonia, dysphagia, and cervical dystonia. In two large Amish-Mennonite families, the gene for DYT6, *THAP1* (THAP [thanatos-associated protein] domain-containing, apoptosis-associated protein 1) was identified on chromosome 8 and is transmitted as an autosomal dominant trait (Fuchs et al. 2009). The onset is in adolescent or in early adult period, and the disease rarely progresses to generalized dystonia. DYT13 has been reported in individuals from one large Italian family, transmitted in an autosomal dominant manner. The phenotype of DYT13 is focal or segmental dystonia with cranial, cervical, or upper limb involvement. Dystonias start with jerky movements of the neck and shoulder at age between 5 years and adulthood, spread variably to cranial and brachial regions. The clinical manifestations were generally mild and slowly progressive. The causative gene locus has been identified on chromosome 1p36.

3.2.3.2 Adult-Onset Primary Dystonia

Most primary dystonias are of adult onset. The adult dystonias are focal or segmental ones, and usually restricted to the first involved muscles. They comprise cervical dystonia (spasmodic torticollis), blepharospasm, oromandibular dystonia, spasmodic dysphonia, and writer's cramp.

Spasmodic torticollis is the most common adult-onset focal dystonia. It occurs at any age, more frequently in women. The neck is sustained to turn, tilt, flex, or extend. The head shifts laterally or anteriorly, and the shoulder is elevated and anteriorly displaced toward the chin. Multiple cervical muscles are involved, such as the sternocleidomastoid, trapezius, splenius, scalenus, and levator scapulae muscles. The torticollis may be relieved by placing a hand or fingers on the cheek, chin, or the back of the head, as the result of a sensory trick.

Blepharospasm is an involuntary contraction of the orbicularis oculi muscles. It usually starts after age 50 years and is more frequent in women. At the beginning, blepharospasm is often noticed by the increased frequency of blinking, followed by the eyelid closure. The symptoms are temporarily relieved during looking down, talking, or singing, whereas the condition exaggerates by bright light and the sun. A sensory trick is placing of a finger just lateral to the orbit. Blepharospasm should not be confused with ptosis, blepharitis, hemifacial spasm, or blinking tics. Blepharospasm can spread to other cranial regions, such as the tongue, jaw, vocal cords, or cervical muscles. The combined state of blepharospasm with other cranial dystonias, especially with oromandibular dystonia, is called *Meige syndrome*.

Spasmodic dysphonia is a voice disorder characterized by dystonic movements or spasms of one or more vocalis muscles during speech. The voice becomes strangled and coarse, often broken up with pauses.

Writer's cramp is a task-specific focal dystonia of the fingers, hand, and forearm. The symptoms first appear only when a person is trying to do a task requiring fine finger movements such as writing. Common symptoms include excessive gripping of a pen, flexing of the wrist, elevation of the elbow, and occasional extension of fingers causing the pen to fall from the hand. The symptoms may progress to affect more general muscles and spread to affect other tasks.

3.2.4 Dystonia-Plus Syndrome

Dystonia-plus syndromes (Asmus and Gasser 2010) represent a heterogeneous group of diseases, where dystonias are accompanied by other neurological features such as parkinsonism or myoclonus, and gene mutations can be detected frequently.

3.2.4.1 Dopa-Responsive Dystonia

Dopa-responsive dystonia (DRD) is a childhood-onset, neurometabolic disorder with two different traits of inheritance.

The autosomal-dominant form of DRD (AD-DRD), often called Segawa disease, is caused by heterozygous mutations of GTP-cyclohydrolase I (GCH1, DYT5) with reduced penetrance (Ichinose et al. 1999). Excellent and sustained response to levodopa is noteworthy. AD-DRD is distinguishable from primary dystonias by the presence of parkinsonism such as bradykinesia, rigidity, and postural instability. Other characteristic and distinctive features of AD-DRD are diurnal fluctuations, with improvement after sleep and worsening toward the evening. The onset age is usually between 6 and 16 years. However, it can appear at infancy resembling cerebral palsy or in adulthood as pure parkinsonism.

In the autosomal-recessive forms of DRD (AR-DRD), homozygous or compound heterozygous mutations of the tyrosine hydroxylase

(TH) or the sepiapterin reductase (SPR) gene cause dystonias. The clinical manifestations of AR-DRD are generally more severe, accompanied by cognitive deficits and developmental delay.

3.2.4.2 Myoclonus-Dystonia

Myoclonus-dystonia (M-D) is caused by heterozygous mutations of the *epsilon-sarcoglycan* gene (Zimprich et al. 2001). In the patients 'lightning-like' myoclonic jerks are the conspicuous symptoms, which can be triggered by complex motor tasks like writing and drawing. The neck and arms are commonly involved, followed by the trunk and bulbar muscles. In contrast, dystonia is generally only mild, and writer's cramp or torticollis could be the only feature. The myoclonic jerks respond to alcohol. Myoclonus and dystonia together with an age at onset below 25 years strongly predict *epsilon-sarcoglycan* gene mutation and differentiate this genetic disease from other 'jerky' dystonias.

3.2.4.3 Other Dystonia-Plus Syndromes

An X-linked recessive hereditary disorder causing dystonia and parkinsonism is designated as DYT3 (Evidente 2005). The mean age of onset in men is 39 years. The clinical course is highly variable with parkinsonism as the initial presenting sign, overshadowed by dystonia as the disease progresses. Features of parkinsonism include resting tremor, bradykinesia, rigidity, postural instability, and shuffling gait. The dystonia develops focally, most commonly in the jaw, neck, trunk, and eyes, and less commonly in the limbs, tongue, pharynx, and larynx, the most characteristic being jaw dystonia often progressing to neck dystonia. Individuals with pure parkinsonism have nondisabling symptoms that are only slowly progressive. Female carriers are mostly asymptomatic. The causative gene has been identified as the TATA-binding protein-associated factor 1 gene, *TAF1* (Makino et al. 2007).

Rapid-onset dystonia-parkinsonism (RDP, DYT12) is a rare disorder with a sudden onset of symptoms over hours to days, prominent bulbar involvement, and parkinsonism with a lack of response to levodopa (Brashear et al. 2007). Patients with this rare phenotype are caused by mutations in the Na(+)/K(+) ATPase alpha3-subunit (*ATP1A3*) gene (de Carvalho Aguiar et al. 2004).

Recently, a novel form of autosomal-recessive early onset dystonia-parkinsonism (DYT16) has been found to be linked to mutations in the *PRKRA* gene (Camargos et al. 2008).

3.2.5 Secondary Dystonia

Secondary dystonia is defined as a dystonic disorder that develops as a result of certain factors that affect the brain or specifically the basal ganglia. Examples of the causes include cerebral palsy, cerebral hypoxia, encephalitis, brain tumor, paraneoplastic syndromes, hypoparathyroidism, toxins such as manganese or cyanide, and certain drugs such as levodopa or dopamine D2 receptor blockers, those are known leading to levodopa-induced dystonia or tardive dystonia (Ekbom et al. 1972), respectively.

3.2.6 Heredodegenerative Dystonia

Neurodegenerative disorders manifesting dystonia as representative features are included in this category. Other neurologic symptoms could be presenting or predominant features. Huntington's disease, Machado–Joseph disease, dentatorubropallidoluysian atrophy, Fahr disease, Wilson's disease, GM1 and GM2 gangliosidoses, juvenile neuronal ceroid lipofuscinosis, metachromatic leukodystrophy, Pelizaeus–Merzbacher disease, or mitochondrial encephalopathy is an example. Parkinsonian syndromes such as progressive supranuclear palsy, multiple system atrophy, or corticobasal degeneration are also included in this category.

3.3 Essential Tremor

Essential tremor is a chronic, progressive neurological disorder that causes a rhythmic tremor of 4–12 Hz, involving the hands, arms, head, voice, or other muscles. The tremor rarely affects the

Table 3.1 ILAE's 1981 international clinical and electroencephalographic classification of epileptic seizures

I. Partial (focal) seizures
A. Simple partial seizures (consciousness not impaired)
1. With motor signs (including jacksonian, versive, and postural)
2. With sensory symptoms (including visual, somatosensory, auditory, olfactory, gustatory, and vertiginous)
3. With psychic symptoms (including dysphasia, dysmensic, hallucinatory, and affective changes)
4. With autonomic symptoms (including epigastric sensation, pallor, flushing, pupillary changes)
B. Complex partial seizures (consciousness is impaired)
1. Simple partial onset followed by impaired consciousness
2. With impairment of consciousness at onset
3. With automatisms
C. Partial seizures evolving to secondarily generalized seizures
II. Generalized seizures of nonfocal origin (convulsive or nonconvulsive)
A. Absence seizures
1. With impaired consciousness only
2. With one or more of the following: atonic components, tonic components, automatisms, autonomic components
B. Myoclonic seizures
Myoclonic jerks (single or multiple)
C. Tonic–clonic seizures (may include clonic–tonic–clonic seizures)
D. Tonic seizures
E. Atonic seizures
III. Unclassified epileptic seizures

legs or feet. The tremor exacerbates during voluntary movements, as in drinking from a glass, writing, shaving, or eating. It may also be present with sustained posture. Neurologic abnormalities other than tremor are not apparent.

Essential tremor can occur at any age but is most common in individuals age 40 and older. About 5 % of patients begin in childhood and are usually familial with an autosomal-dominant trait. However, no causative gene has been identified so far.

Although usually not a devastating condition, essential tremor worsens over time and can be severe in some patients. The tremor is aggravated by emotional stress, caffeine intake, and certain medications, whereas many patients note that tremor is suppressed by drinking alcohol.

3.4 Epilepsy

3.4.1 Definition of Epilepsy and Seizure

A Task Force of the International League Against Epilepsy (ILAE) formulated conceptual definitions of "seizure" and "epilepsy" in 2005 as follows: "Epilepsy is a disorder of the brain characterized by an enduring predisposition to generate epileptic seizures, and by the neurobiological, cognitive, psychological, and social consequences of this condition. The definition of epilepsy requires the occurrence of at least one epileptic seizure. An epileptic seizure is a transient occurrence of signs and/or symptoms due to abnormal excessive or synchronous neuronal activity in the brain."

3.4.2 Classification of Seizures and Epilepsy

The classification of epileptic seizures is primarily based on clinical observation. ILAE published the last official update of the classification for seizures in 1981 (Table 3.1) (Commission on Classification and Terminology of the International League Against Epilepsy. 1981), and the last official update for the epilepsies in 1989 (Table 3.2) (Commission on Classification and Terminology of the International League Against Epilepsy. 1989). Although there continues to be efforts to develop revisions, especially to incorporate growing evidence of genetic contributions, the 1981 and 1989 updates still form the currently accepted standards.

Table 3.2 ILAE's 1989 international classification of epilepsies and epileptic syndromes

1. Localization-related epilepsies and syndromes
1.1. Idiopathic
Benign childhood epilepsy with centrotemporal spikes
Childhood epilepsy with occipital paroxysms
Primary reading epilepsy
1.2. Symptomatic
Chronic progressive epilepsia partialis continua of childhood (Kojewnikow's syndrome)
Syndromes characterized by seizures with specific modes of precipitation
Temporal lobe epilepsies
Frontal lobe epilepsies
Parietal lobe epilepsies
Occipital lobe epilepsies
1.3. Cryptogenic
2. Generalized epilepsies and syndromes
2.1. Idiopathic
Benign neonatal familial convulsions
Benign neonatal convulsions
Benign myoclonic epilepsy in infancy
Childhood absence epilepsy
Juvenile absence epilepsy
Juvenile myoclonic epilepsy
Epilepsy with GTCS on awakening
Other generalized idiopathic epilepsies not defined above
Epilepsies with seizures precipitated by specific modes of activation
2.2. Cryptogenic or symptomatic
West syndrome
Lennox–Gastaut syndrome
Epilepsy with myoclonic-astatic seizures
Epilepsy with myoclonic absences
2.3. Symptomatic
2.3.1. Nonspecific etiology
Early myoclonic encephalopathy
Early infantile epileptic encephalopathy with suppression burst
Other symptomatic generalized epilepsies not defined above
2.3.2. Specific syndromes
Diseases in which seizures are a presenting or predominant feature
3. Epilepsies and syndromes undetermined whether focal or generalized
3.1. With both generalized and focal seizures
Neonatal seizures
Severe myoclonic epilepsy in infancy
Epilepsy with continuous spike waves during slow wave sleep
Acquired epileptic aphasia (Landau–Kleffner syndrome)
Other undetermined epilepsies not defined above
3.2. Without unequivocal generalized or focal features (i.e. Sleep related GTCS; when the EEG shows both focal and generalized ictal or interictal discharges, and when focal or generalized onset cannot be determined clinically)
4. Special syndromes
4.1. Situation-related seizures
Febrile convulsions
Isolated seizures or isolated status epilepticus
Seizures occurring only when there is an acute metabolic or toxic event (alcohol, drugs, eclampsia, nonketotic hyperglycemia)

3.4.3 Symptoms of Seizures

Seizures can be basically categorized into two types (Bazil and Pedley 2010). One is *partial or focal seizures* those are with onset restricted to a part of one cerebral hemisphere, and the other is *generalized seizures* those involve the brain diffusely from the beginning.

Partial seizures are subdivided into *simple partial seizures* and *complex partial seizures*. Consciousness is preserved in the former and lost in the latter. Generalized seizures are also subdivided on the presence or the absence of ictal motor seizures and their character. Simple partial seizures may progress to complex partial seizures, and further evolve into secondarily generalized seizures.

In *simple partial seizures* the ictal discharges are limited in a small area of cerebral cortex. This is the epileptogenic focus. The symptoms, realized by the patients as '*aura*', vary and depend on the site of the epileptogenic focus, including elementary motor, unilateral sensory disturbance, an epigastric rising sensation, fear, a feeling of unreality, déjà vu and jamais vu, and olfactory hallucinations. The patients can interact with the environment normally.

Complex partial seizures are partial seizures with impairment of consciousness. They may start as simple partial seizures and evolve into complex partial seizures, or may begin as complex partial seizures with impairment of consciousness at the onset of the seizure. Automatisms, such as lip smacking and repeated swallowing may be concomitant with loss of consciousness. Postictal confusional states are usually present for several minutes.

In *generalized tonic–clonic seizures*, the patients first lose consciousness abruptly and extend the trunk and the bilateral limbs (*tonic phase*), accompanied by a loud vocalization (*ictal cry*). The pupils become dilated, the eyes deviate upwards, and the mouth is forcefully closed which may result in a tongue bite. The upper extremities abduct and flex at the elbows, while the lower extremities may briefly flex and then extend and adduct with the toes pointed. The respiratory muscles are also involved and the patient becomes cyanotic. These tonic seizures are followed by synchronous jerking of limbs (*clonic phase*). Gasping respirations and urinary incontinence may occur. In some patients only a tonic or a clonic phase is apparent. Postictally, the patients are confused, lethargic, and falling in sleep. Epileptic prodromes are nonspecific symptoms such as ill-defined anxiety, irritability, decreased concentration, and headache. The patients realize these feelings for minutes to several hours before a generalized tonic–clonic seizure. These are not aura.

Absence seizures are characterized by sudden-onset, brief, temporary loss of consciousness, accompanied by motion arrest and staring. Mild myoclonic jerks of the facial muscles and automatisms may accompany longer absence seizures. The end of the seizures is also abrupt. There is no aura or prodromal symptoms, nor postictal confusion. In contrast, the term *atypical absence seizures* is applied if the beginning and the end of 'absence seizures' are less distinct, or if tonic and autonomic components are included in the events. Atypical absences are seen in the Lennox–Gastaut syndrome or in developmentally delayed children with epilepsy.

Myoclonic seizures are generalized seizures characterized by rapid, brief, irregular muscle jerks of the head, trunk, or limbs. They can occur bilaterally or unilaterally, synchronously or asynchronously. The extent and intensity of myoclonic jerks vary, from isolated movements of face or arm muscles to massive simultaneous spasms involving the whole body. They tend to occur close to sleep onset and upon awakening from sleep. Myoclonic seizures can be a feature of juvenile myoclonic epilepsy, myoclonic-astatic epilepsy, Lafora disease, and infantile spasms. Consciousness is not impaired and there is no postictal confusion with isolated myoclonic jerks. Myoclonic seizures can occur in clusters and evolve into generalized tonic–clonic seizures.

Atonic seizures, also called *drop attacks*, are characterized by sudden loss of muscle tone, leading to a head drop, a limb drop, or a drop of the whole body resulting in a fall. A brief loss of consciousness is accompanied, resulting in injuries to the face. Drop attacks last less than 5 s, and postictal confusion is minimal. When atonic seizures are preceded by a brief myoclonic jerk or tonic spasm, an acceleratory force is added to the fall, resulting in the high rate of self-injury of the face or the head.

3.4.4 Symptoms of Epilepsy

In diagnosing the patients with ictal event, neurological history taking and examinations are the first steps in order to determine whether the episode is epileptic. Disorders that must be differentiated from epilepsy include syncope, transient ischemic attacks, migraine, and non-epileptic pseudoseizure (psychogenic seizures). Once the ictal event is determined to be epileptic, the next step is searching for underlying causes. Diagnostic appraisal then focuses on determining what types of seizures occurred, whether the disorder would be considered as primary or secondary, and whether the clinical features constitute a recognized epileptic syndrome.

The clinical manifestations of epileptic syndromes are highly variable and depend on the cortical areas involved. Among them, surgically remediable epileptic syndromes (Engel et al. 2007) include mesial temporal lobe epilepsy, discrete neocortical lesions, diffuse hemispheric disturbances, drop attacks as the most disabling seizure type, and others such as Landau–Kleffner syndrome and medically refractory gelastic epilepsy.

3.4.4.1 Mesial Temporal Lobe Epilepsy (MTLE)

MTLE is a form of temporal lobe epilepsy associated with hippocampal sclerosis. This is often refractory to antiepileptic drugs and is most commonly referred for epilepsy surgery. Thus, MTLE is the prototype of a surgically remediable syndrome. The age of onset is usually in the first decade of life, but the seizures commonly do not become medically intractable until adolescence or later. Patients often had history of complicated febrile convulsions or other cerebral insults before age 5. Aura is usually present for several seconds. The most common aura is an epigastric sensation (a rising sensation, butterflies, nausea). Others include fear, olfactory hallucinations, gustatory sensation, lightheadedness, and déjà vu. Complex partial seizure often begins with arrest and stare, followed by oroalimentary automatisms, lasting 1–2 min. Posturing of one upper extremity and head turn may occur contralateral to the ictal discharges. Secondarily generalized seizures are infrequent. Postictally, disorientation, recent memory deficit, and amnesia for the event are noted. Neurological examinations usually reveal no abnormality, but may disclose recent memory deficit. Interictal behavioral disturbance, most commonly depression, can develop.

3.4.4.2 Epilepsy with Discrete Neocortical Lesions

Patients with medically intractable partial seizures caused by discrete neocortical structural lesions, such as neoplasms, scars, vascular malformations, cysts, focal cortical dysplasia, and other localized congenital aberrations in accessible brain areas also have a surgically remediable syndrome.

The symptoms vary and depend on the site of the lesion.

Frontal lobe seizures are usually brief, being less than 30 s, can occur several times a day in clusters, and often have minimal or no postictal confusion. The clinical symptoms generally include an abrupt onset of stereotyped hyperkinetic behavior, vocalizations, gestural or sexual automatisms, and pedaling or bicycling automatisms of the legs.

Detailed ictal symptoms of frontal lobe seizures vary depending on what region of the frontal lobe is involved.

Seizures originating from the mesial frontal region or supplementary motor area (SMA) are characterized by vocalizations and abrupt tonic asymmetric extension of the proximal extremities. Consciousness is unusually retained, and postictal confusion is minimal. Lateral dorsal frontal lobe seizures are characterized by speech arrest, forced thinking, contraversive head and eye deviation, and automatisms such as laughing, crying, sniffing, chewing, or kicking. Orbitofrontal seizures are characterized by prominent autonomic symptoms such as flushing, mydriasis, and tachycardia, in addition to automatisms and loud vocalizations. Cingulate gyrus seizures are similar to SMA seizures but also involve behavioral arrest, oroalimentary automatisms, gestural or sexual automatisms, mood changes, and sometimes urinary incontinence.

Frontal lobe seizures are often misdiagnosed as pseudoseizures because of their bizarre symptoms.

Parietal lobe seizures manifest somatosensory symptoms, most commonly in the face and hand, contralateral to the epileptic focus. Somatosensory symptoms include paresthesia and numbness, pain, a vague head sensation, and genital sensations. In dominant-side parietal lobe seizures, patients may develop language dysfunction. On the other hand, in nondominant parietal lobe seizures, patients can have spatial neglect of the contralateral body or environment, and somatosensory illusions.

Occipital lobe seizures are characterized by elementary visual hallucinations of fixed or moving flashing white or colored lights. They start in the contralateral visual field and spread to the entire visual field. The eyes may deviate contralaterally, and the eyelids may rapidly blink. If the seizure spreads to the posterior temporal region, which is known as the area of visual association cortex, complex visual hallucinations may occur.

3.4.4.3 Epilepsy with Diffuse Hemispheric Disturbances

Infants and young children with diffuse hemispheric disturbances such as Rasmussen's encephalitis, vascular malformations, Sturge–Weber syndrome, hemimegalencephaly, and large congenital porencephalic cysts may develop frequent unilateral or generalized motor seizures. In case the patients already have severe hemiparesis, hemispherectomy can suppress seizures in 70–80 % of patients and reverse the developmental delay, without inducing further neurological deficit.

3.4.4.4 Drop Attacks as the Most Disabling Seizure Type

Drop attacks, or atonic seizures, are characterized by a sudden loss of muscle tone, leading to a drop of the whole body (see above). Drop attacks are commonly experienced in the symptomatic generalized epilepsies, such as Lennox-Gastaut syndrome. Drop attacks are medically intractable but can be eliminated by corpus callosotomy.

References

Ashour R, Tintner R, Jankovic J (2005) Striatal deformities of the hand and foot in Parkinson's disease. Lancet Neurol 4:423–431

Asmus F, Gasser T (2010) Dystonia-plus syndromes. Eur J Neurol 17(Suppl 1):37–45

Baba T, Kikuchi A, Hirayama K et al (2012) Severe olfactory dysfunction is a prodromal symptom of dementia associated with Parkinson's disease: a 3 year longitudinal study. Brain 135:161–169

Bazil CW, Pedley TA (2010) Epilepsy. In: Rowland LP, Pedley TA (eds) Merrit's neurology, 12th edn. Lippincott Williams & Wilkins, Philadelphia, pp 927–948

Brashear A, Dobyns WB, de Carvalho Aguiar P et al (2007) The phenotypic spectrum of rapid-onset dystonia-parkinsonism (RDP) and mutations in the ATP1A3 gene. Brain 130:828–835

Camargos S, Scholz S, Simón-Sánchez J et al (2008) DYT16, a novel young-onset dystonia-parkinsonism disorder: identification of a segregating mutation in the stress-response protein PRKRA. Lancet Neurol 7:207–215

Commission on Classification and Terminology of the International League Against Epilepsy (1981) Proposal for revised clinical and electroencephalographic classification of epileptic seizures. Epilepsia 22:489–501

Commission on Classification and Terminology of the International League Against Epilepsy (1989) Proposal for revised classification of epilepsies and epileptic syndromes. Epilepsia 30:389–399

de Carvalho Aguiar P, Sweadner KJ, Penniston JT et al (2004) Mutations in the Na+/K+ -ATPase alpha3 gene ATP1A3 are associated with rapid-onset dystonia parkinsonism. Neuron 22:169–175

Ekbom K, Lindholm H, Ljungberg L (1972) New dystonic syndrome associated with butyrophenone therapy. Z Neurol 202:94–103

Engel J Jr, Cascino GD, Shields WD (2007) Surgically remediable syndromes. In: Engel J, Pedley TA, Aicardi J (eds) Epilepsy: a comprehensive textbook, 2nd edn. Lippincott Williams & Wilkins, Philadelphia, pp p1761–p1769

Evidente VGH (2005) X-linked dystonia-parkinsonism. In: Pagon RA, Adam MP, Bird TD, Dolan CR, Fong CT, Stephens K (eds) GeneReviews™ [Internet]. University of Washington, Seattle, pp p1993–p2013

Fahn S, Bressman S (2010) Dystonia. In: Rowland LP, Pedley TA (eds) Merrit's neurology, 12th edn. Lippincott Williams & Wilkins, Philadelphia, pp p738–p748

Fahn S, Przedborski S (2010) Parkinson disease. In: Rowland LP, Pedley TA (eds) Merrit's neurology, 12th edn. Lippincott Williams & Wilkins, Philadelphia, pp p751–p769

Ford B, Pfeiffer RF (2005) Pain syndromes and disorders of sensation. In: Pfeiffer RF, Bodis-Wollner I (eds) Parkinson's disease and nonmotor dysfunction. Humana Press, Totowa, pp p255–p267

Frucht S, Rogers JD, Greene PE et al (1999) Falling asleep at the wheel: motor vehicle mishaps in persons taking pramipexole and ropinirole. Neurology 52:1908–1910

Fuchs T, Gavarini S, Saunders-Pullman R et al (2009) Mutations in the THAP1 gene are responsible for DYT6 primary torsion dystonia. Nat Genet 41:286–288

Heiman GA, Ottman R, Saunders-Pullman RJ et al (2004) Increased risk for recurrent major depression in DYT1 dystonia mutation carriers. Neurology 63:631–637

Ichinose H, Suzuki T, Inagaki H et al (1999) Molecular genetics of dopa-responsive dystonia. Biol Chem 380:1355–1364

Jankovic J, Schwartz KS, Ondo W (1999) Re-emergent tremor of Parkinson's disease. J Neurol Neurosurg Psychiatry 67:646–650

Makino S, Kaji R, Ando S et al (2007) Reduced neuron-specific expression of the TAF1 gene is associated with X-linked dystonia-parkinsonism. Am J Hum Genet 803:393–406

McKeith IG, Galasko D, Kosaka K et al (1996) Consensus guidelines for the clinical and pathologic diagnosis of dementia with Lewy bodies (DLB): report of the consortium on DLB international workshop. Neurology 47:1113–1124

Ozelius LJ, Hewett JW, Page CE et al (1997) The early-onset torsion dystonia gene (DYT1) encodes an ATP-binding protein. Nat Genet 17:40–48

Tassorelli C, Furnari A, Buscone S et al (2012) Pisa syndrome in Parkinson's disease: clinical, electromyographic, and radiological characterization. Mov Disord 27:227–235

Voon V, Fernagut PO, Wickens J et al (2009) Chronic dopaminergic stimulation in Parkinson's disease: from dyskinesias to impulse control disorders. Lancet Neurol 8:1140–1149

Zimprich A, Grabowski M, Asmus F et al (2001) Mutations in the gene encoding epsilon-sarcoglycan cause myoclonus-dystonia syndrome. Nat Genet 29:66–69

Intraoperative Microelectrode Recording

4

Kazutaka Kobayashi and Yoichi Katayama

4.1 Electrodes for Extracellular Recording

Extracellular recordings measure the current flowing in the extracellular regions neighboring the cell membrane rather than the cell membrane potential itself. In other words, these extracellular recordings measure the potential difference (extracellular potential) between an extracellular electrode placed in the extracellular space and a distant indifferent electrode. Two types of extracellular potential exist between cells: (1) action potentials generated by cell bodies, dendrites, axons, and other cellular components and (2) synaptic potentials. Microelectrode recording (MER) measures the electrical activity of cell bodies, dendrites, axons, and other cellular components.

MER properties differ according to the resistance and diameter of the microelectrode tip. A fine microelectrode with a small contact area and high resistance (Fig. 4.1) can more readily record single-unit activity, whereas a larger diameter semimicroelectrode with a larger contact area and lower resistance can more readily record multiunit activity. Nevertheless, even the smallest electrodes used for clinical treatment can record multiunit activity, whereas semimicroelectrodes can record single-unit activity if used properly. Unlike action potentials, a local field potential (LFP) represents a complex potential composed of both the synaptic potential and action potentials from cell bodies, dendrites, and other cellular components. Because multiunit activity and LFP have different frequency bands, they can be simultaneously recorded with the same electrode if it has a large contact area and the recording system uses a filter to separate the two signals.

4.2 MER Devices, Electrodes, and Recording Systems

The LeadPoint® (Medtronic, Japan; Fig. 4.2a) is one of the best known recording systems manufactured specifically for use in DBS surgery. Similar to most systems, the LeadPoint® incorporates a special microelectrode drive and micromanipulator to advance the electrodes in fine increments (microTargeting™ drive, Medtronic; Fig. 4.2b). This system can be adapted for simultaneous multitrack recording, which is described below. Medtronic recording electrodes (Fig. 4.1) typically have a resistance of 1.0 MΩ (at 1,000 Hz) and a diameter of 10 μm at the tip. MER is performed using the tip of the microelectrode sheath (length 1 mm) as the indifferent electrode, which can also be used as the stimulating electrode for intraoperative test stimulation.

K. Kobayashi, MD, PhD (✉) • Y. Katayama, MD, PhD
Division of Neurosurgery,
Department of Neurological Surgery,
Nihon University School of Medicine, Tokyo, Japan
e-mail: kobayashi.kazutaka@nihon-u.ac.jp

T. Itakura (ed.), *Deep Brain Stimulation for Neurological Disorders: Theoretical Background and Clinical Application*, DOI 10.1007/978-3-319-08476-3_4,

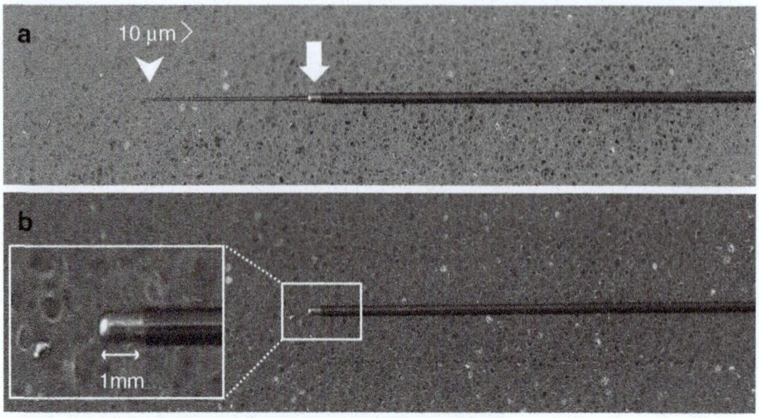

Fig. 4.1 Electrodes used for microelectrode recording (MER). (**a**) MER performed using the electrode tip (*arrowhead*) as the recording electrode and the tip of the outer sheath (*arrow*) as the indifferent electrode. (**b**) The recording electrode has been withdrawn, leaving only the outer sheath. The tip of this sheath is used as the stimulating electrode for intraoperative stimulation

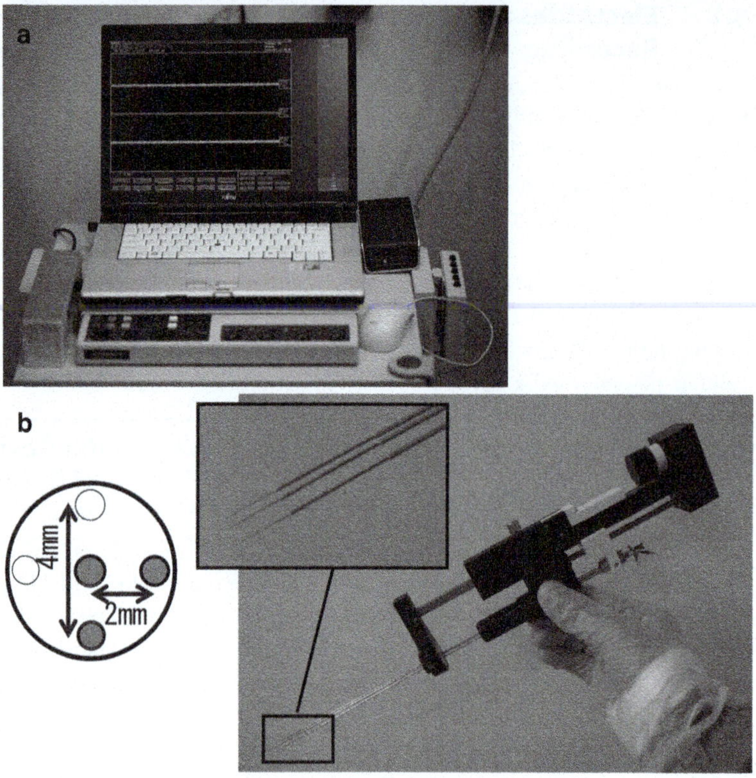

Fig. 4.2 Microelectrode recording (MER) system. (**a**) External appearance of the LeadPoint® system (Reprinted with the permission of Alpine Biomed ApS). (**b**) *Right:* MicroTargeting™ Drive system comprising an electrode holder and a micromanipulator for inserting the electrode. *Top left:* Pattern diagram of multitrack electrodes. In addition to a central electrode, other electrodes can be simultaneously inserted in the 0, 3, 6, and 9 o'clock positions. In this example, three electrodes (the central electrode and two others at 3 and 6 o'clock positions) have been fitted in the holder (Reprinted with the permission of FHC, Inc.)

4.3 Target Identification for MER

MER is performed while using a manipulator to gradually advance the microelectrode toward the target sites identified prior to the surgery. Typically, the microelectrode is advanced to its final location from a point approximately 10–20 mm away the target site. To decrease the risk of hemorrhage, the recommended speed of microelectrode advancement is ≤ 0.5 mm/s (Binder et al. 2005). The target sites are confirmed by using neurophysiological factors such as the background activity level, changes in neuronal discharge patterns, and neural activity in response to peripheral sensory stimulation. The target sites for DBS typically include the cortex–basal ganglia

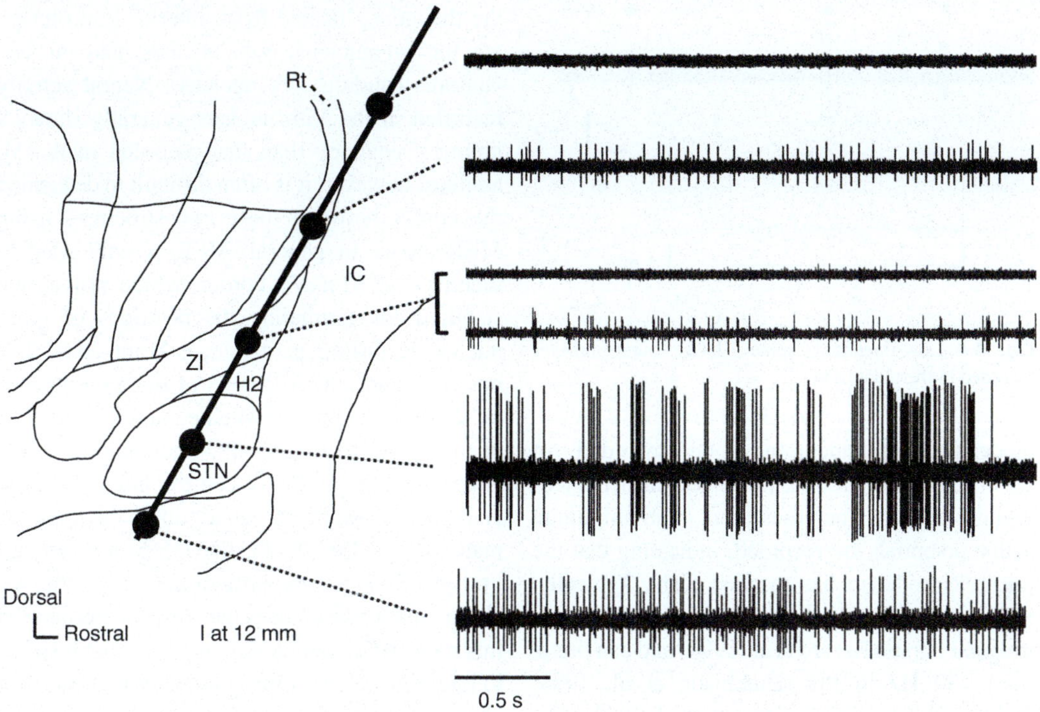

Fig. 4.3 Neural activity recorded along the insertion route to the subthalamic nucleus superimposed on a sagittal section (12-mm lateral) from the Schaltenbrand–Wahren atlas. *H2* H2 field of Forel, *IC* internal capsule, *Rt* reticular thalamic nucleus, *STN* subthalamic nucleus, *ZI* zona incerta

pathways. Because the neural activity in the basal ganglia varies with different disorders, the characteristics of neural activity identified using MER also will differ depending on the disease.

4.3.1 Subthalamic Nucleus (STN) (Fig. 4.3)

STN is commonly targeted for DBS treatment of Parkinson's disease (PD). When the recording microelectrode is targeted toward STN at an angle of 50–60° to the anterior commissure (AC) and the posterior commissure (PC) line (viewed in a sagittal section), it typically passes through the thalamus, zona incerta (ZI), H2 field of Forel, STN, and substantia nigra pars reticulata (SNr). ZI is dorsally surrounded by the thalamic fasciculus (the H1 field of Forel) and ventrally surrounded by the lenticular fasciculus (H2 field of Forel). Because the cell density is higher in STN than in these other structures, STN can be identified using MER because of its high background activity and frequent spontaneous discharges. A microelectrode targeting STN also will pass through the thalamic subnuclei, including the nucleus reticularis and the nucleus ventralis oralis (Vo nucleus), where irregular firing at approximately 10–30 Hz is evident. Compared with the nucleus ventralis intermedius (Vim nucleus), there is little spontaneous discharge in these thalamic subnuclei, and their amplitudes are low. When the angle of insertion viewed in a sagittal plane is small (when insertion is performed from the front), the electrode does not pass through the thalamus but through the internal capsule, where few action potentials are recorded because of the dense white matter. In the thalamus, low-threshold spike (LTS) bursts are often recorded (Kim et al. 2009; Kobayashi et al. 2009) (Fig. 4.4). After exiting the thalamus and entering the white matter of ZI/H2 field of Forel, both background activity and spontaneous neuron discharge decrease. Spontaneous discharges with

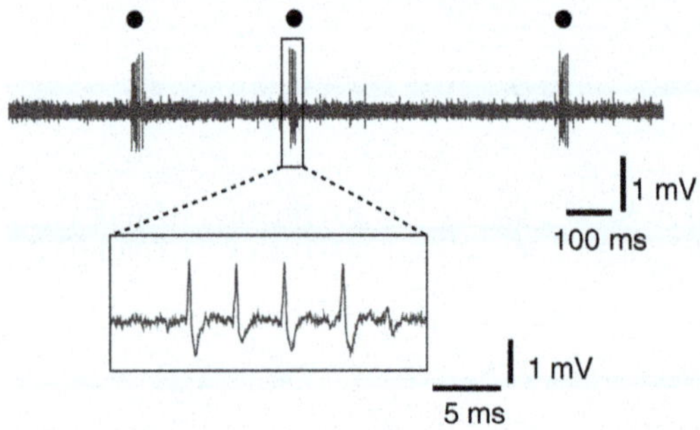

Fig. 4.4 Low-threshold spike (LTS) burst (*circle*) recorded in the thalamus

moderate amplitudes may be recorded in ZI. When the electrode is advanced further, background activity increases and high-amplitude action potentials are recorded, indicating that the microelectrode tip has reached STN. Typically, STN neurons have high spontaneous activity with irregular bursts (Bezard et al. 1999) and can fire at rates >30 Hz in PD (Hutchison et al. 1998; Steigerwald et al. 2008; Schrock et al. 2009). The dorsolateral region of STN is a sensorimotor region that receives input from the primary motor area of the cerebral cortex. STN neurons in this region respond with a change in firing frequency to passive joint movement of the contralateral limbs, and they are somatotopically arranged into regions for the upper and lower limbs, arranged from the lateral to the medial side (Rodriguez-Oroz et al. 2001). This neural organization is helpful for assessing the microelectrode position in the lateromedial direction (*X*-axis). After the microelectrode passes through STN, it reaches the white matter on the dorsal side of SNr, which is indicated by a decrease in background activity in MER. This white matter is only a few hundred microns thick (up to approximately 3 mm) and is often not identified before the electrode enters SNr. Although it may be difficult to distinguish between SNr and STN, SNr exhibits a somewhat higher firing frequency (50–70 Hz) than STN and shows a regular discharge pattern with few bursts.

4.3.2 Thalamus

The thalamus is often the target in DBS for the treatment of tremors. On the ventrolateral part of the thalamus, located from anterior to posterior, are the Vo nucleus, Vim nucleus, and nucleus ventralis caudalis (Vc nucleus). Neural activity recorded in the Vim nucleus generally shows a greater frequency than that recorded in the Vo nucleus; however, it is often difficult to determine the border between these two structures using MER alone. In general, MER is only used to identify the Vim–Vc border, which provides a standard for estimating the positions of other nuclei, according to a human brain atlas. The posterior and anterior limits of the Vim nucleus on the AC–PC line are situated at 2/12 and 3/12 of the length of the AC–PC line, anterior to PC (Benabid et al. 1996). When the microelectrode is inserted toward PC at an angle of approximately 45° to the AC–PC line (viewed in the sagittal plane), it passes through the Vim to the Vc along a path that crosses the Vim–Vc border. On this path, MER can identify neurons that respond to joint movement of the contralateral limbs (by a change in firing frequency) and discharge rhythmically at the same frequency as tremors are recorded in the Vim nucleus. Neurons that fire rhythmically at the same frequency as tremors are known as "tremor cells" (Fig. 4.5) and are thought to be associated with the generation of tremors. They are often recorded within the Vim nucleus of the thalamus but may also be recorded in the Vc and Vo nuclei (Lenz et al. 1994; Katayama et al. 2005). In terms of the somatotopy of neurons responding to joint movement, this somatic localization is distributed into regions for the upper and lower limbs arranged from the medial to the lateral side (Lenz et al. 1988). Further advancement of the microelectrode reveals MER from neurons responding to light tactile stimulation of the skin, which indicates that the electrode has entered the Vc nucleus, which receives input from the medial lemniscus. The Vim–Vc border is physiologically defined as the most anterior neuron along a length of trajectory in which more than one-half of the neurons located posteriorly were neurons responding to sensory stimulation (Hua and Lenz 2005) (Fig. 4.6). Somatotopy within the Vc nucleus is similar to that within the Vim nucleus, with the lower limb region located on the lateral side, the upper limb region located medially.

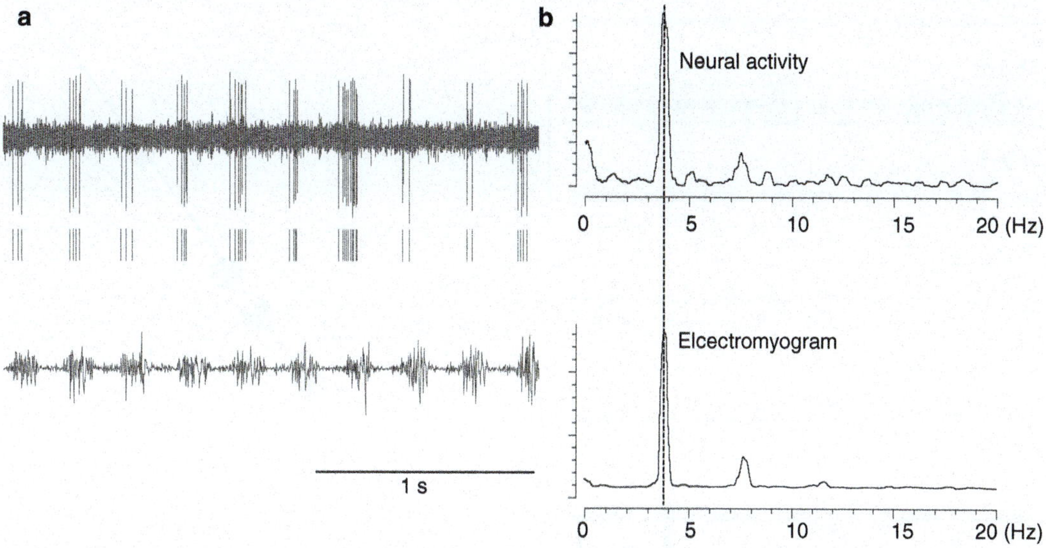

Fig. 4.5 Neurons recorded in the thalamus that fire at the same frequency as tremors (tremor cells). (**a**) *Top:* Neural activity. *Middle:* Raster display of neuron firing. *Bottom:* Electromyogram (EMG) of tremors recorded simultaneously. (**b**) Power spectrum of timing of neuron firing (*top*) and the frequency of electromyogram (EMG) of tremors (*bottom*). They both peaked with the same frequency (3.8 Hz)

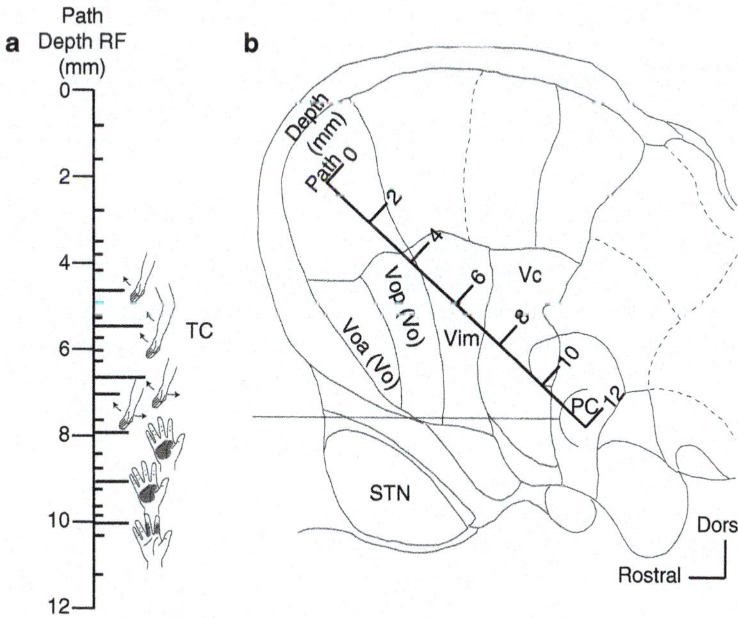

Fig. 4.6 Identification of the border between the Vim and Vc nuclei (Vim–Vc border). The Vim–Vc border is physiologically defined as the most anterior neuron along a length of trajectory in which more than one-half of the neurons located posteriorly were sensory neurons (Hua and Lenz 2005). (**a**) Body parts that respond to peripheral sensory stimulation on the insertion route (receptor field: *RF*). *Short line:* sites where neuron activity was recorded. *Long line:* the neurons responding to joint movement or neurons responding to tactile stimulation of the skin. *TC* tremor cell. (**b**) A insertion route superimposed on a sagittal section (14.5-mm lateral) from the Schaltenbrand–Wahren atlas. *Voa* nucleus ventralis oralis anterior, *Vop* nucleus ventralis oralis posterior, *Vim* nucleus ventralis intermedius, *Vc* nucleus ventralis caudalis, *STN* subthalamic nucleus

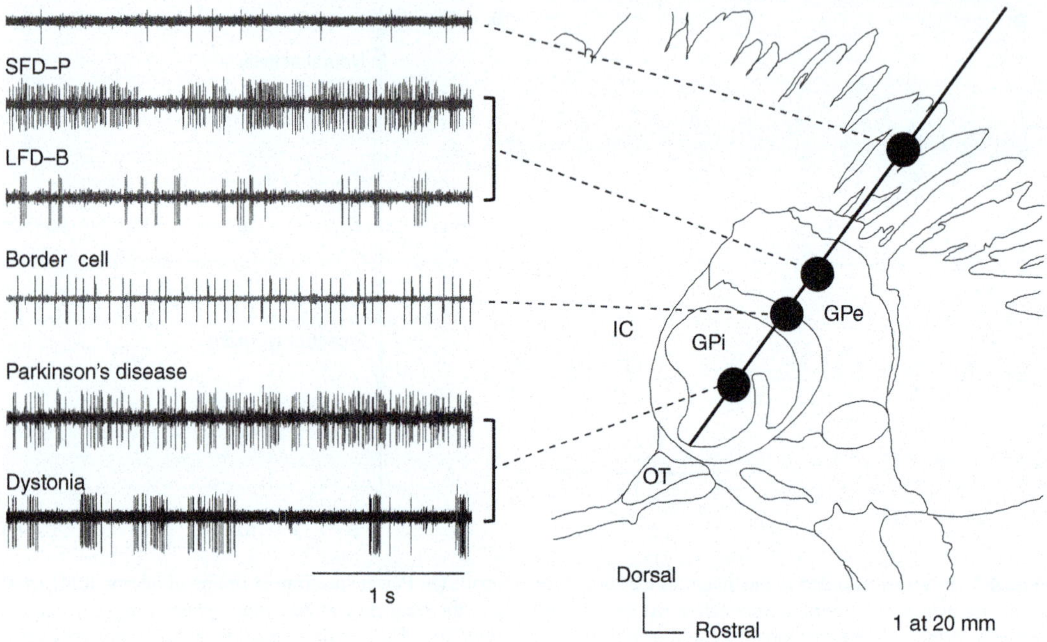

Fig. 4.7 Neural activity recorded along the insertion route toward the globus pallidus internus (GPi) superimposed on a sagittal section (20-mm lateral) from the Schaltenbrand–Wahren atlas. *GPe* globus pallidus externus, *GPi* globus pallidus internus, *IC* internal capsule, *LFD-B* low-frequency discharge with bursts, *SFD-P* slow-frequency discharge with pauses, *Str* striatum

4.3.3 Globus Pallidus Internus (GPi) (Fig. 4.7)

The GPi is a target site for DBS treatment of PD and dystonia. The frequency and pattern of neural discharges in pallidum are thought to vary with different diseases and etiology. Dystonia can be categorized into primary or secondary according to the etiology and as focal, segmental, multifocal, hemi-, and general according to the regions of the body showing symptoms, with varying underlying pathologies. Therefore, MER findings also can differ by the type of dystonia. Here, we focus on primary general dystonia (hereafter simply "dystonia"), which is the type most frequently treated with DBS.

4.3.3.1 Striatum

The insertion route into pallidum begins with the identification of the striatum. Compared with pallidum, striatal cells exhibit low-amplitude and low-frequency (≤10 Hz) neural activity (Holloway et al. 2008). As the microelectrode is advanced, neural activity and firing frequency increase from the striatum to the external segment of globus pallidus externus (GPe), which indicates its boundary with the striatum.

4.3.3.2 GPe

GPe contains two neuron types with different firing patterns. The first type pauses during sustained firing (firing frequency 10–100 Hz), whereas the other type discharges with a low frequency (10–30 Hz) and exhibits bursts of activity.

4.3.3.3 "Border Cells"

In some cases, neurons called "border cells" that discharge with regular bursts around 30–50 Hz can be recorded at the boundary between GPi and GPe (Hutchison 2004; Holloway et al. 2008). Border cells are thought to be cells that have migrated from the nucleus basalis of Meynert. Recordings from these border cells indicate the boundary between GPe and GPi.

4.3.3.4 GPi

The spontaneous firing frequency of GPi neurons during "off" periods in PD is 70–100 Hz, and many of these neurons display a sustained firing pattern. In primary general dystonia, however, the spontaneous firing frequency is lower than that observed in PD and healthy monkeys (Sanghera et al. 2003; Starr et al. 2005), and an inverse correlation between firing frequency and severity has been reported (Lenz et al. 1998; Starr et al. 2005). Patients with dystonia are frequently administered propofol during surgery to prevent movements, and it has been pointed out that this decrease in the spontaneous firing frequency in GPi may be due to the effect of propofol (Hutchison et al. 2003). In our experience and as per previous reports, however, the firing frequency of GPi neurons recorded in patients with primary general dystonia under local anesthesia is 40–50 Hz, which is lower than that observed in PD (Sanghera et al. 2003; Starr et al. 2005). Analysis of the relationship between the spontaneous firing frequency of GPi neurons in dystonia, blood propofol concentration, and level of anesthesia revealed that propofol had no effect (Steigerwald et al. 2005). Taking all these into consideration, although the decrease in spontaneous firing frequency may have been caused by propofol, it is difficult to regard this as the main reason. Although many neurons exhibit irregular but sustained firing patterns in PD, the firing pattern of GPi neurons in dystonia is characterized by many neurons exhibiting irregular firing, with both bursts of firing and long pauses.

4.3.3.5 Sensorimotor Region

The posteroventral portion of pallidum is a sensorimotor region, with GPe and GPi having their own respective somatotopy in which the areas representing the upper and lower limbs are distributed from the ventral to the dorsal side in primate (DeLong et al. 1985; Baron et al. 2002). In dystonia, the receptor fields of the affected body parts are thought to be enlarged (Lenz et al. 1998; Vitek et al. 1998).

4.3.3.6 Identification of the Optic Tract (OT)

OT is located in the ventral GPi. If the DBS electrode is placed close to OT, photesthesia may occur as a side effect during stimulation. To avoid this side effect, responses in reaction to photostimulation in a darkened room should be observed and recorded using MER. Therefore, either OT should be identified or it should be confirmed that it is not close to the microelectrode insertion route.

4.3.4 Subthalamic Area (SA)

The posterior SA (PSA) has been the target site for ablation surgery, however, in recent years, it also has become one of the target sites selected for DBS treatment of tremors. PSA is generally regarded as comprising the white matter region below the thalamus, including the prelemniscal radiations (PRL) and part of ZI. When performing MER, PRL are located approximately 1–2 mm inferior to the AC–PC line and pass through the thalamus. Because PRL consist of white matter, they can be identified by their low amplitude and quiet background activity (Jimenez et al. 2000). Moderate-amplitude spontaneous firing of approximately 4–20 Hz can be observed in ZI (Merello et al. 2006).

4.4 Target Confirmation by Intraoperative Stimulation

Intraoperative test stimulation is broadly evaluated by two points: the first is the assessment of the stimulation-induced improvement in symptoms, whereas the second is the assessment of stimulation-induced side effects. With the Medtronic electrodes, intraoperative test stimulation can be performed using the tip of the outer sheath of the microelectrode (Fig. 4.1b). This sheath electrode has a large contact area, indicating that it delivers macrostimulation rather than microstimulation. Although macrostimulation lacks the spatial resolution of microstimulation, it applies an electrical stimulus through an electrode that is close to the size of the actual DBS electrode, which more effectively indicates whether the site is appropriate for DBS placement.

Table 4.1 Stimulation-induced side effects and stimulated structures surrounding the target site

Target site	Side effects	Stimulated structures surrounding the target site	Positional relation to the target site
STN	Oculomotor disturbance (diplopia)	Fibers of the oculomotor nerve	Medioventral
	Concomitant deviation (gaze palsy)	Corticospinal tract (internal capsule)	Anteriolateral
	Muscle contraction	Corticospinal tract (internal capsule)	Anteriolateral
	Dysarthria	Corticospinal tract (internal capsule)	Anteriolateral
	Paresthesia	Medial lemniscus	Posterior
Thalamus (Vim nuclei)	Muscle contraction	Corticospinal tract (internal capsule)	Lateral
	Dysarthria	Corticospinal tract (internal capsule)	Lateral
	Paresthesia	Vc nuclei	Posterior
Pallidum (GPi)	Muscle contraction	Corticospinal tract (internal capsule)	Medial
	Dysarthria	Corticospinal tract (internal capsule)	Medial
	Photesthesia	Optic tract	Posteroventral

4.4.1 Assessment of Stimulation-Induced Improvement in Symptoms

Symptoms that do not immediately respond to electrical stimulation cannot be easily evaluated during the short duration of surgery. For example, it is frequently difficult to observe improvement in dystonia symptoms as a result of intraoperative stimulation. Its effect on tremors and rigidity, however, can be assessed during the surgery. Symptoms frequently improve or resolve due to the lesions produced with electrode insertion, even without stimulus application. In this case, it may be difficult to assess the effect of electrical stimulation on improving symptoms during the operation, but as it is important to evaluate the lesion effect immediately, as this suggests that it is the optimum insertion path from the perspective of improving symptoms, stimulation-induced side effects should be assessed.

4.4.2 Assessment of Stimulation-Induced Side Effects

The side effects that should be considered vary depending on the structures surrounding the target site. Table 4.1 presents typical target sites and easily induced side effects for these sites. For almost all these side effects, increasing the stimulation intensity increases the extent of current spread and the region affect by stimulation, which often causes these side effects to appear. It should therefore be confirmed that side effects do not appear at a stimulus intensity below that required to achieve adequate improvement of symptoms.

4.5 Simultaneous Multitrack Recording

Multitrack MER, in which several microelectrodes are simultaneously inserted, has recently become feasible. In this method, a maximum of five electrodes can be simultaneously inserted in an arrangement where a central electrode is surrounded by electrodes in the 0, 3, 6, and 9 o'clock positions (Fig. 4.2b). Multitrack MER has advantages over single-track recording because multiple tracks enable target site identification in less time, allow three-dimensional information, and allow simple comparison of intraoperative stimulation. Furthermore, during single-track recording, removing the electrode may cause the brain to tilt; however, when inserting multiple electrodes simultaneously, the electrodes play an anchoring role and help to prevent this tilting.

However, because several electrodes are simultaneously inserted, there are concerns of increased risk of hemorrhage. Although no association has been found between the number of recording electrodes inserted and the risk of hemorrhage (Terao et al. 2003; Binder et al. 2005; Sansur et al. 2007), the number of microelectrodes used should not be increased without careful consideration, and it may be necessary to carefully analyze the number actually required. In our hospital, when identifying STN, we simultaneously insert a total of three electrodes, with one of the two extra electrodes being lateral and the other one being posterior to the central electrode. We use posterior tracking to take into account brain shifting in the posterior direction (with gravity) due to the flow of cerebrospinal fluid (Obuchi et al. 2008). It goes without saying that the use of contrast MRI during planning to ensure adequate insertion space on the brain surface (Binder et al. 2005), avoiding the superficial veins, and the performance of sufficient simulation of the insertion route to the target site are vital in order to reduce the risk of hemorrhage.

References

Baron MS, Wichmann T, Ma D et al (2002) Effects of transient focal inactivation of the basal ganglia in parkinsonian primates. J Neurosci 22:592–599

Benabid AL, Pollak P, Gao D et al (1996) Chronic electrical stimulation of the ventralis intermedius nucleus of the thalamus as a treatment of movement disorders. J Neurosurg 84:203–214

Bezard E, Boraud T, Bioulac B et al (1999) Involvement of the subthalamic nucleus in glutamatergic compensatory mechanisms. Eur J Neurosci 11:2167–2170

Binder DK, Rau GM, Starr PA (2005) Risk factors for hemorrhage during microelectrode-guided deep brain stimulator implantation for movement disorders. Neurosurgery 56:722–732; discussion 722–732

DeLong MR, Crutcher MD, Georgopoulos AP (1985) Primate globus pallidus and subthalamic nucleus: functional organization. J Neurophysiol 53:530–543

Holloway KL, Baron MS, Oberlander E et al (2008) Pallidal stimulation for Parkinson's disease. In: Starr P, Barbaro NB, Larson PS (eds) Functional neurosurgery (Neurosurgical operative atlas), 2nd edn. Thieme Medical Publishers, New York, pp 188–194

Hua SE, Lenz FA (2005) Posture-related oscillations in human cerebellar thalamus in essential tremor are enabled by voluntary motor circuits. J Neurophysiol 93: 117–127

Hutchison WD (2004) Electrophysiological findings in Gpe and Gpi. In: Israel Z, Burchiel K (eds) Microelectrode recording in movement disorder surgery. Thieme Medical Publishers, New York, pp 72–81

Hutchison WD, Allan RJ, Opitz H et al (1998) Neurophysiological identification of the subthalamic nucleus in surgery for Parkinson's disease. Ann Neurol 44:622–628

Hutchison WD, Lang AE, Dostrovsky JO et al (2003) Pallidal neuronal activity: implications for models of dystonia. Ann Neurol 53:480–488

Jimenez F, Velasco F, Velasco M et al (2000) Subthalamic prelemniscal radiation stimulation for the treatment of Parkinson's disease: electrophysiological characterization of the area. Arch Med Res 31:270–281

Katayama Y, Kano T, Kobayashi K et al (2005) Difference in surgical strategies between thalamotomy and thalamic deep brain stimulation for tremor control. J Neurol 252(Suppl 4):IV17–IV22

Kim JH, Ohara S, Lenz FA (2009) Mental arithmetic leads to multiple discrete changes from baseline in the firing patterns of human thalamic neurons. J Neurophysiol 101:2107–2119

Kobayashi K, Winberry J, Liu CC et al (2009) A painful cutaneous laser stimulus evokes responses from single neurons in the human thalamic principal somatic sensory nucleus ventral caudal – Vc. J Neurophysiol 101: 2210–2217

Lenz FA, Dostrovsky JO, Tasker RR et al (1988) Single-unit analysis of the human ventral thalamic nuclear group: somatosensory responses. J Neurophysiol 59:299–316

Lenz FA, Kwan HC, Martin RL et al (1994) Single unit analysis of the human ventral thalamic nuclear group. Tremor-related activity in functionally identified cells. Brain 117(Pt 3):531–543

Lenz FA, Suarez JI, Metman LV et al (1998) Pallidal activity during dystonia: somatosensory reorganisation and changes with severity. J Neurol Neurosurg Psychiatry 65:767–770

Merello M, Tenca E, Cerquetti D (2006) Neuronal activity of the zona incerta in Parkinson's disease patients. Mov Disord 21:937–943

Obuchi T, Katayama Y, Kobayashi K et al (2008) Direction and predictive factors for the shift of brain structure during deep brain stimulation electrode implantation for advanced Parkinson's disease. Neuromodulation 11:302–310

Rodriguez-Oroz MC, Rodriguez M, Guridi J et al (2001) The subthalamic nucleus in Parkinson's disease: somatotopic organization and physiological characteristics. Brain 124:1777–1790

Sanghera MK, Grossman RG, Kalhorn CG et al (2003) Basal ganglia neuronal discharge in primary and secondary dystonia in patients undergoing pallidotomy. Neurosurgery 52:1358–1370; discussion 1370–1373

Sansur CA, Frysinger RC, Pouratian N et al (2007) Incidence of symptomatic hemorrhage after stereotactic electrode placement. J Neurosurg 107:998–1003

Schrock LE, Ostrem JL, Turner RS et al (2009) The subthalamic nucleus in primary dystonia: single-unit discharge characteristics. J Neurophysiol 102:3740–3752

Starr PA, Rau GM, Davis V et al (2005) Spontaneous pallidal neuronal activity in human dystonia: comparison with Parkinson's disease and normal macaque. J Neurophysiol 93:3165–3176

Steigerwald F, Hinz L, Pinsker MO et al (2005) Effect of propofol anesthesia on pallidal neuronal discharges in generalized dystonia. Neurosci Lett 386:156–159

Steigerwald F, Potter M, Herzog J et al (2008) Neuronal activity of the human subthalamic nucleus in the parkinsonian and nonparkinsonian state. J Neurophysiol 100:2515–2524

Terao T, Takahashi H, Yokochi F et al (2003) Hemorrhagic complication of stereotactic surgery in patients with movement disorders. J Neurosurg 98:1241–1246

Vitek JL, Zhang J, Evatt M et al (1998) GPi pallidotomy for dystonia: clinical outcome and neuronal activity. Adv Neurol 78:211–219

Instrument of Brain Stimulation 5

Takamitsu Yamamoto, Chikashi Fukaya,
Atsuo Yoshino, and Yoichi Katayama

5.1 Chronic Brain Stimulation System

Deep brain stimulation (DBS) and motor cortex stimulation (MCS) are the best known applications of chronic brain stimulation with surgically implanted stimulation systems. DBS (Hosobuchi et al. 1973) and MCS (Tsubokawa et al. 1993) have been applied for the treatment of intractable pain, movement disorders (Benabid et al. 1996; Yamamoto et al. 2004; Limousin et al. 1998; Krauss et al. 1999), motor weakness (Brown et al. 2006; Levy et al. 2008; Harvey et al. 2009; Yamamoto et al. 2011), psychiatric disorders (Nuttin et al. 1999; Mayberg et al. 2005), epilepsy (Hodaie et al. 2002), and prolonged unconsciousness (Tsubokawa et al. 1990; Schiff et al. 2007; Yamamoto et al. 2010). Hosobuchi et al. (1973) were the first to report chronic DBS employing an implanted depth electrode in 1973. They applied this technique for the treatment of intractable pain, and the target of the stimulation point was the sensory thalamus. Subsequently, chronic DBS was mainly applied for the treatment of intractable pain (Hosobuchi et al. 1977; Adams et al. 1974; Mazars 1975), and Medtronic Co. commercially released the DBS system in 1976. Motor cortex stimulation was first reported by Tsubokawa et al. (1991) in 1991, for the treatment of poststroke pain.

The first DBS system was an Extrel type, consisting of an external transmitter, an antenna, a receiver with an extension cable, and a stimulation electrode (Fig. 5.1). The external transmitter was an analog type at first (model 3523, Medtronic Co, Minneapolis, USA) and developed into a digital type (model 3425 and 3210, Medtronic Co, Minneapolis, USA) (Fig. 5.2a, b). The external transmitter contains the circuitry and power source (an alkaline battery) and is connected with an antenna. The antenna was placed on the skin located over the implanted receiver and was connected with the implanted stimulation electrode. The energy evoked by the external transmitter was transmitted through the antenna using a radio-frequency-coupled link, and the subcutaneous receiver decoded the radio frequency signal and delivered it to the stimulation electrode. The Extrel system had the advantage that it did not use implanted batteries or other life-limiting components, and so pulse generator replacement was not routinely required.

T. Yamamoto, MD, PhD (✉) • C. Fukaya, MD, PhD
Division of Applied System Neuroscience,
Department of Neurological Surgery,
Nihon University School of Medicine, Tokyo, Japan
e-mail: yamamoto-takamitsu@nihon-u.ac.jp

A. Yoshino, MD, PhD • Y. Katayama, MD, PhD
Division of Neurosurgery,
Department of Neurological Surgery,
Nihon University School of Medicine, Tokyo, Japan

T. Itakura (ed.), *Deep Brain Stimulation for Neurological Disorders: Theoretical Background and Clinical Application*, DOI 10.1007/978-3-319-08476-3_5,

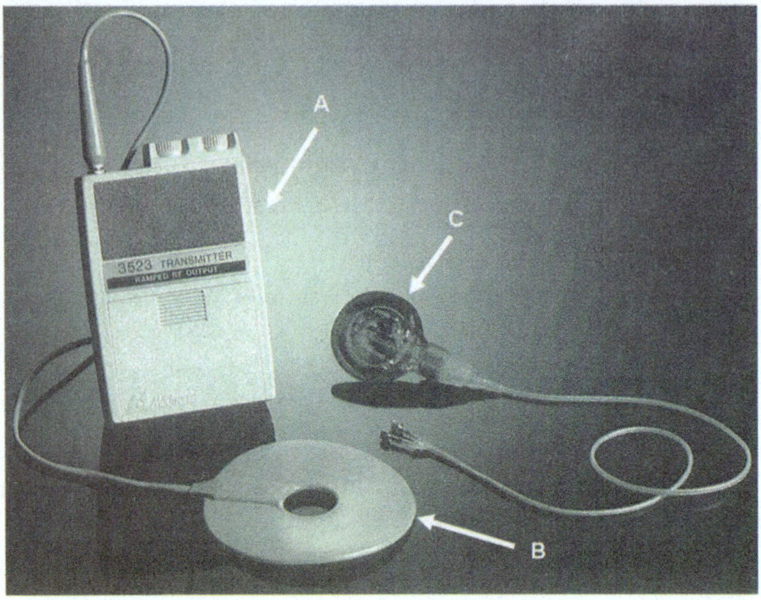

Fig. 5.1 Extrel type DBS system. (**a**) External transmitter (model 3523). (**b**) Antenna. (**c**) Receiver (model 3360). (**d**) Stimulation electrode (Reprinted with the permission of Medtronic, Inc. © 1991)

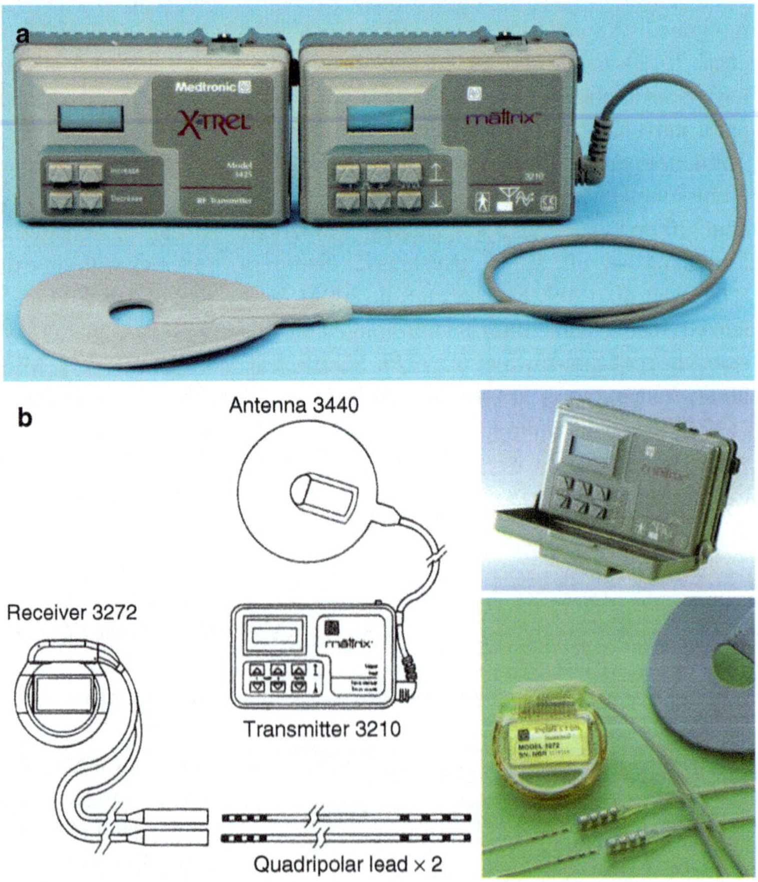

Fig. 5.2 (**a**) Extrel type transmitter. One channel (*left*) and two channel (*right*) transmitter. (**b**) Two channel Extrel type stimulation system (Reprinted with the permission of Medtronic, Inc. © 1994, 1996)

The patient felt inconvenienced, however, by the need to wear an external device, and variable coupling between the external antenna and the receiver could lead to fluctuations in the stimulation amplitude.

Later, the Itrel type DBS system was developed. The Itrel type DBS system consists of an implantable pulse generator (IPG) which contains its own battery, extension cable, and stimulation electrode. Thus, the DBS system became completely internalized. The patient receiving the DBS was no longer inconvenienced by the need to wear an external device. Recently, the IPG was developed further, such that one of the new IPG devices contains a rechargeable battery. The rechargeable battery is useful for the prolongation of battery life and has extended the time before IPG replacement is required up to 9 years.

5.2 DBS and MCS Electrode

The early DBS electrodes were quite different from the present DBS electrodes. There were four stimulation points as with recent electrodes, but the most distal stimulation point was ring shaped and the body of electrode was twisted as shown in Fig. 5.3. For the implantation of this electrode, the most distal ring-shaped part was hooked by a pointed guide needle and advanced toward the target. After that procedure, the guide needle was pulled out slowly so as not to move the tip of the implanted electrode.

The present DBS electrode is also quadripolar, but the surface of the electrode is smooth and the tip of electrode is domelike in shape. This coaxial electrode has a central stylet, and the central stylet is pulled out after the electrode is advanced toward the target. Two types of DBS electrode (models 3387 and 3389, Medtronic Co, Minneapolis, USA) are commonly used, and both have a 1.27-mm diameter. Each individual contact is 1.5-mm high, and the difference between the two models is the spacing between the contacts. The contact edge-to-edge space is 1.5 mm in the model 3387 and 0.5 mm in model 3389. Therefore, the distances from the tip of the most distal contact point to the top of the most proximal contact point for these two electrode models are 10.5 and 7.5 mm, respectively (Fig. 5.4). The design of these DBS electrodes is shown in Fig. 5.5, and the device specifications for the leads are presented in Table 5.1. In addition, other DBS electrodes such as the Medtronic model 3387 IES (diameter, 1.27 mm; contact length, 3 mm; inter-electrode spacing, 4 mm) and model 3887 (diameter, 1.3 mm; contact length, 3 mm; inter-electrode spacing, 4 mm) have been developed to cover relatively wider target areas such as the anterior limb of the internal capsule for the treatment of obsessive compulsive disorder.

The DBS electrodes are fixed into place with a combination of a plastic burr-hole ring and burr-hole cap contained in the DBS electrode package made by Medtronic Co. The burr-hole ring has a slit with a width of several mm, and small ring holes are located bilaterally beside the slit. It is

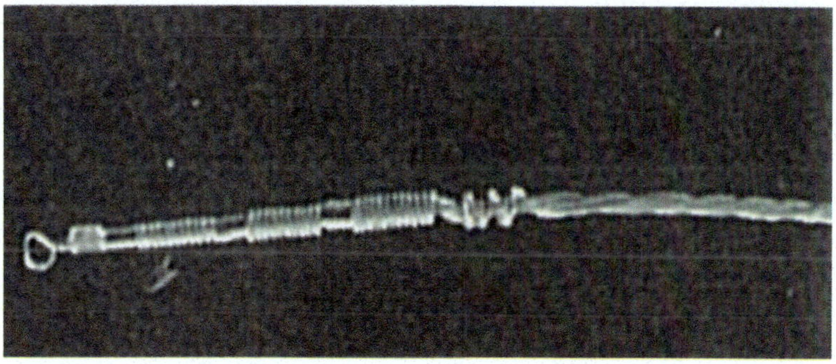

Fig. 5.3 The early DBS electrode (model 3380). This platinum–iridium electrode is composed of a distal loop and three other active contact points, each approximately 2-mm long

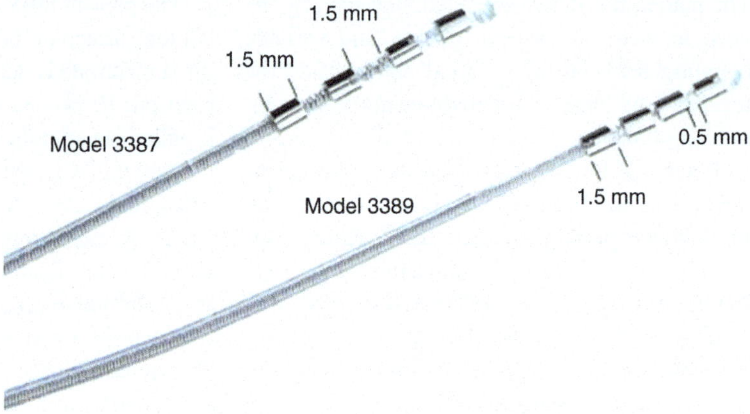

Fig. 5.4 The recent DBS electrodes. The Medtronic 3387 model has 1.5-mm contact spacing and the 3389 model has 0.5-mm spacing. Each individual contact is 1.5-mm high. Both electrodes are quadripolar and have a 1.27-mm diameter (Reprinted with the permission of Medtronic, Inc. © 2012)

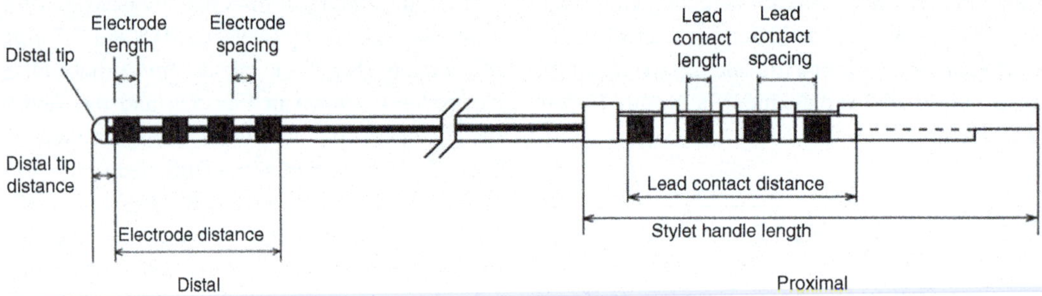

Fig. 5.5 The design of recent DBS electrode (electrode, lead contact, and stylet) (Reprinted with the permission of Medtronic, Inc.)

possible to make the slit smaller by closing the bilateral small ring holes using pointed forceps, temporarily decreasing the diameter for placement into the perforated burr hole; once in place, the ring is released and expands in diameter to fix tightly to the burr-hole edge in the skull bone. The burr-hole ring also contains two grooves, which serve to fix the DBS electrodes. After that, the burr-hole cap is fixed to the burr-hole ring. The DBS electrodes are fixed in the groove of burr-hole ring and covered by the burr-hole cap (Yamamoto et al. 2003) (Fig. 5.6).

Tsubokawa et al. (1991) first applied MCS for poststroke pain and used the RESUME II electrode (Medtronic Co, Minneapolis, USA). The RESUME II electrode is a paddle type, single quadripolar column (1×4) electrode (Fig. 5.7). Recently, many more kinds of paddle-type electrodes have been developed, with different numbers of contact points (4–20 points) and columns (1–5), and different length and width paddles (Fig. 5.7).

5.3 Implantable Pulse Generator

In recent years, the Extrel type stimulation system, consisting of an external pulse generator, an antenna, and a receiver which contains the transmitter has become clinically obsolete. The Itrel type pulse generator, which is totally implanted and powered by an internal battery, is now the clinical standard. In an Itrel type pulse generator, both nonrechargeable and rechargeable pulse generators are available for clinical use. The rechargeable pulse generator must be periodically recharged with an external radiofrequency antenna, and the advantage of this system is longer duration of the batteries (up to 9 years) without need for replacement. At present, Medtronic Co. has released four types of IPGs for clinical use, namely, the Activa-PC-3761, Activa-RC-37612, Activa-SC-37602, and Activa-SC-37603. The Activa-PC-3761 and Activa-RC-37612 are multi-programmable devices that deliver stimulation through one or two leads while Activa-SC-37602

Table 5.1 The device specifications for recent DBS electrodes 3387 and 3389

Description	Model 3387	Model 3389
Connector	Quadripolar, in-line	Quadripolar, in-line
Shape	Straight	Straight
Conductor resistance[a]	<100 Ω	<100 Ω
Length	10–50 cm	10–50 cm
Diameter	1.27 mm	1.27 mm
Distal end		
Number of electrodes	4	4
Electrode shape	Cylindrical	Cylindrical
Electrode length	1.5 mm	1.5 mm
Electrode spacing	1.5 mm	0.5 mm
Electrode distance	10.5 mm	7.5 mm
Distal tip distance	1.5 mm	1.5 mm
Proximal end		
Lead contact length	2.3 mm	2.3 mm
Lead contact spacing	4.3 mm	4.3 mm
Lead contact distance	16.6 mm	16.6 mm
Stylet handle length	40.1 mm	40.1 mm

Reprinted with the permission of Medtronic, Inc.
[a]Electrical resistance is proportional to lead length

and Activa-SC-37603 are multiprogram devices that deliver stimulation through only one lead. Only Activa-RC-37612 is a rechargeable type IPG, and the other three types are nonrechargeable type IPGs.

5.3.1 Activa® PC (Activa-PC-37601)

The Activa PC neurostimulator is a multiprogrammable device that delivers stimulation through one or two leads. The stimulation settings are stored as "programs" with specific pulse width, pulse rate, and pulse amplitude settings acting on a specific combination of electrodes. Up to four programs can be combined into a group. When using more than one program, the pulses are delivered sequentially—first a pulse from one program, then a pulse from the next program. Pulse width, amplitude, and electrode polarity for each program within the group can have different values. Rate, rate limits, SoftStart/Stop, and cycling for each program within the group have the same values (Fig. 5.8 and Table 5.2).

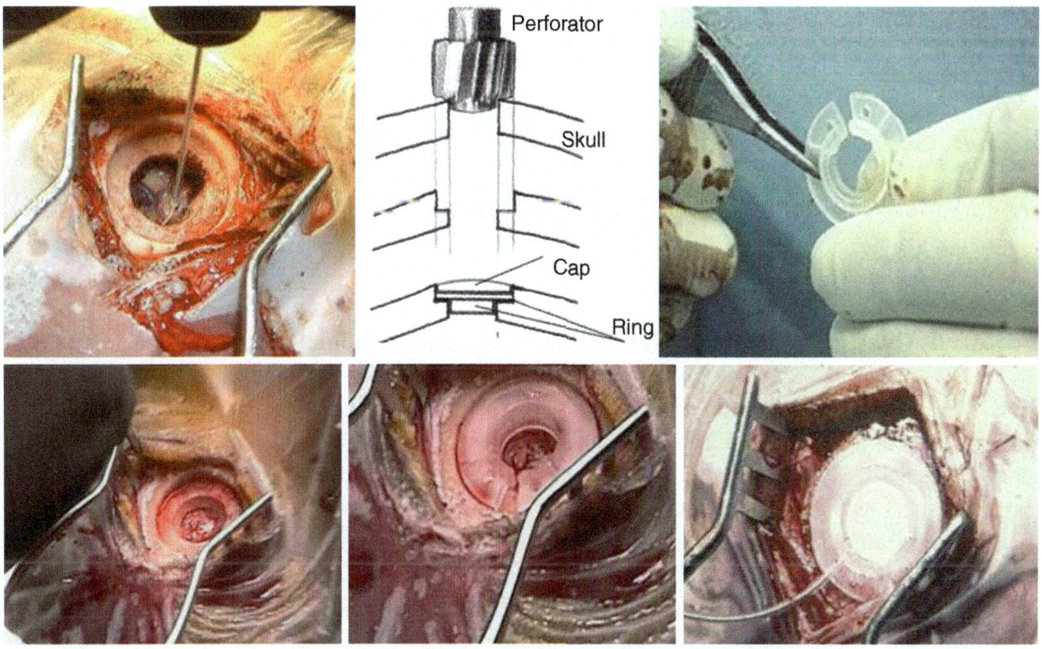

Fig. 5.6 Burr-hole ring and burr-hole cap. The DBS electrode is fixed by the burr-hole ring and burr-hole cap. We have also reported the dual floor burr-hole method, which is convenient for fixation (Yamamoto et al. 2003)

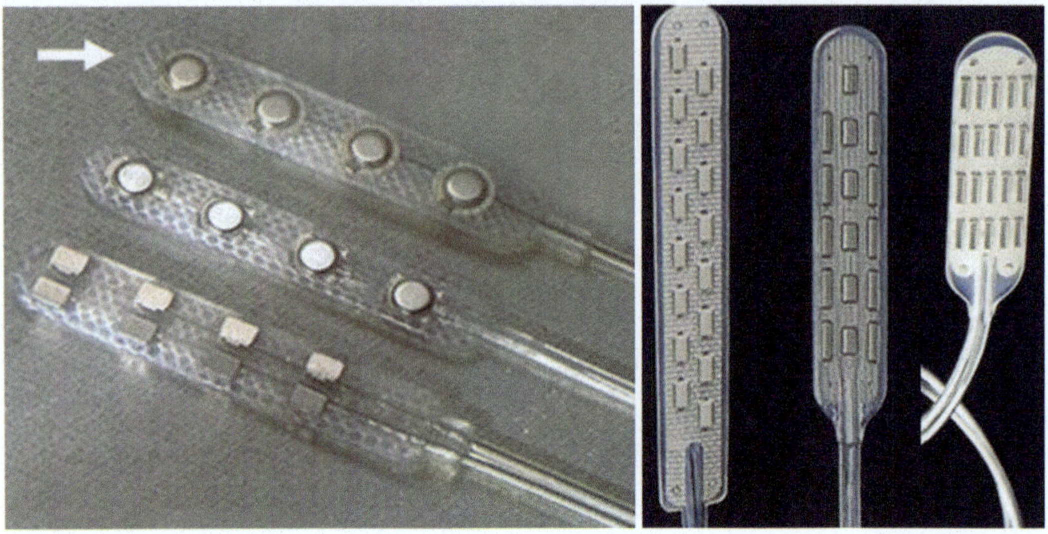

Fig. 5.7 The RESUME II electrode and other paddle type electrodes. RESUME electrode is a paddle type consisting of a single quadripolar column (1 × 4) electrode. The diameter of each stimulation point is 4 mm, and each stimulation point is separated by 6.2 mm (→). The number of contact points (4–20 points) and columns (1–5), and the length and width of the paddle are different in each electrode

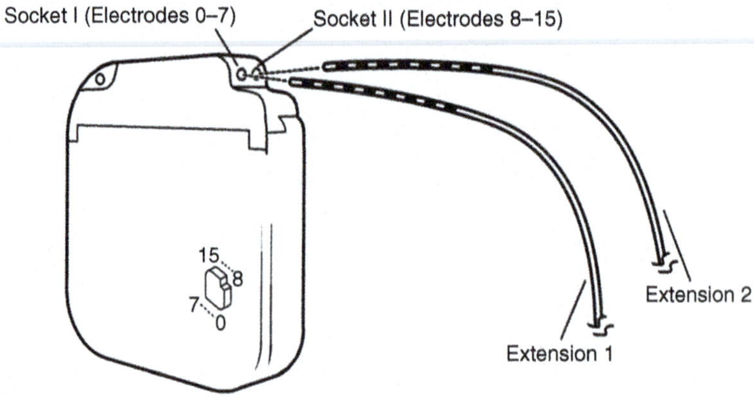

Fig. 5.8 Figure of Activa® PC (Activa-PC-37601) with connection to the stimulating electrode (Reprinted with the permission of Medtronic, Inc. © 2012)

5.3.2 Activa® RC (Activa-RC-37612)

The Activa RC is a multiprogrammable, rechargeable device that delivers stimulation through one or two leads. The stimulation settings are stored as "programs," with specific pulse width, pulse rate, and pulse amplitude settings acting on a specific combination of electrodes. Up to four programs can be combined into a group, with a maximum of two programs per lead. When using more than one program, the pulses are delivered sequentially—first a pulse from one program, then a pulse from the next program. Pulse width and amplitude and electrode polarity for each program within the group can have different values. Rate, rate limits, ramping, and cycling for each program within the group have the same values (Fig. 5.9 and Table 5.3).

5.3.3 Activa® SC (Activa-SC-37602)

This Activa SC is a multiprogram device that delivers stimulation through one lead. The stimulation settings are stored as "programs," with specific pulse width, pulse rate, and pulse amplitude settings acting on a specific electrode combination. Up to two programs can be combined into a group. When using more than one program, the pulses are delivered sequentially—first a pulse from one program, then a pulse from the next program. Pulse width and amplitude and electrode polarity for each program within the group can have different values. Rate, rate limits, SoftStart/Stop, and Cycling for each program

Table 5.2 Device specifications for Activa® PC (Activa-PC-37601)

Description	Value
Connector type	Octapolar, in-line 2.8 mm (0.110 in.) spacing
Height	65.0 mm (2.6 in.)
Length	49.0 mm (1.9 in.)
Thickness	
Case	15.0 mm (0.6 in.)
Connector	15.0 mm (0.6 in.)
Weight	67.0 g (2.4 oz)
Volume	39.0 cm^3
Power source	6.3 Amp hours, 3.2 V HCSVO[a] cell
Storage temperature	−18° to +52 °C (0° to +126 °F)
Serial number model designator[b]	NKM
Radiopaque Identification (ID) code	NKD

Reprinted with the permission of Medtronic, Inc.
[a]Hybrid combined silver vanadium oxide
[b]The serial number is the model designator followed by a number. The clinician programmer displays the entire serial number beginning with the model designator

Table 5.3 Device specifications for Activa® RC (Activa-RC-37612)

Description	Value
Connector type	Octapolar, in-line 2.8-mm (0.110-in.) spacing
Height	54 mm (2.1 in.)
Length	54 mm (2.1 in.)
Thickness	
Case	9 mm (0.4 in.)
Connector	11 mm (0.4 in.)
Weight	40 g (1.6 oz)
Volume	22 cm^3
Battery life	9 years
Power source[a]	Lithium ion rechargeable battery
Storage temperature	−18° to +52 °C (0° to +126 °F)
Serial number model designator[b]	NKG
Radiopaque Identification (ID) code	NKG

Reprinted with the permission of Medtronic, Inc.
[a]The neurostimulator is not shipped with a full battery charge. Refer to the charging system user manual for neurostimulator charging instructions
[b]The serial number is the model designator followed by a number. The clinician programmer displays the entire serial number beginning with the model designator

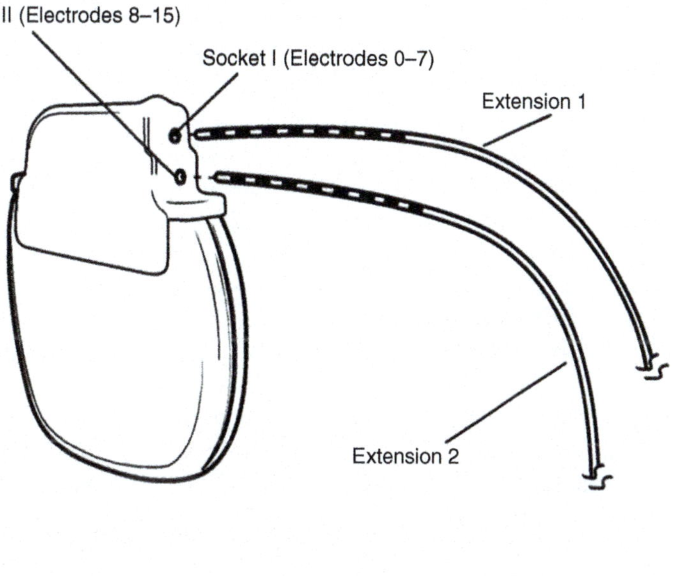

Fig. 5.9 Figure of Activa® RC (Activa-RC-37612) with connection to the stimulating electrode (Reprinted with the permission of Medtronic, Inc. © 2012)

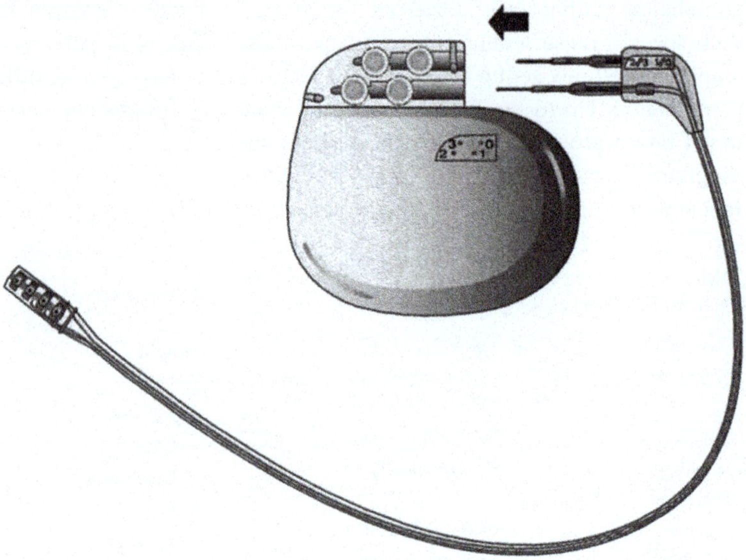

Fig. 5.10 Figure of Activa® SC (Activa-SC-37602) with connection to the stimulating electrode (Reprinted with the permission of Medtronic, Inc. © 2012)

within the group have the same values (Fig. 5.10 and Table 5.4).

5.3.4 Activa® SC (Activa-SC-37603)

This Activa SC is a multiprogram device that delivers stimulation through one lead. The stimulation settings are stored in programs. A program is a specific combination of pulse width, pulse rate, and pulse amplitude settings acting on a specific electrode combination. Up to two programs can be combined into a group. When using more than one program, the pulses are delivered sequentially—first a pulse from one program, then a pulse from the next program. Pulse width and amplitude and electrode polarity for each program within the group can have different values. Rate, rate limits, SoftStart/Stop, and Cycling for each program within the group have the same values (Fig. 5.11 and Table 5.5).

Table 5.4 Device specifications for Activa® SC (Activa-SC-37602)

Description	Value
Connector type	Quadrapolar, two bore[a]
Height	55 mm (2.2 in.)
Length	60 mm (2.4 in.)
Thickness	11 mm (0.4 in.)
Weight	45 g (1.6 oz)
Volume	28 cm^3
Power source	4.5 Amp hours, 3.2 V HCSVO[b] cell
Temperature limitation	−18° to +52 °C (0° to +126 °F)
Serial number model designator[c]	NLA
Radiopaque identification (ID) code	NLA

Reprinted with the permission of Medtronic, Inc.
[a]Compatible with two-pronged extension
[b]Hybrid combined silver vanadium oxide
[c]The serial number is the model designator followed by a number. The clinician programmer displays the entire serial number beginning with the model designator

5.4 Clinician Programmer (N'VISION)

The N'Vision (model 8840, Medtronic Co.) is the clinician programmer (Fig. 5.12), and the application card (model 8870) is a handheld device for programming Medtronic devices for neuromodulation therapies. The programmer is used to review and program device parameters using telemetry, a radio-frequency (RF) communication. The programmer is also used to set limits for the patient control devices.

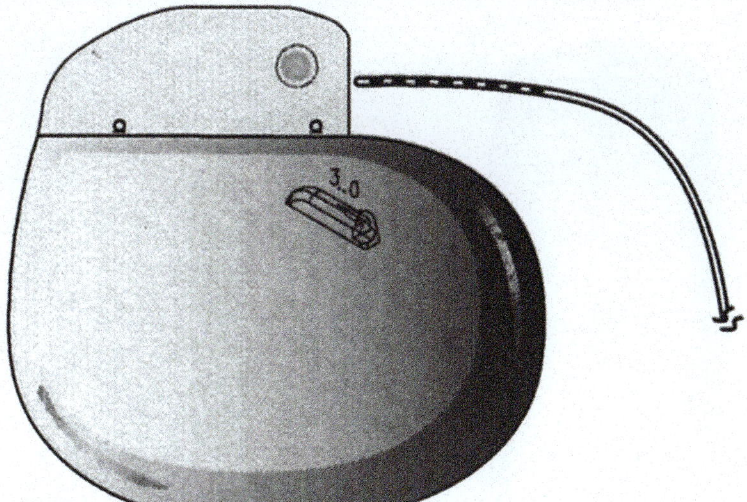

Fig. 5.11 Figure of Activa® SC (Activa-SC-37603) with connection to the stimulating electrode (Reprinted with the permission of Medtronic, Inc. © 2012)

Table 5.5 Device specifications for Activa® SC (Activa-SC-37603)

Description	Value
Connector type	Octapolar, one bore[a,b]
Height	55 mm (2.2 in.)
Length	60 mm (2.4 in.)
Thickness	11 mm (0.4 in.)
Weight	44 g (1.6 oz)
Volume	27 cm^3
Power source	4.5 Amp hours, 3.2 V HCSVO[c] cell
Temperature limitation	−18° to +52 °C (0° to +126 °F)
Serial number model designator[d]	NLB
Radiopaque identification (ID) code	NLB

Reprinted with the permission of Medtronic, Inc.
[a]Compatible with 8-4 extension
[b]Four contacts active
[c]Hybrid combined silver vanadium oxide
[d]The serial number is the model designator followed by a number. The clinician programmer displays the entire serial number beginning with the model designator

5.5 Patient Programmer

The Activa® PC Model 37601, Activa® RC Model 37612, Activa® SC Model 37602, and Activa® SC Model 37603 can be controlled by the Patient Programmer (model 37642, Medtronic Co.) (Fig. 5.13). The patient programmer is used to control and monitor the implanted neurostimulator. The patient programmer can (1) turn the switch of the IPG on or off, (2) check the neurostimulator and patient programmer battery status, (3) alert the patient when the status of the neurostimulator battery needs to be checked, and (4) change therapy settings within the range established by the doctor.

The patient programmer communicates with the implanted IPG by sending signals to and receiving signals from the implanted IPG. When patients use the patient programmer, they must hold it directly over the implanted IPG so that the programming screen faces out. The back of the patient programmer must be placed close to the implanted IPG.

5.6 Charge Density

A survey of literature regarding electrical stimulation of neural tissue suggests that damage may occur at levels above 30 $\mu C/cm^2$/phase. In voltage mode, the delivered current depends on the therapy impedance. In the Medtronic DBS system, the maximum programmable amplitude is 10.5 V (25.5 mA) and the maximum programmable pulse width is 450 μs. The curved lines in

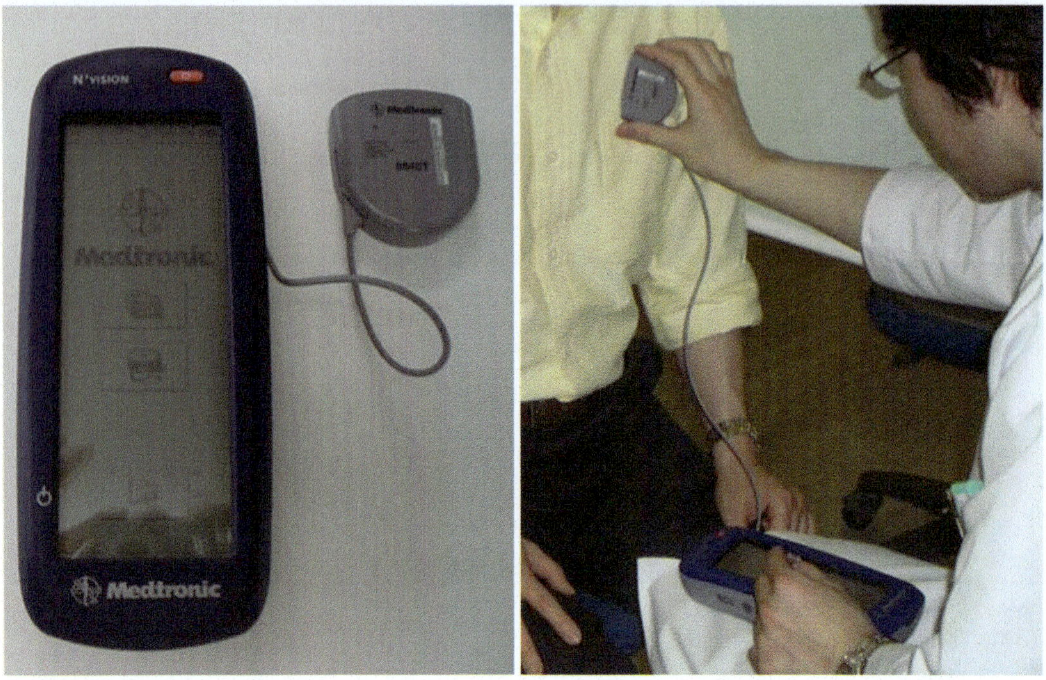

Fig. 5.12 The N'Vision (model 8840, Medtronic Co.). The programmer is used to review and program device parameters. The programmer is also used to set limits for the patient control devices

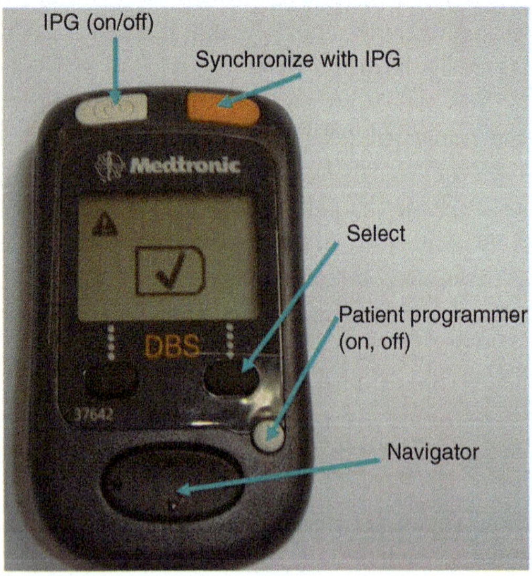

Fig. 5.13 Patient Programmer (model 37642, Medtronic Co.). The patient programmer is used to control and monitor the implanted neurostimulator or neurostimulators

Fig. 5.14 represent a charge density of 30 μC/cm^2/phase at various impedance measurements, calculated for the electrode surface area of the DBS Model 3387 Lead and DBS Model 3389 Lead. The mean impedances found in the clinical studies were as follows: (1) Parkinson's disease clinical studies (all targets), 1,294 Ω (range, 415–1,999 Ω); (2) Parkinson's disease clinical studies (GPi), 1,161 Ω (range, 415–1,967 Ω); and (3) Parkinson's disease clinical studies (STN), 1,177 Ω (range, 628–1,926 Ω).

In voltage mode, the charge density is determined by plotting a point corresponding to the pulse width setting (x-axis) and the amplitude setting (y-axis). If this point is below the appropriate impedance curve, then the charge density is below 30 μC/cm^2/phase. Points above the curve indicate a charge density above 30 μC/cm^2/phase. The shaded area of Fig. 5.14 indicates a charge density above 30 μC/cm^2/phase at the conservative impedance estimate

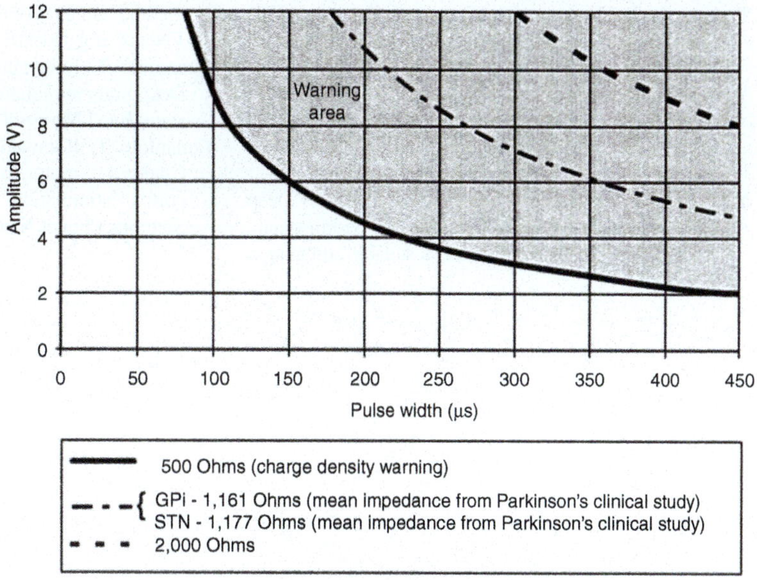

Fig. 5.14 Charge density using clinical studies impedance values. The amplitude and pulse-width limits were computed for impedances ranging from 500 to 2,000 Ω, an electrode surface area of 0.06 cm², and a charge density threshold of 30 μC/cm²/phase (Reprinted with the permission of Medtronic, Inc.)

of 500 Ω. If the selected stimulation parameters exceed the threshold, (indicated by the shaded area of the graph), a warning stating that the charge density may be high enough to cause tissue damage appears on the screen of N'Vision.

References

Adams JE, Hosobuchi Y, Fields HL (1974) Stimulation of internal capsule for relief of chronic pain. J Neurosurg 41:740–744

Benabid AL, Pollak P, Gao D et al (1996) Chronic electrical stimulation of the ventralis intermedius nucleus of the thalamus as a treatment of movement disorders. J Neurosurg 84:203–214

Brown JA, Lutsep HL, Weinand M et al (2006) Motor cortex stimulation for the enhancement of recovery from stroke: a prospective, multicenter safety study. Neurosurgery 58:456–473

Harvey RL, Winstein CJ, Everest Trial Group (2009) Design for the Everest randomized trial of cortical stimulation and rehabilitation for arm function following stroke. Neurorehabil Neural Repair 23:32–44

Hodaie M, Wennberg RA, Dostrovsky JO (2002) Chronic anterior thalamus stimulation for intractable epilepsy. Epilepsia 43:603–608

Hosobuchi Y, Adams JE, Rutkin B (1973) Chronic thalamic stimulation for the control of facial anesthesia dolorosa. Arch Neurol 29:158–161

Hosobuchi Y, Adams JE, Linchitz R (1977) Pain relief by electrical stimulation of the central gray matter in humans and its reversal by naloxone. Science 197(4299):183–186

Krauss JK, Pohle T, Weber S et al (1999) Bilateral stimulation of globus pallidus internus for treatment of cervical dystonia. Lancet 354:837–838

Levy R, Ruland S, Weinard M et al (2008) Cortical stimulation for the rehabilitation of patients with hemiparetic stroke: a multicenter feasibility study of safety and efficacy. J Neurosurg 108:707–714

Limousin P, Krack P, Pollak P et al (1998) Electrical stimulation of the subthalamic nucleus in advanced Parkinson's disease. N Engl J Med 339:1105–1111

Mayberg HS, Lozano AM, Voon V et al (2005) Deep brain stimulation for treatment-resistant depression. Neuron 45:651–660

Mazars GJ (1975) Intermittent stimulation of nucleus ventralis posterolateralis for intractable pain. Surg Neurol 4:93–95

Nuttin B, Cosyns P, Demeulmeester H et al (1999) Electrical stimulation in anterior limbs of internal capsules in patients with obsessive-compulsive disorder. Lancet 354(9189):1526

Schiff ND, Giacino JT, Kalmar K et al (2007) Behavioural improvements with thalamic stimulation after severe traumatic brain injury. Nature 448:600–603

Tsubokawa T, Yamamoto T, Katayama Y et al (1990) Deep-brain stimulation in a persistent vegetative state: follow-up results and criteria for selection of candidates. Brain Inj 4:315–327

Tsubokawa T, Katayama Y, Yamamoto T et al (1991) Chronic motor cortex stimulation for the treatment of central pain. Acta Neurochir Suppl (Wien) 52:137–139

Tsubokawa T, Katayama Y, Yamamoto T et al (1993) Chronic motor cortex stimulation in patients with thalamic pain. J Neurosurg 78:393–401

Yamamoto T, Katayama Y, Kobayashi K et al (2003) Dual-floor burr hole adjusted to burr-hole ring and cap for implantation of stimulation electrodes. Technical note. J Neurosurg 99:783–784

Yamamoto T, Katayama Y, Kano T et al (2004) Deep brain stimulation for the treatment of parkinsonian, essential, and post-stroke tremor: a suitable stimulation method and changes in effective stimulation intensity. J Neurosurg 101:201–209

Yamamoto T, Katayama Y, Kobayashi K et al (2010) Deep brain stimulation for the treatment of vegetative state. Eur J Neurosci 32:1145–1151

Yamamoto T, Katayama Y, Watanabe M et al (2011) Changes in motor function induced by chronic motor cortex stimulation in post-stroke pain patients. Stereotact Funct Neurosurg 89:381–389

6 Surgical Technique of Brain Stimulation

Hiroki Nishibayashi and Toru Itakura

6.1 Introduction

Deep brain stimulation (DBS) is a well-established treatment for movement disorders, such as Parkinson's disease (PD), essential tremor, and dystonia. The best clinical effect depends on precise placement of the electrode in the motor territory of the target nucleus by stereotactic neurosurgery. Stereotactic neurosurgery was developed by the pioneers Sir Victor Horsley, Clarke, Spiegel and Wycis (Spiegel et al. 1947), and others. To ensure accuracy and safety, surgical techniques have been improved according to the accumulated clinical results. However, surgical techniques are not uniform and differ slightly between countries as well as between institutes in the same country. The results from a recent survey evaluated procedures and apparatus used in institutes performing DBS surgery (Abosch et al. 2013). Frequently used stereotactic frames include Leksell or CRW. The preferred procedures are as follows: imaging by computed tomography (CT) after head-frame fixation, combined AC(anterior commissure)–PC(posterior commissure)-based and direct visual targeting, microelectrode recording setup, and macrostimulation. Combinations of procedures also differ slightly between institutes. In the past, we used to determine tentative targets using ventriculography and CT, however, since 2001, we have been using CT-magnetic resonance imaging (MRI) fusion-guided targeting by Leksell's frames. Here we describe our procedure with reviewing literatures (Starr 2002; Kramer et al. 2010).

6.2 Patient Selection

Patient selection is an important criterion. At our institute, neurologists and neurosurgeons discuss diagnosis, surgical indication, target, and DBS tuning. A diagnosis of Parkinson's disease is essential for good surgical results. Medical treatments, the coexistence of visual hallucinations, and higher cortical dysfunction are discussed. To select the optimal target, the patients' symptoms are also discussed. If unilateral tremor is main symptom, ventral intermediate(Vim) thalamic-DBS is offered, and marked drug-induced dyskinesia for internal segment of globus pallidus (GPi)-DBS, wearing off, fluctuations in Parkinson's symptoms for subthalamic nucleus (STN)-DBS. The patient's age and duration of disease are also important factors. If intracerebral microbleedings are apparent on T2*-weighted images (T2*WI), careful surgical

H. Nishibayashi, MD, PhD (✉)
Department of Neurological Surgery, Wakayama Medical University Hospital, Wakayama, Japan

T. Itakura, MD, PhD
Department of Neurological Surgery, Koyo Hospital, Wakayama, Japan

T. Itakura (ed.), *Deep Brain Stimulation for Neurological Disorders: Theoretical Background and Clinical Application*, DOI 10.1007/978-3-319-08476-3_6,

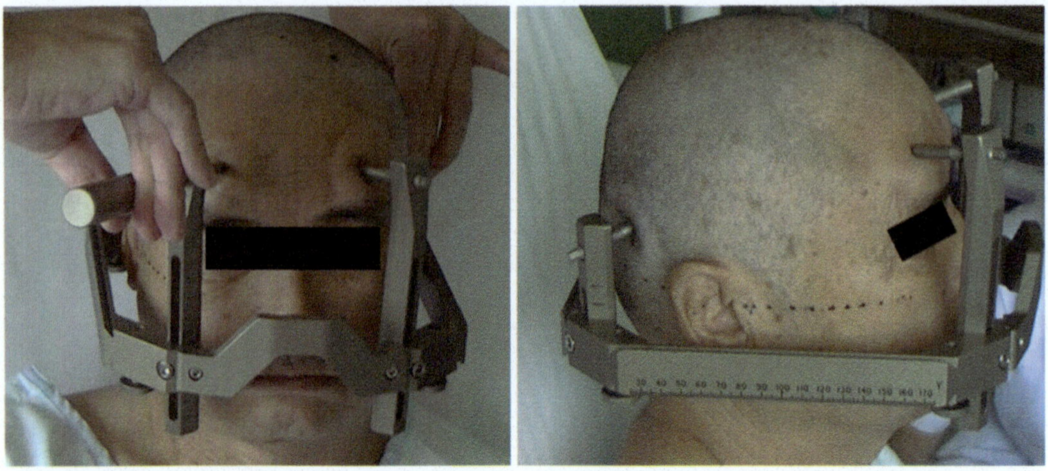

Fig. 6.1 Frame placement procedures using the Leksell Stereotactic System model G (Elekta Instrument AB, Sweden). The stereotactic frame is placed and fixed parallel to the Frankfurt line joining the inferior orbital rim and the upper limit of external auditory canal. The length of the frame pole is adjusted for individuals so that it is not too close to the shoulders. Pin lengths are adjusted according to head shape. The two diagonal pins are tightened simultaneously, followed by the other pair of diagonal pins. Drivers are held by the thumb and index or middle finger, and pins are tightened using maximum power. During pin tightening, care should be taken to avoid frame rotation. Therefore, the correct framing from three directions should be repeatedly verified

interventions and microelectrode recordings are necessary (Terao et al. 2003; Gorgulho et al. 2005; Ben-haim et al. 2009). Bilateral GPi-DBS is performed in primary dystonia (Krause et al. 2004) or tardive dystonia, whereas ventrooralis thalamotomy is performed in unilateral focal dystonia. Aggressiveness of the involuntary movement is discussed because in dystonic cases or in children, general anesthesia is required for frame placement, and while verifying optimal targeting, a staged operation is required (Starr et al. 2006; Air et al. 2011; Cif et al. 2012). Past history, preoperative screening tests, laboratory data, and cardiorespiratory functions are also assessed.

6.3 Presurgical Medication

Medications are interrupted on the night before surgery, if possible. Several dopamine agonists have prolonged antiparkinsonian effects. For suitable targeting, macrostimulation effects for involuntary movements are critical, particularly in Vim thalamotomy or thalamic DBS.

6.4 Stereotactic Frame Placement

Considering the application accuracy, Leksell's frame or CRW is widely used for stereotactic surgery (Maciunas et al. 1994). Here we describe frame placement procedures using the Leksell Stereotactic System model G (Elekta Instrument AB, Sweden). Frame fixation should be parallel to the Frankfurt line joining the inferior orbital rim and the upper limit of external auditory canal. Shaving of hair is not necessary (Miyagi et al. 2002), but hair should be tied to perceive head shape easily. Before stereotactic frame fixation, an intravenous line is obtained. Sedative drugs are not preferable because they modify intraoperative involuntary movements, consciousness, and neurological findings. However, they can be used if the patient has anxiety, intolerance during procedures, or hyperkinetic involuntary movements that disturb accurate frame placement. Blood pressure is monitored intermittently at approximately 10-min intervals. An antihypertensive agent is injected intravenously when blood pressure increases above

140/90 mmHg. Pain at the pin site or a sitting position may cause vasovagal reflex. Care should be taken for hypotension, bradykinesia, and autonomic signs such as sleepiness, yawns, or cold sweat. Syncope or convulsive syncope may sometimes occur. A supine position or rapid hydration may improve symptoms and vital signs. A patient is positioned on bed, which is elevated at 60–70°. A cushion is placed under shoulders and upper back. Ear bars are used to prevent head roll and yaw. Inserting a sponge in the external auditory meatus prevents ear pain or discomfort. A stereotactic frame is placed and fixed parallel to the Frankfurt line joining inferior orbital rim and upper limit of external auditory canal (Fig. 6.1). The frame is intended to be parallel to the AC–PC line. However, the AC–PC line varies in length and gradient among individuals; therefore, we adjust individually using preoperative images. Three people check to ensure the frame is parallel with the head from three directions. The pin tightening location is selected 6–7 cm above the Frankfurt line. Care is taken that head pins do not slip because of the forehead curve. The length of the frame pole is adjusted for individuals so that it is not too close to the shoulders. Pin lengths are adjusted according to head shape. Local anesthesia is performed using 4–5 mL of 1 % lidocaine. The skin surface, galea, and periosteum are anesthetized sufficiently. Patients feel no pain but head tightness after frame fixation. Two diagonal pins are tightened simultaneously, followed by the other pair of diagonal pins. Drivers are held by the thumb and index or middle finger, and pins are tightened using maximum power. During pin tightening, care should be taken to avoid frame rotation. Therefore, the correct framing from three directions should be repeatedly verified.

6.5 Imaging Acquisition

Historically, tentative targets had been identified using ventriculography or CT-guided targeting, but MRI-guided targeting is being used recently (Kawashima et al. 1992; Alexander et al. 1995; Kondziolka and Flickinger 1996; Starr et al. 1999). A previous report comparing ventriculography and CT-guided stereotactic neurosurgery concluded that ventriculography has no advantage over CT-guided targeting, although no cases of STN ablation were observed (Hariz and Bergenheim 1990). MRI-guided targeting has advantages of high spatial resolution, noninvasiveness, and no exposure to radiation. However, spatial distortion (Sumanaweera et al. 1994) and long acquisition times are disadvantageous. The image fusion method has resolved these problems (Alexander et al. 1995). A CT-MRI fusion method overcomes spatial distortion in MRI-guided targeting. This method is also advantageous because speedy CT scanning after fixation of stereotactic frame relieves the burden on the patient. Among several targeting methods, we describe here a CT-MRI fusion, MRI-guided targeting using Framelink (Medtronics, USA).

6.5.1 MRI Acquisition on the Preoperative Day

An MRI is performed on the preoperative day. We use a 1.5 Tesla MRI system and obtain three-dimensional T1-MPRAGE (Siemens, Germany) with gadolinium enhanced images (field of view 240, voxel size 256×256, slice thickness 1.5, TE 4 ms, and TR 4.7 ms). Data are imported to recordable media. T2 turbo spin-echo or inversion recovery sequences demarcate the STN or pallido-internal capsule border (Starr et al. 2002; Air et al. 2011) (Fig. 6.2). Images using 3 T MRI may offer reliable targeting for STN-DBS surgery (Toda et al. 2009; Patil et al. 2012). Segmentation of thalamic nucleus and identification of Vim is tried by diffusion tensor imaging (Coenen et al. 2011). The best method for correct targeting is under debate (Shin et al. 2010; Thani et al. 2011; Pezeshkian et al. 2011). A combination of these methods may approach the optimal target (Brouenberg et al. 2011) and achieve a better clinical outcome.

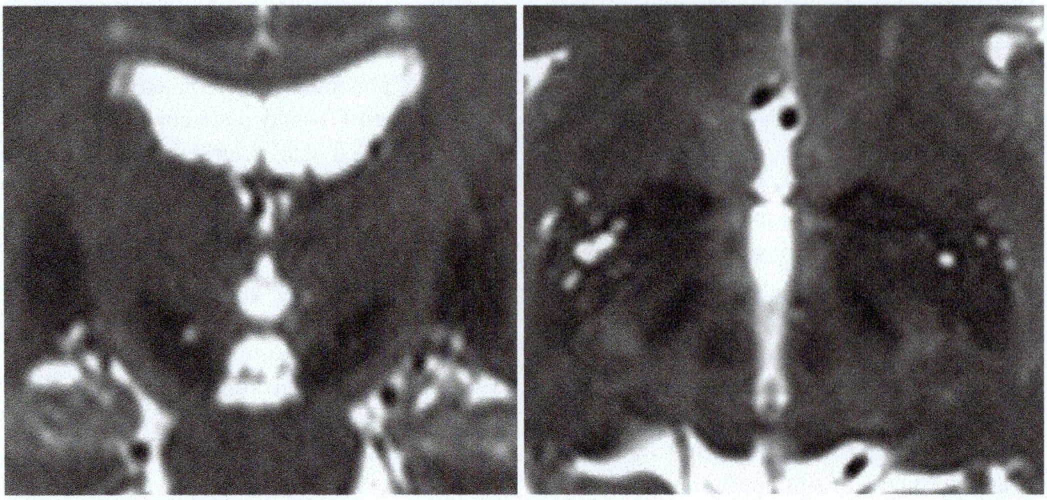

Fig. 6.2 T2 fast spin-echo images by 3T MRI demarcate the subthalamic nucleus or pallido-internal capsule border, which may offer reliable targeting

6.5.2 CT Image Acquisition on the Operative Day

On the operating day, CT images are acquired after stereotactic frame fixation. Care should be taken to avoid respiratory failure due to overflexion or extension of the neck by frame fixation during the CT scan, even during short acquisition times. After proper setting of the CT adapter, the Leksell frame is fixed to it. The frame indicator of the midline and horizontal line should match the laser beam of the CT gantry. If a gap appears, flexion, extension, and lateral tilt are adjusted using a wrench driver. We use the GE Signa CT system. Image sequences are obtained by 1.25 mm slice thickness. After verifying that the CT images show CT indicators, the data are recorded in recordable media. The patient is released from the CT adapter and transported to the operating room.

6.6 Operating Room Setting

Neurophysiological examination is important for correct targeting and for suitable local anesthesia. Patients with violent, aggressive involuntary movement such as dystonia or drug-induced dyskinesia, or those with dysphagia or upper respiratory tract problems may be suitable for general anesthesia. Rigid neck fixation may be intolerable in some cases; thus, sedative drugs should be prepared. Propofol is preferable because its effects on microelectrode recordings and evaluation of the effects of macrostimulation are less than other anesthetics. The patient is fixed to the stereotactic frame adapter for the operating table. Overflexion of the neck may cause respiratory failure and dysphagia, as well as aspiration pneumonia; therefore, frame adaptation is very important for future procedures. The upper body is elevated to 30° to prevent continuous cerebrospinal fluid (CSF) leak. Electrocardiography is set up. A sphygmomanometer is put on the upper limb of the one side, and an oximetry is placed on the index finger of the same upper limb. To examine neuronal activity by passive joint movement or macrostimulation effects for involuntary movement, the monitoring setup during surgery is changed to the contralateral upper limb according to the circumstances. These monitoring devices are particularly useful in patients who need mild sedation because of anxiety or restlessness. Blood pressure should be maintained lower than 120/90 mmHg by intravenous bolus or continuous injection of antihypertensive drugs. Transparent draping is preferable because the

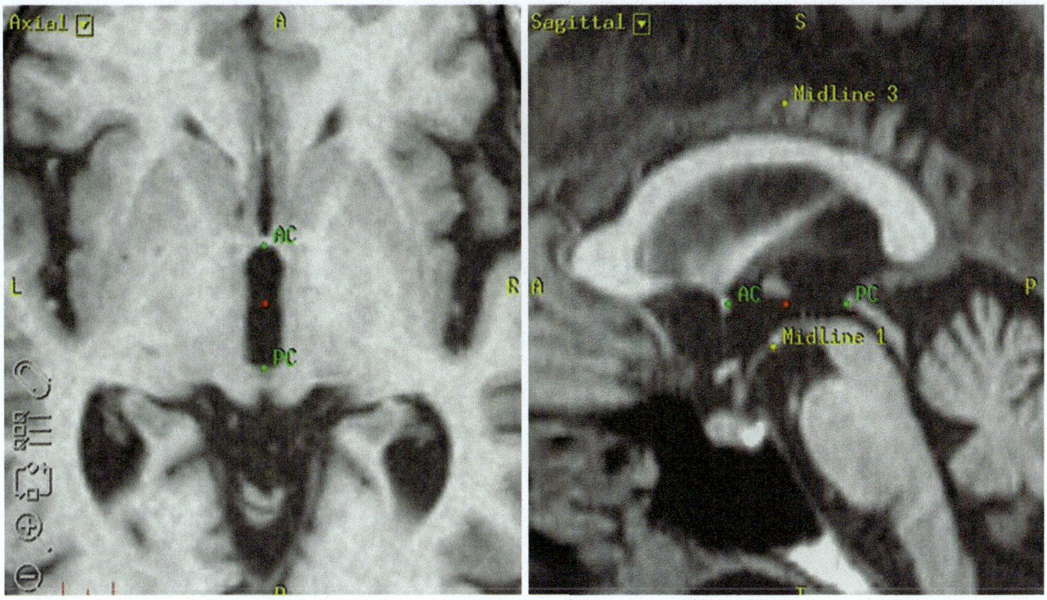

Fig. 6.3 The anterior commissure and the posterior commissure are verified using the MRI working images. The border of each commissure and the third ventricle are selected. Three other midline landmarks such as the pituitary stalk, inter-mammillary body, midbrain aqueduct, or cingulate cortex are also selected. The tentative target can be decided by AC–PC based indirect method

surgeon can observe the patient's landmark, consciousness, and neurological findings. The intraoperative fluoroscopy C-arm is set up, and a simulation is performed to determine if the tip of electrode can be observed. Apparatus for neurophysiological examinations and the computer workstation are placed near the surgeon to ensure trajectory and unit recording.

6.7 Preoperative Targeting

Preoperative frameless MRI is fused to CT images with stereotactic frame. Using this method, AC–PC-based targeting (indirect targeting) and MRI-image guided targeting (direct targeting) are developed. Image data are imported to the workstation (Framelink, Medtronics, USA) by recordable media. CT images are used as reference images and MRI images as working images, and then fused on the workstation. We use 3D T1-MPRAGE with gadolinium-enhanced images as our working images because they show the cortical and sulcal vessels that should be avoided during electrode insertion. Reference CT images are selected in which nine indicators are arranged with almost equal distances. Next, all indicators are registered from the right lower to the left lower in a counterclockwise manner. The anterior commissure and the posterior commissure are verified using the MRI working images (Fig. 6.3). The border of each commissure and the third ventricle are selected. Three other midline landmarks such as the pituitary stalk, inter-mammillary body, midbrain aqueduct, or cingulate cortex are also selected. The tentative target is decided by indirect or direct methods, or a combination of both. Our strategy is AC–PC-based indirect targeting, modified according to the patient's AC–PC length, with confirmed optical points by neurophysiological examinations. We set the *X*, *Y*, and *Z* coordinates of the tentative target (indirect target) by Schaltenbrand Wahren atlas (Schaltenbrand and Wahren 1977) for STN (10 mm lateral, 2.5 mm posterior, and 4 mm ventral from the mid-commissural point), GPi (20 mm lateral, 3 mm anterior, and 4 mm ventral from the mid-commissural point), and Vim (12 mm lateral, 5 mm posterior, and 0 mm from the mid-commissural point). The

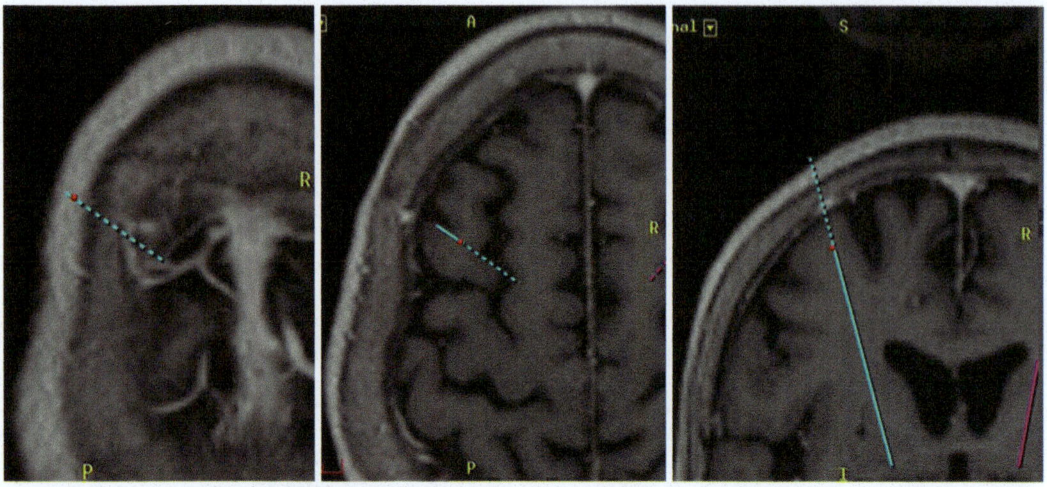

Fig. 6.4 Three-dimensional T1-MPRAGE images with gadolinium-enhanced images are used for planning trajectory. They show the cortical and sulcal vessels that should be avoided during electrode insertion. The trajectory is verified virtually to avoid penetration into the sulci, cortical vessels, or lateral ventricle

red nucleus-based targeting in an axial plane or the nigrocapsular angle in a sagittal plane is also used for indirect targeting of STN (Brouenberg et al. 2011). The dorsal border of optic tract is a landmark for indirect GPi targeting (Starr et al. 2002). On the background of extended application of DBS for involuntary movements and psychiatric disorders, neuroimaging-guided electrode placement under general anesthesia without neurophysiological examination or frameless DBS using intraoperative CT and microelectrode recording has been performed with favorable outcomes (Burchiel et al. 2013; Smith and Bakay 2011).

6.8 Preoperative Trajectory

The standard trajectory is 60° to the AC–PC line. In practice, ventricle shape and size can be asymmetrical, and inter-individual differences cannot be disregarded. We must modify the trajectory to the lateral side to avoid ventricular penetration, which may increase hemorrhage risk and electrode malposition (Zrinzo et al. 2009). Additionally, cortical vessels or sulci should be avoided. MRI images showing visible vessels, 3D T1-weighted images may assist in avoiding these complications (Fig. 6.4). The Leksell Multi Arc is set to the frame. The *Y* and *Z* scales are confirmed by two nonsterile assistants and fixed. The *X* scale is confirmed by two sterile surgeons. The scale of arc (lateral rotation) and ring (anterior–posterior rotation) is input to the workstation. The probe is set at the presumed burr hole, and the trajectory is verified virtually to avoid penetration into the sulci, cortical vessels, or lateral ventricle. The scale of arc and ring is modified if necessary. The design of the presumed burr holes and skin incisions is marked.

6.9 Skin Incision, Burr Hole Making, Corticotomy

Antibiotic drug is dripped intravenously prior to skin incision. Skin incisions are made in semicircular shape bilaterally after local anesthesia with 1 % lidocaine. Burr holes are made at the center of the skin incision. Insufficient anesthesia may induce pain due to scalp clip or skin rotation. We select the side of initial trajectory on the basis of the patient's symptoms. We start from the contralateral hemisphere to the limbs in patients with more severe symptoms because the first trajectory is less influenced by brain shift. As operating time progresses, accurate placement becomes more difficult than the first track. Skin hemostasis is completed by electrocoagulation and a scalp clip. Skin flap is opened using a retractor. Burr holes are made by a trepanator, and inner bone is removed by curate. Bleeding from epidural space and bone edge is controlled by gel form, surgical cotton, and bone wax. These procedures prevent air embolism because of head elevation. To prevent cortical vessels injury, approximately 14–16-mm size burr hole is necessary. In case of thick bone, more bone removal and widening of burr hole would be required for suitable trajectory. We usually make burr holes at 1 cm anterior to the coronal suture and 3 cm lateral from the midline. Cross-dural incision is performed, and edge of dura is electrocoagulated to widen corridor for trajectory. Prior to making trajectories, arachnoid membrane is electrocoagulated to the minimum extent necessary for trajectory. If arachnoid membrane is thickened, it should be cut with scalpel to prevent electrode bending. CSF leak is prevented using fibrin glue or gel form. Continuous CSF leak may cause difficulties in correct targeting during surgery, also lead malposition due to recovery from brain shift (Munckhof et al. 2010). Care is taken regarding the patient's neurological findings. Venous injury or cortical damage may cause convulsive seizures. In such a situation, the guide cannula should be removed and cortical surface irrigated with cold saline, and then the operation should be interrupted to check head CT.

6.10 Intraoperative Neurophysiological Examinations

6.10.1 Microelectrode Recordings

A microelectrode driver is set to the arc. Verify whether each part is constructed and not loose. Insert a microelectrode guide cannula gently to 30 mm above the target. Next, remove inner probe and insert microelectrode (high-impedance (0.1–1.0 MΩ at 1,000 Hz), tungsten-coated stainless steel microelectrode with a 15–25 μm tip diameter, FC1002, Medtronic, USA). Cables

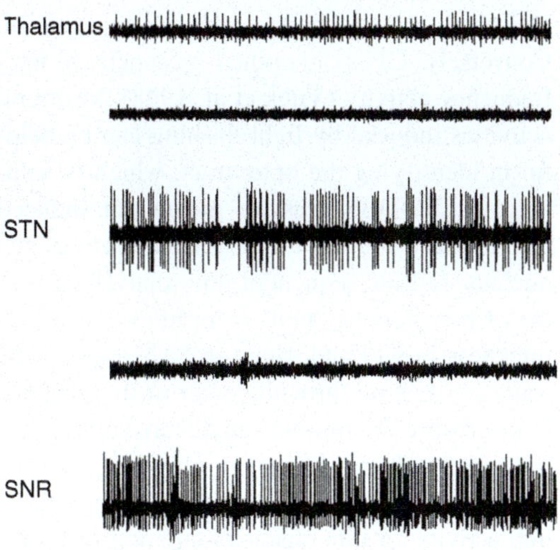

Fig. 6.5 In STN-DBS, STN neurons are identified by irregular firing, and the ventral border is identified by the absence of unitary activity and appearance of regular high frequency activity by SNr. *SNr* substantia nigra

are connected between a microelectrode and amplifier (Leadpoint 9033A0315, Medtronic, USA). A ground earth is set at the outer cannula or the retractor. Check baseline neuronal activity and contamination with artifactual noises. For safety and stable unit recordings, a microdriver should be handled with gentle manipulation with slow but continuous rotation. If large unit activities are recorded, remove the fingers gently from the microdriver and observe unit firing pattern. Stable recordings are not easy, but make efforts to record approximately 10 ~ 20 s per unit activity. Care should be taken against artifact contamination during unit recording, such as passive movement, intracranial pulsatile pressure, cardiorespiratory activity, and audio signals. When assessing neuronal activities by passive movements, multiunit recordings are more suitable than single unit recordings. A semimicroelectrode with relatively low impedance (20–100 kΩ) is preferable in such cases. In STN-DBS, STN neurons are identified by irregular firing, and the ventral border is identified by absence of unitary activity and appearance of regular high frequency activity by substantia nigra (Fig. 6.5). In GPi-DBS, external segment of the globus pallidus (GPe)/GPi border, or ventral GPi border, is identified by absence of unitary activity. GPe is identified by a burst and pause pattern. Conversely, GPi is identified by repetitive high frequency activity (Vitek et al. 1998). Multiunit activities induced by light flashing can be helpful in identifying the optic tract, which is valuable in GPi-DBS. Passive movement induced activity may suggest motor-related areas of the nucleus. Offline sequential unit analysis is useful. Characteristic unit recordings of 6-mm thickness in GPi and 4-mm in STN suggest the trajectory passed through center of the nucleus. If macrostimulation-induced adverse effects are not observed, a permanent electrode can be implanted in the same target. If low, infrequent unit activity, or thin characteristic unit activities are observed, the coordinate is changed within 2 mm to either side with reference to results of macrostimulation. It is important to consider brain shift when moving the target. When unilateral trepanation is performed, brain shift tends to occur unilaterally and the target may shift posteriorly. For example, when Vim-DBS is performed, the target should be modified 2 mm posterior and 2 mm lateral, because the internal capsule is located more laterally if the coordinate is modified posteriorly. When a contralateral trajectory is performed after a unilateral lead placement, brain tends to sink posteriorly and shift to the contralateral side (Miyagi et al. 2007). Thus, MER or permanent electrode can penetrate more medially and anteriorly than expected. There is a risk for ventricular penetration in cases of ventriculomegaly. Intraoperative neurophysiological testing may not always provide proper guidance for the optimal point. In such cases, we transiently implant the permanent electrode and then plan a staged operation after verifying the electrode location and clinical effects. Multitrack targeting by Bengun has the advantage wherein the microelectrodes prevent brain sinking when exchanging the electrode demonstrating the most optimal track to the permanent electrode. A single microelectrode recording may cause a gap to the optimal target during electrode exchange.

Patient selection for MER is important to prevent adverse effects. In cases of Vim thalamotomy, MER is less valuable than STN-DBS or GPi-DBS. The optimal target is well detected by the macrostimulation effect. MER may have some value to detect the bottom of the Vim. The dentate-thalamo-cerebellar tract shows convergence at the ventral thalamus; therefore, a more ventral site is effective for inhibiting the tract. Microelectrodes with fine tips can cause intraparenchymal hemorrhage more than macrostimulation with dull tips. Regardless of gentle manipulation, unexpected hemorrhages may occur. Preoperative T2* images can detect microbleeding, which may easily suggest the subcortical gray and white matter bleeding. In particular, in elderly patients over 70 years of age, MER should be avoided or considered according to individual conditions.

6.10.2 Macrostimulation

Custom-made microelectrodes can be used for macrostimulation. Bipolar stimulation is possible using the outer cannula of microelectrode, with a tip of the electrode selected as a cathode contact; a constant current is delivered through the lead-point. Muscle twitch by the pyramidal tract is evaluated by 2 Hz (1 ms duration) rectangular stimulation. Aggravation of involuntary movements is assessed by 5 Hz (1 ms duration) stimulation. Dysesthesia by medial lemniscus or ventral posterolateral nucleus is assessed by 20 Hz (1 ms duration) stimulation. Inhibition of involuntary movements is assessed by stimulation by 100 Hz (100 μs duration). In constant voltage stimulation test, 2 Hz and 1–1.5 V muscle twitching may be a good target. However, <0.5 V indicates near the pyramidal tract and no response >5 V indicates far from the pyramidal tract. Paresthesia at the mouth, labial commissure, thumb, and index finger <1 V indicate proximity to the sensory system (medial lemniscus or ventral posterolateral nucleus). Tremor aggravation at 5 or 20 Hz, and cessation at 100 Hz, 0.5–1 V may be a good target for Vim-DBS. Permanent electrodes may also be used in verifying adverse effects or clinical effects during surgery. Stimulation parameters are similar to the postoperative ones, therefore, we can exactly predict postoperative effects.

6.11 Lead Fixation

Exchange of the microelectrode and permanent electrode is performed under intraoperative fluoroscopy. Confirm the microelectrode tip points to the crosshair of the indicator by fluoroscopy. The tip of the microelectrode is barely detected by fluoroscopy. Next, remove the microelectrode and insert the permanent electrode. Ensure the tip contact of the permanent electrode is located at the center of the indicator because brain shift may occur during the short period of the exchange. The inner guide wire is pulled out, and the outer cannula is then removed slowly. Continuous fluoroscopy is useful for preventing the electrode from being inserted to a depth beyond the target. Several methods are proposed for lead fixation as burr hole cap (Ray 1981) or titan plate (Falve et al. 1996). We fix a lead at a burr hole edge by a titan plate tight enough so that it does not fall while performing fluoroscopy. A custom-made burr hole cap is widely used. A dual-floor burr hole may be cosmetic (Yamamoto et al. 2003). After fixation, impedance of a permanent electrode should be checked. After skin closure, the head frame is removed. On the same day, implantable pulse generators (IPG) are implanted under general anesthesia. In cases requiring test stimulation, disposable connecters are guided via a subcutaneous tunnel out of the skin, apart from the skin incisions. A lead is tightly fixed to skin by 2-0 silk, which prevents CSF leak. After 1 week, staged implantation is performed.

6.12 Lead and IPG Implantation

IPG implantation is also not uniform. Bilateral subclavicular chests are selected, in majority. Subaxillar or upper abdomen is also included in selected cases. Unilateral subclavicular implantation is another option. Neck is rotated to the contralateral side, and an approximately 2-cm skin incision is made at the postauricular scalp, where the lead is relayed. An approximately 5 cm linear or semicircular skin incision is made at the subclavicular chest. To implant IPG on the major pectoralis muscle, blunt exfoliation is performed. Thin chest skin and hyperkinetic involuntary movement may cause wound erosion. Thus, implantation sites should be selected on the basis of individual patient's condition to prevent delayed wound complication or infection (Oh et al. 2002; Sillay et al. 2008; Fenoy and Simpson 2012). IPG is fixed to the fascia by 3-0 silk not to sink via gravitational force. Skin closure is performed by subcutaneous anti-infectious absorbable suture. Surgical tape is sufficient and suitable for cosmetic aspects. The relay site should be at the postauricular site. High convex is risky for skin erosion and the neck for lead fracture by involuntary movement. Dystonia or violent drug-induced dyskinesia should be monitored for skin trouble. After IPG implantation, dressing of the implantation site for 2–3 weeks is necessary for wound healing in such hyperkinetic disorders.

6.13 Stereotactic Ablation

DBS has advantages in reversibility and adjustment, but disadvantages in device implantation. Efficacy of stereotactic ablation is established in essential tremor or focal dystonia. We prefer Vim thalamotomy for controlling unilateral disabling tremor in essential tremor or Parkinson's disease. Prior to thermocoagulation, observation of the macrostimulation effect is necessary. We evaluate the distance to the internal capsule by muscle twitch in the contralateral arm with low frequency stimulation. Next, dysesthesia in the contralateral mouth, thumb, and index finger is evaluated by 5–20-Hz stimulation. If muscle twitch is elicited by ~1.5 V, and dysesthesia by above 1.5 V, thermocoagulation can be safely achieved avoiding adverse effects on the pyramidal tract and ventral posterolateral nucleus. After verifying tremor aggravation at 5–20 Hz and cessation at high-frequency stimulation, thermocoagulation is performed at 60 °C for 60 s. During ablation, the patient is asked to elevate both arms and make a posture that enhances tremor. Once cessation of tremor and no motor paresis is verified without sensory disturbance, additional thermocoagulation at 70 °C for 90 s is performed. Additional ablation is performed at the site 3–4 mm above the tentative target if involuntary movements recur in a few minutes. Rapid thermocoagulation may induce vessel rupture via the popping effect, followed by intracerebral hemorrhage.

6.14 Dystonia Case

In case of aggressive involuntary movement such as dystonia, frame placement is also performed under general anesthesia (Starr et al. 2006; Air et al. 2011). The patient is anesthetized using propofol and vecuronium, and transoral intubation is performed. After rapid induction, stereotactic frame is placed. The operating table is elevated at 30°. Cushions are put under the shoulders. Placement of the frame parallel to the midline and Frankfurt line is verified. Diagonal two pins are tightened followed by the other pair of diagonal pins. If MRI-guided targeting is planned, no metal should remain on the patient. Spiral intubation tubes are not preferable because they cause artifacts during MRI image acquisition. The patient is transported to CT room by manually ventilating using an air bag. After image acquisition, the patient is transported to the operating room and fixed to the frame adapter. Vital sign monitors are put on. We implant the electrode in the bilateral posteroventral GPi in dystonia cases. Unlike cases of Parkinson's disease, microelectrode recording is less applicable under general anesthesia. Even under light intravenous sedation, unitary activity would decrease. The macrostimulation effect is informative for the distance to corticospinal and corticobulbar tracts. Contralateral muscle twitch is elicited by 3–5 mA with 2 Hz constant current for 1 ms, and proper targeting is suggested. In cases of no response, we intentionally plan staged surgery. Electrodes are implanted according to indirect targeting, and the position of the electrode is confirmed by MRI after the operation. If the electrode is placed at the posteroventral GPi, permanent IPG implantation is performed under general anesthesia. If the electrode is located medially or laterally, a new coordinate is set using references to the previous electrode, and no adverse effects by macrostimulation are verified. In children or patients with mental illness, scratching of the wound site and aggressive movement may disturb wound healing; therefore, prolonged wound care is necessary. If the skin is thin at the subclavicle, IPGs are intentionally implanted in the upper abdomen with an extended electrode.

References

Abosch A, Timmermann L, Bartley S et al (2013) An international survey of deep brain stimulation procedural steps. Stereotact Funct Neurosurg 91:1–11

Air EL, Ostrem JL, Sanger TD et al (2011) Deep brain stimulation in children: experience and technical pearls. J Neurosurg Pediatr 8:566–574

Alexander E III, Kooy HM, Herk M et al (1995) Magnetic resonance image-directed stereotactic neurosurgery: use of image fusion with computerized tomography to enhance spatial accuracy. J Neurosurg 83:271–276

Ben-haim S, Assad WF, Gale JT et al (2009) Risk factors for hemorrhagic microelectrode-guided deep brain stimulation and the introduction of an improved microelectrode design. Neurosurgery 64:754–763

Brouenberg EJL, Platel B, Hofman PAM et al (2011) Magnetic resonance imaging techniques for visualization of subthalamic nucleus. J Neurosurg 115:971–984

Burchiel KJ, MaCartney S, Lee A et al (2013) Accuracy of deep brain stimulation electrode placement using intraoperative computed tomography without microelectrode recording. J Neurosurg 119:301–306

Cif L, Gonzalez-Martinez V, Vasques X et al (2012) Staged implantation of multiple electrodes in the internal globus pallidus in the treatment of primary generalized dystonia. J Neurosurg 116:1144–1152

Coenen VA, Madler B, Schiffbauer H et al (2011) Individual fiber anatomy of the subthalamic region revealed with diffusion tensor imaging: a concept to identify the deep brain stimulation target for tremor suppression. Neurosurgery 68:1069–1076

Falve J, Taha JM, Steel T (1996) Anchoring of deep brain stimulation electrodes using a microplate. J Neurosurg 85:1181–1183

Fenoy AJ, Simpson RK (2012) Management of device-related wound complications in deep brain stimulation surgery. J Neurosurg 116:1324–1332

Gorgulho A, DeSalles AAF, Frighetto L et al (2005) Incidence of hemorrhage associated with electrophysiological studies performed using macroelectrodes and microelectrodes in functional neurosurgery. J Neurosurg 102:888–896

Hariz MI, Bergenheim T (1990) A comparative study on ventriculographic and computerized tomography-guided determinations of brain targets in functional stereotaxis. J Neurosurg 73:565–571
Kawashima Y, Chen HJ, Takahashi A et al (1992) Application of magnetic resonance imaging in functional stereotactic thalamotomy for the evaluation of individual variations of the thalamus. Stereotact Funct Neurosurg 58:33–38
Kondziolka D, Flickinger J (1996) Use of magnetic resonance imaging in stereotactic surgery. Stereotact Funct Neurosurg 66:193–197
Kramer DR, Halpern CH, Bounacore DL et al (2010) Best surgical practice: a stepwise approach to the University of Pennsylvania deep brain stimulation protocol. Neurosurg Focus 29(2):E3. doi:10.3171/2010.4.FOCUS10103
Krause M, Fogel W, Kloss M et al (2004) Pallidal stimulation for dystonia. Neurosurgery 55:1361–1370
Maciunas RJ, Galloway RL, Latimer JM (1994) The application accuracy of stereotactic frames. Neurosurgery 35:682–695
Miyagi Y, Shima F, Ishido K (2002) Implantation of deep brain stimulation electrodes in unshaved patients. J Neurosurg 97:1476–1478
Miyagi Y, Shima F, Sasaki T (2007) Brain shift: an error factor during implantation of deep brain stimulation electrodes. J Neurosurg 107:989–997
Munckhof P, Contarino MF, Bour LJ et al (2010) Postoperative curving and upward displacement of deep brain stimulation electrodes caused by brain shift. Neurosurgery 67:49–54
Oh MY, Abosch A, Kim SH et al (2002) Long-term hardware-related complications of deep brain stimulation. Neurosurgery 50:1268–1276
Patil PG, Conrad EC, Aldridge JW (2012) The anatomical and electrophysiological subthalamic nucleus visualized by 3-T magnetic resonance imaging. Neurosurgery 71:1089–1095
Pezeshkian P, Desalles AAF, Gorgulho A et al (2011) Accuracy of frame-based stereotactic magnetic resonance imaging vs frame-based stereotactic head computed tomography fused with recent magnetic resonance imaging for postimplantation deep brain stimulator lead localization. Neurosurgery 69:1299–1306
Ray CD (1981) Burr-hole ring-cap and electrode anchoring device. J Neurosurg 55:1004–1006
Schaltenbrand G, Wahren W (1977) Atlas for stereotaxy of human brain, 2nd edn. Georg Thieme, Stuttgart
Shin M, Penholate MF, Lefaucheur JP et al (2010) Assessing accuracy of the magnetic resonance imaging-computed tomography fusion images to evaluate the electrode positions in subthalamic nucleus after deep-brain stimulation. Neurosurgery 66:1193–1202
Sillay KA, Larson PS, Starr PA (2008) Deep brain stimulator hardware-related infections: incidence and management in a large series. Neurosurgery 62:360–367
Smith AP, Bakay RAE (2011) Frameless deep brain stimulation using intraoperative O-arm technology. J Neurosurg 115:301–309
Spiegel EA, Wysis HT, Marks M et al (1947) Stereotaxic apparatus for operations on the human brain. Science 106:349–350
Starr PA, Vitek JL, Delong M et al (1999) Magnetic resonance imaging-based stereotactic localization of the globus pallidus and subthalamic nucleus. Neurosurgery 44:303–314
Starr PA (2002) Placement of deep brain stimulators into the subthalamic nucleus or globus pallidus internus: technical approach. Stereotact Funct Neurosurg 79:118–145
Starr PA, Christine CW, Theodosopoulos PV et al (2002) Implantation of deep brain stimulators into the subthalamic nucleus: technical approach and magnetic resonance imaging-verified lead locations. J Neurosurg 97:370–387
Starr PA, Turner RS, Rau G et al (2006) Microelectrode-guided implantation of deep brain stimulation into globus pallidus internus for dystonia, techniques, electrode locations, and outcomes. J Neurosurg 104:488–501
Sumanaweera TS, Adler JR, Napel S et al (1994) Characterization of spatial distortion in magnetic resonance imaging and its implications for stereotactic surgery. Neurosurgery 35:696–704
Terao R, Takahashi H, Yokochi F et al (2003) Hemorrhagic complication of stereotactic surgery in patients with movement disorders. J Neurosurg 98:1241–1246
Thani NB, Bala A, Swann GB (2011) Accuracy of postoperative computed tomography and magnetic resonance image fusion for assessing deep brain stimulation electrodes. Neurosurgery 69:207–214
Toda H, Sawamoto N, Hanakawa T et al (2009) A novel composite targeting method using high-field magnetic resonance imaging for subthalamic nucleus deep brain stimulation. J Neurosurg 111:737–745
Vitek JL, Bakay RAE, Hashimoto T et al (1998) Microelectrode-guided pallidotomy: technical approach and its application in medically intractable Parkinson's disease. J Neurosurg 88:1027–1043
Yamamoto T, Katayama Y, Kobayashi K et al (2003) Dual-floor burr hole adjusted to burr-hole ring and cap for implantation of stimulation electrodes. J Neurosurg 99:783–784
Zrinzo L, van Hurzen AL, Gorgulho AA et al (2009) Avoiding the ventricle: a simple step to improve accuracy of anatomical targeting during deep brain stimulation. J Neurosurg 110:1283–1290

Stimulation of Subthalamic Nucleus for Parkinson's Disease

7

Takashi Agari and Isao Date

7.1 Introduction

Stereotactic neurosurgery of the basal ganglia and thalamus deep in the brain is a long-employed surgical treatment for Parkinson's disease (PD). Previously, surgical procedures only involved destructive surgery, but since deep brain stimulation (DBS) was reported by Benabid et al. (1987) as a treatment for PD tremors, this has now become the treatment of choice because of its safety and reliability.

According to a study of PD models, the subthalamic nucleus (STN) forms an indirect pathway and plays an important role in the appearance of symptoms in PD, which is caused by the abnormal activity of STN inhibitory neurons (Alexander et al. 1986). Therefore, this has been examined as a target for stereotactic neurosurgery, although there was initial hesitation in destroying the STN because of the risk of adverse effects such as hemiballism. Benabid et al. (1994) have targeted the STN in PD patients and demonstrated that bilateral stimulation was safe and highly effective. Till date, a number of clinical studies have examined the STN and reported that STN stimulation is effective for managing motor symptoms such as motor fluctuations and dyskinesia in PD patients. In Japan, DBS was listed in the insurance system in 2000; since then, it rapidly spread as a surgical procedure for PD and is now an established procedure.

In order to maximize the usefulness of DBS, appropriate surgical indications, precise surgery, and appropriate adjustment of stimuli are necessary. A deeper understanding of the effects of STN-DBS is also necessary. This paper explains the clinical characteristics of STN-DBS.

7.2 Surgical Indications of STN-DBS

Appropriate patient selection is crucial for effective STN-DBS treatment. A positive outcome of STN-DBS can only be expected in patients with idiopathic PD, and this procedure is essentially off-label for other diseases that exhibit Parkinsonism, such as multiple system atrophy (Tarsy et al. 2003; Shih and Tarsy 2007). STN-DBS has numerous indications. These include motor fluctuations and dyskinesia in advanced PD, where control is difficult to achieve with drug therapy alone; the wearing-off phenomenon; and levodopa-induced dyskinesia. It is also indicated when adequate drug therapy is not possible because of adverse effects and in cases of drug therapy-resistant tremors. The best therapeutic effect is anticipated when the response to

T. Agari, MD, PhD (✉) • I. Date, MD, PhD
Department of Neurological Surgery,
Okayama University Graduate School of Medicine,
Dentistry and Pharmaceutical Sciences,
Okayama, Japan
e-mail: agarit@cc.okayama-u.ac.jp

T. Itakura (ed.), *Deep Brain Stimulation for Neurological Disorders: Theoretical Background and Clinical Application*, DOI 10.1007/978-3-319-08476-3_7,

levodopa is very good, the patient is of a younger age, there are no or only mild axial symptoms that respond poorly to levodopa, there is a mild or no decline in cognitive function, and there are well-controlled or no psychiatric symptoms.

The most important factor when considering surgical indications is prior response to levodopa (Charles et al. 2002; Kleiner-Fisman et al. 2006). However, patients that must spend most of the day in an off-period because of significant wearing-off phenomena exhibit the best surgical outcomes. Studies examining prognostic predictors have shown that levodopa response is a significant predictor of a favorable prognosis (Charles et al. 2002; Kleiner-Fisman et al. 2006; Welter et al. 2002; Piboolnurak et al. 2007; Tsai et al. 2009; Smeding et al. 2011). Many facilities have conducted levodopa challenge tests in accordance with the Core Assessment Program for Surgical Interventional Therapies in PD (CAPSIT-PD) protocol (Defer et al. 1999) and found that a ≥30 % improvement in the Unified Parkinson's Disease Rating Scale (UPDRS-III) after levodopa loading is a useful indicator of levodopa response. However, no absolute indications exist. Response to levodopa is an important short-term predictor, but this is not necessarily translated into the long-term (Piboolnurak et al. 2007; Tsai et al. 2009). Drug therapy-resistant tremors do not conform to this rule.

The main targets of treatment are bradykinesia, rigidity, tremors, gait disturbance, and motor fluctuations and dyskinesia. Lang and Widner (2002) reported that patients who are severely impaired by the cardinal symptoms of PD during the off-period and are independent during the on-period are the best surgical cases.

Age is also an important factor. STN-DBS may be effective in patients of any age, but younger patients typically exhibit better outcomes compared with older patients (Charles et al. 2002; Welter et al. 2002; Tsai et al. 2009; Smeding et al. 2011; Ory-Magne et al. 2007). Many facilities require an age of ≤70 years, but there is no clear limit. Indeed, elderly individuals leading younger lifestyles can also be suitable for treatment. However, good prognoses after surgery are less likely in the elderly, and a decline in cognitive function can apparently occur after STN-DBS (Welter et al. 2002; Smeding et al. 2011). Some reports also state that elderly individuals are more likely to experience serious surgical complications such as intracerebral hemorrhage (Ory-Magne et al. 2007). It is essential to be mindful of the risks of cognitive and intracerebral hemorrhage when considering indications for surgery in the elderly (Sansur et al. 2007; Saint-Cyr et al. 2000).

In contrast, STN-DBS is not indicated for patients with a severe decline in cognitive function or psychiatric symptoms (Defer et al. 1999; Lang and Widner 2002; Lopiano et al. 2002; Bronstein et al. 2011). In addition, hemorrhagic diathesis; high risk of intracranial hemorrhage (ICH); marked cerebrovascular disease or cerebral atrophy, particularly with severe underlying atherosclerotic disease; severe heart disease; systemic or local infection that cannot be actively controlled; malignant tumors; and short prognosis are also considered off-label indications.

Sustained long-term improvement after STN-DBS cannot be expected after a poor response to drug therapy or a severe decline in cognitive function. Furthermore, in patients with marked cerebral atrophy, accurate electrode placement during surgery is often difficult; therefore, surgical indications should be carefully determined after taking other factors into account.

7.3 Timing of STN-DBS Initiation

DBS is more effective when it is performed soon after disease onset, i.e., if the disease duration is short or the symptoms are mild. DBS in PD patients with a short disease duration is reportedly very effective in improving quality of life (QOL) (Schüpbach et al. 2007; Espay et al. 2010; Schuepbach et al. 2013).

DBS is generally initiated between 10 and 15 years after disease onset, when significant motor fluctuations and dyskinesia make it difficult to implement appropriate drug therapy. Kleiner-Fisman et al. (2006) compared a 10- to 13-year disease duration group and a ≥14-year group in a meta-analysis on the effectiveness of

DBS according to disease duration. They found that the improvement rate in the UPDRS-III score was significantly better in the ≥14-year disease duration group. Therefore, we cannot definitively claim that the early initiation of DBS is always optimal. Furthermore, when performing surgery within 5 years of disease onset, we must be cautious of the possibility of erroneously performing DBS in patients with Parkinsonism rather than PD. Regardless of the effectiveness of the earlier initiation of DBS, follow-up drug therapy should be conducted for at least 4–5 years. Currently, there is no evidence suggesting that early DBS has specific neuroprotective effects.

The recent EARLYSTIM trial (multicenter randomized controlled trial) reported in Europe divided 251 early PD patients (≥4 years since onset; mean disease duration, 7.5 years; stage 1–3 on the Hoehn and Yahr scale) into an STN-DBS group and drug therapy only group. This trial revealed a significant improvement in QOL in the STN-DBS group after 2 years (Schuepbach et al. 2013). DBS was noted as a possible treatment option for PD patients with early development of motor fluctuations and dyskinesia, suggesting that the early initiation of DBS should be considered by doctors (Schüpbach et al. 2007; Espay et al. 2010).

7.4 Factors Pertaining to the Surgical Procedure for DBS

DBS requires a DBS electrode lead and an implantable stimulation device. Four platinum electrodes are placed at 0.5- or 1.5-mm intervals on the tip of the stimulation electrode lead, enabling stimulation via any of the electrodes.

The STN is very small and responds to projections from the cerebral cortex and the external segment of the globus pallidus (GPe). The motor territory projecting into the two output structures of the basal ganglia, namely the internal segment of the GP (GPi) and substantia nigra pars reticulate (SNr), is located dorsolaterally to the STN (Benarroch 2008). Electrodes need to be inserted into this motor territory to maximize the effectiveness of STN-DBS. When placing a 1-mm wide stimulating electrode in the 3–4-mm STN motor territory, the slightest displacement of the electrode can cause stimulation to spread to the surrounding tissue, resulting in undesirable stimulus-induced effects. Therefore, correct electrode placement is essential to minimize these adverse effects.

In magnetic resonance imaging (MRI)-guided targeting, the STN can be identified from T2 hyposignals. The STN is often located symmetrically to the anterior–posterior commissure (AC-PC) line. However, because the bilateral STNs can also be located asymmetrically, high-resolution MRI-guided direct targeting is recommended (Patel et al. 2008; Andrade-Souza et al. 2005; Toda et al. 2009). The entry point of the electrode trajectory on the brain surface is plotted and planned to follow a route that does not pass through the lateral ventricle and avoids the surface blood vessels and the cerebral sulcus. If the electrode trajectory passes through the lateral ventricle, the increased risk of hemorrhage from the ependymal blood vessels and resulting outflow of cerebrospinal fluid can cause intraoperative brain shift, with a risk of lead migration after therapeutic electrode placement. The STN can be confirmed by performing semi-microelectrode recording and monitoring the neural firing pattern and kinesthetic response (López-Flores et al. 2003; Gross et al. 2006). Anatomically, the STN is an isolated nucleus surrounded by nerve fibers; therefore, the semi microelectrode recording reaches the STN via the thalamus and zona incerta, resulting in a comparatively rapid increase in background activity when the electrode is inserted. This allows recording of the burst-like neural activity within the STN. A kinesthetic response is confirmed in the dorsolateral motor territory of the STN (Benazzouz et al. 2002; Starr et al. 2003).

Clinical improvements and stimulation-induced adverse effects are observed via intraoperative stimulation tests that help in determining the optimal electrode position (Pollak et al. 2002). Amelioration of motor symptoms such as rigidity and tremor can be easily confirmed, but limitations based on patient immobility during surgery hinder

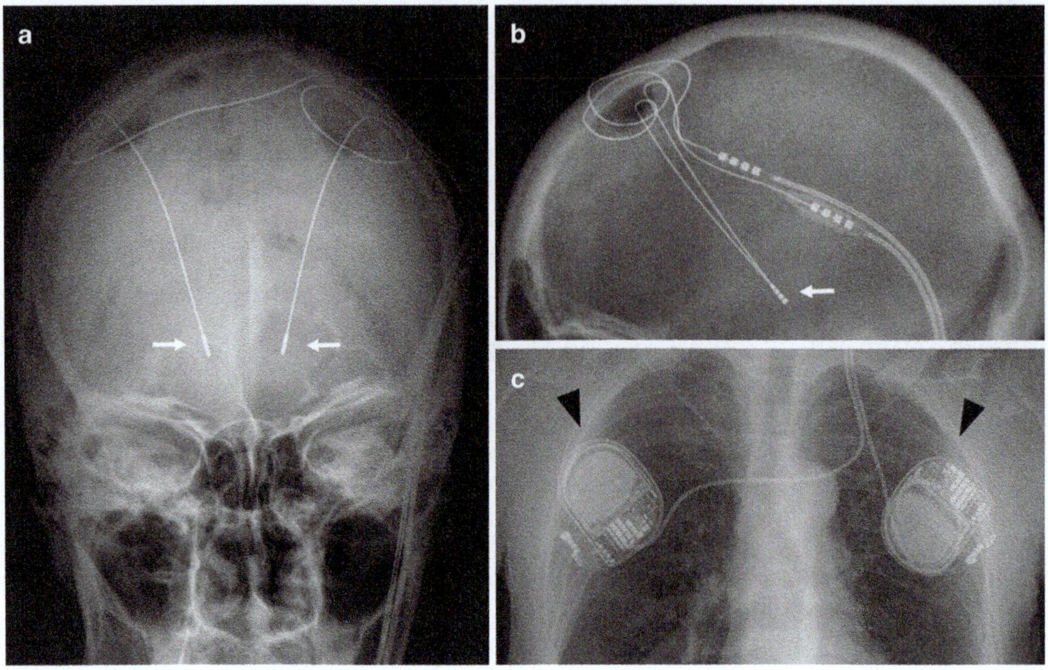

Fig. 7.1 Postoperative radiograph example of subthalamic deep brain stimulation (STN-DBS). (**a**, **b**) Skull X-ray demonstrates electrode leads for STN-DBS (*white arrow*). (**c**) Chest X-ray demonstrates implantable pulse generators in the bilateral anterior chest (*black arrowhead*)

a complete assessment. Symptomatic improvement can occur regardless of test stimuli because of micro-lesion effects occurring after semi-microelectrode recording. Meanwhile, adverse effects can be easily assessed with stable tests. It is possible to estimate the location of the active contact site in the STN from the anatomical relationship of the STN with the surrounding nerve fibers. When double vision and motor contraction occur at a low threshold, electrode placement should be re-examined because stimulation cannot be performed after initiating STN-DBS until the intensity required for clinical effects is reached.

When using electrodes (3389, Medtronic) at 0.5-mm intervals, three contact electrodes are often placed in the STN. Contacts in the STN are placed as follows: zero at the base; one in the middle; two dorsolaterally; and three superiorly and externally. Postoperative computed tomography is performed, and the electrode contact position should always be confirmed by fused preoperative or postoperative MRI images (see Figs. 7.1 and 7.2) (Shin et al. 2007).

7.5 DBS Control After Surgery

After surgery, signals can be sent to the stimulation device from outside the body using a dedicated programmer. This allows changes to be made to the stimulation conditions and sites. Adjustments are necessary so that benefits can be optimized. The electrode position must be known when programming DBS, and intraoperative data and postoperative images are useful for electrode selection. Furthermore, thorough assessment of both the stimulus and adverse effects of all electrodes during initial programming makes subsequent electrode adjustments easier (Bronstein et al. 2011; Volkmann et al. 2006). Stimulating from the center of the STN to the dorsolateral area (contact 1 or 2) is effective for the cardinal symptoms of PD. An immediate effect is seen on rigidity as a result of stimulation, followed by a slightly delayed effect on tremors. The effect on bradykinesia is more individualized and is often observed over time. Stimulation is often initiated days or weeks after surgery because of unstable symptoms

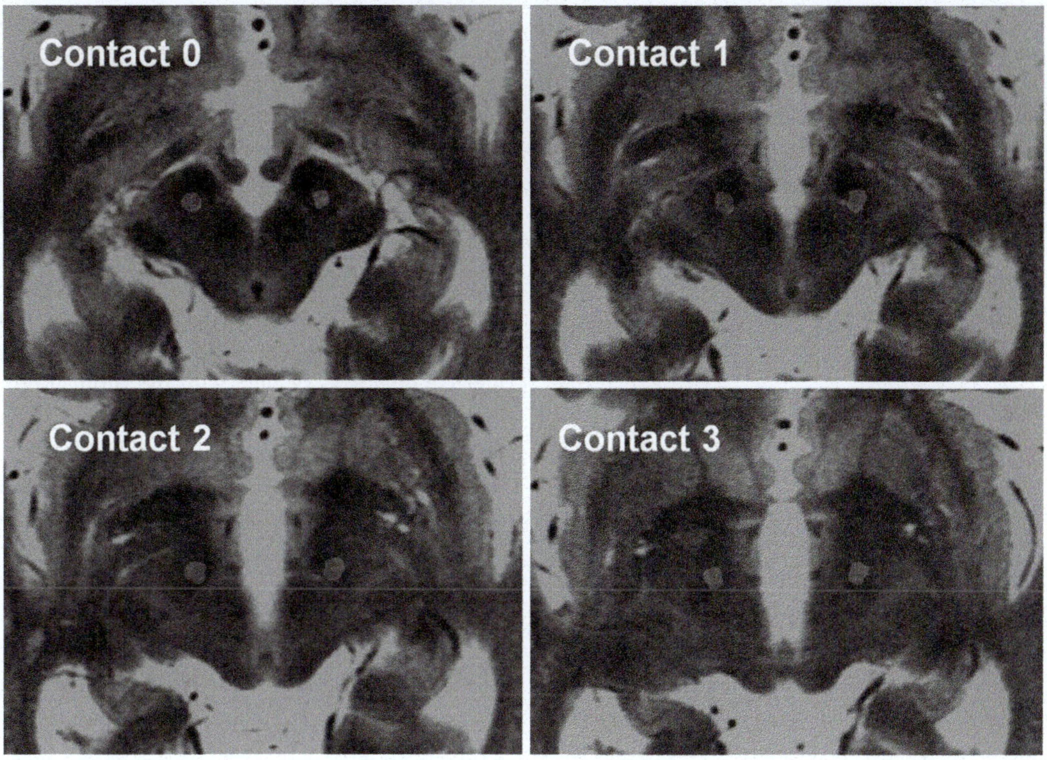

Fig. 7.2 Postoperative CT-preoperative MRI fusioned image shows artifacts of the electrodes placed within the STN

caused by postoperative drug adjustments, changes in resistance levels caused by environmental changes around the electrode, and microlesion effects caused by the surgical procedure.

Recent improvements in stimulation devices have enabled constant current stimulation (Okun et al. 2012) from the early postoperative period. After initiation of stimulation, its conditions (frequency, pulse width, stimulation intensity) are adjusted to eliminate bilateral symptom differences and gradually increase intensity with the aim of improving the off-period condition (Volkmann et al. 2006). Drugs are then tapered as appropriate according to dyskinesia. Some advanced PD patients have a very narrow therapeutic window for levodopa. These patients can be in an off-period condition during the daytime, with constant dyskinesia during the on-period. In some patients, the STN stimulation itself causes further exacerbation of dyskinesia.

When dyskinesia makes it difficult to adjust STN-DBS stimulation, control can be achieved by the selection of electrodes with a narrow distance between poles in active contact or by electrode configuration that enables direct stimulus application to the pallidofugal fibers outside and above the STN (Katayama et al. 2006). Some patients require regular stimulus frequency changes after surgery, but by 3–6 months, the need for further adjustment should be minimal.

Decreasing the amount of drug intake is often possible after STN-DBS initiation in many subjects. However, adjustments must carefully maintain the delicate balance between drug therapy and DBS. Dopaminergic medications should be tapered gradually and should not be excessively tapered at an early stage to avoid depression or apathy (Czernecki et al. 2008; Thobois et al. 2010). Witt et al. (2006) assessed the effects of the single levodopa challenge test and STN-DBS on depression and hedonic tone and found that both the single levodopa challenge test and STN-DBS ameliorated depression, whereas only levodopa ameliorated hedonic symptoms. This suggests that the excessive postoperative tapering of dopaminergic medication may cause anhedonia. Okun et al. (2009) performed the Cognition and Mood in Parkinson's disease in STN versus GPi-DBS (COMPARE) trial and reported that subjects became confused, less energetic, less euphoric, and sad when the ventral STN was stimulated. Therefore, if these symptoms appear, the stimulation site should be changed to a more dorsolateral region.

7.6 Surgical Outcomes of STN-DBS

7.6.1 Effectiveness of STN-DBS

STN-DBS ameliorates the cardinal symptoms of PD, including bradykinesia, rigidity, and tremors, and activities of daily living (ADL). It primarily ameliorates motor symptoms and ADL during drug off-periods, shortens drug off-periods, allows dose tapering, and ameliorates dyskinesia, and improves QOL (Limousin et al. 1998; Kumar et al. 1998, 1999; Burchiel et al. 1999; Moro et al. 1999; Molinuevo et al. 2000; Deep-Brain Stimulation for Parkinson's Disease Study Group 2001; Pinter et al. 1999; Houeto et al. 2000; Katayama et al. 2001; Simuni et al. 2002; Herzog et al. 2003; Kleiner-Fisman et al. 2003; Krack et al. 2003; Rodriguez-Oroz et al. 2004). Kleiner-Fisman et al. (2006) performed a systematic review of 37 cohort studies including 921 cases and reported that UPDRS ADL scores (UPDRS-II) and motor scores (UPDRS-III) improved by 50 and 52 %, respectively, when comparing postoperative off-periods and stimulation on-periods and preoperative drug off-periods. Levodopa dosage, dyskinesia, and daytime off-periods decreased by 55.9, 69.1, and 68.2 %, respectively. A 34.5 % improvement was observed in the PD questionnaire (PDQ-39).

Till date, three randomized controlled trials have compared drug therapy alone with STN-DBS for advanced PD. Deuschl et al. (2006) divided 156 PD patients aged ≥75 years into an STN-DBS group ($n=78$) and a drug therapy alone group ($n=78$) and compared their prognoses after 6 months using PDQ-39 and UPDRS-III. These outcomes significantly improved in the STN-DBS group compared with those in the drug therapy alone group. Weaver et al. (2009) divided 255 PD patients into a DBS group [STN ($n=60$) or GPi ($n=61$)] and a drug therapy alone group ($n=134$) and compared symptoms during the on-period after 6 months. Their results revealed improved on-periods without dyskinesia or motor function problems and improved QOL in the DBS group. However, adverse effects associated with the surgical procedure were observed, with serious adverse effects being more common in the DBS group. These studies observed STN-DBS over short 6-month periods, whereas the PD-SURG trial, a large randomized trial evaluating the role of surgery as therapy for PD, compared treatment outcomes and complications after 1 year. Williams et al. (2010) allocated 366 PD patients to surgery ($n=183$; STN-DBS group: 174 patients) or drug therapy alone ($n=183$) and assessed their PDQ-39 scores after 1 year (PD-SURG trial). Improvements in the PDQ-39 summary index, mobility domain, ADL domain, and bodily discomfort domain were significantly greater in the STN-DBS group than in the drug therapy alone group. Complications associated with surgery were observed in 36 patients, with one procedure-related death. Twenty patients in the STN-DBS group and 13 in the drug therapy group experienced serious adverse effects associated with PD. The results indicated that STN-DBS was more effective than drug therapy alone.

7.6.2 The Characteristics of STN-DBS

The primary effect of STN-DBS is a significant decrease in the off-period duration. The treatment also affects the on-period, although less significantly. In patients with marked motor fluctuations with a good preoperative on-period state, the good state can be maintained after DBS (see Fig. 7.3, Case A). Conversely, in patients with advanced PD who already exhibit a poor response to levodopa, good outcomes are unlikely

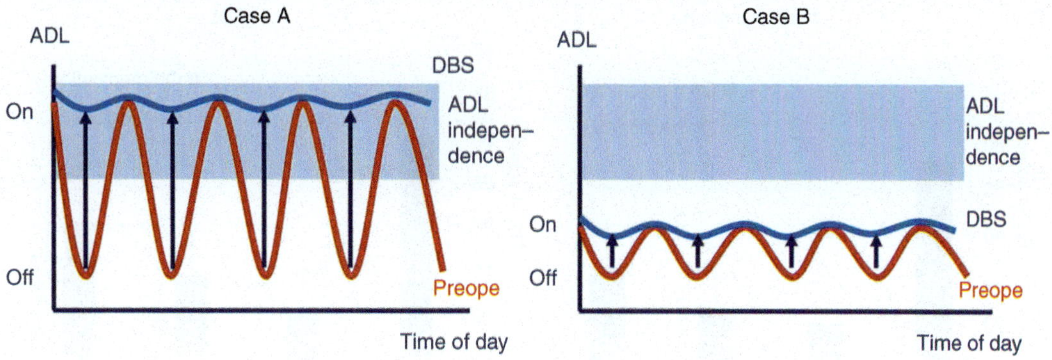

Fig. 7.3 Illustration of improvement of motor fluctuation in activities of daily living in the patients treated with STN-DBS

despite a slightly improved response to DBS (see Fig. 7.3, Case B). This applies equally to the long-term, where off-period improvements are maintained for a comparatively long period. However, even if an improvement is seen in the on-period, levels quickly return to their preoperative state, and there is often a subsequent exacerbation (Deuschl et al. 2006; Rodriguez-Oroz et al. 2005; Moro et al. 2010).

Levodopa dosage or the levodopa-equivalent dosage can be decreased after STN-DBS (Tavella et al. 2002; Thobois et al. 2002; Vingerhoets et al. 2002). While the extent of dose reduction varies among reports, most state that STN-DBS can decrease the dosage of anti-PD drugs. However, this effect is not significant for GPi-DBS (Scotto di Luzio et al. 2001; Volkmann et al. 2001; Anderson et al. 2005; Minguez-Castellanos et al. 2005; Weaver et al. 2005; Valldeoriola et al. 2002). In addition, amelioration of levodopa-induced dyskinesia can be expected, which is thought to be due to decreased dyskinesia resulting from anti-PD dose reductions (Deuschl et al. 2006; Anderson et al. 2005; Weaver et al. 2005; Valldeoriola et al. 2002). A direct effect has also been reported (Katayama et al. 2006).

7.6.3 The Long-Term Effect of STN-DBS

Several prospective studies with 3- to 5-year follow-up periods have examined the long-term effects of STN-DBS. Sustained improvements are observed in ADL, motor symptoms, rigidity, bradykinesia, and dose reductions (see Fig. 7.4) (Krack et al. 2003; Rodriguez-Oroz et al. 2005; Schüpbach et al. 2005; Østergaard and Aa Sunde 2006; Volkmann et al. 2009; Moro et al. 2010). The results of 8- or 10-year follow-ups have also been reported, and while tremors remain controlled in the long-term, there appears to be a decline in the effect on axial symptoms (Fasano et al. 2010; Castrioto et al. 2011).

7.6.4 Symptoms for Which DBS Is Inadequate

DBS tends to be inadequate in patients with levodopa resistant symptoms such as weakness, dysarthria, freezing of gait, and postural instability. Axial symptoms (particularly in the on-period) can be difficult to control. STN-DBS mainly ameliorates motor symptoms during the off-period (Deuschl et al. 2006; Anderson et al. 2005; Weaver et al. 2005), and axial symptoms such as postural instability and freezing of gait observed in the preoperative on-period often fail to ameliorate after surgery and appear during long-term follow-up of STN-DBS therapy (Welter et al. 2002; Tsai et al. 2009; Davis et al. 2006).

In a meta-analysis by St George at al. that was based on 11 articles, postural instability and gait disturbance deteriorated within 2 years, regardless of postoperative improvement, and tended to fall

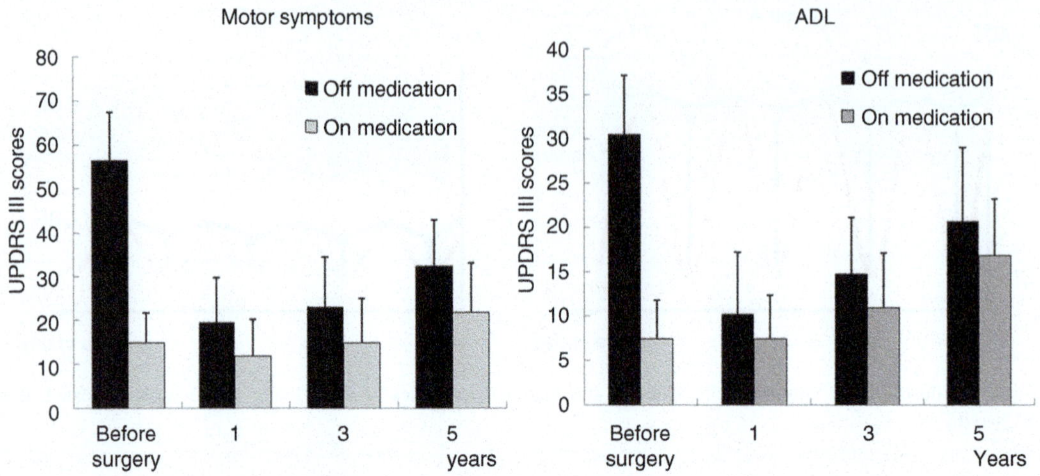

Fig. 7.4 Long-term effects of STN-DBS in motor UPDRS III subscore and ADL UPDRS II subscore in 132 PD patients who underwent bilateral STN-DBS in our institution. Significant improvement of off-medication state sustained up to 5 years after surgery

below preoperative levels (St George et al. 2010). In a 7-year follow-up reported by Muniz et al. (2010), freezing of gait (on initiation of walking) occurred more readily in the STN-DBS group than in the drug therapy alone group. In a study that examined the long-term effects of STN-DBS over 8–10 years, axial symptoms were the first to deteriorate (Fasano et al. 2010; Castrioto et al. 2011). Axial symptoms such as freezing and postural instability and related gait disturbance are motor symptoms that are difficult to control with STN-DBS, and their management is a topic for future study.

7.7 Complications of STN-DBS

DBS-induced adverse effects usually disappear when stimulation is discontinued, and they can be controlled by changing the stimulation conditions. Nevertheless, device-related issues such as disconnection or complications such as infection can occur. The most serious complication is ICH, which occurs in 3.9 % patients according to a systematic review by Kleiner-Fisman et al. (2006). Deuschl et al. (2006) reported that while life-threatening adverse effects such as ICH were more common with DBS than with drug therapy, overall treatment-related adverse effects were more common with drug therapy alone.

Previous studies have reported minor or transient complications related to cognitive and affective function that rarely affect ADL in a significant manner (Saint-Cyr et al. 2000; Kumar et al. 1999; Moro et al. 1999; Molinuevo et al. 2000; Pillon et al. 2000; Woods et al. 2002; Funkiewiez et al. 2004; Morrison et al. 2004). However, cognitive and behavioral dysfunction and psychiatric symptoms have recently been highlighted as consequences of STN-DBS. In a systematic review of 1,398 patients from 82 articles by Temel et al. (2006), cognitive dysfunction occurred in 41 % patients, depression in 8%, and hypomania in 4 %. In addition, a meta-analysis by Parsons et al. (2006) that was based on 612 patients from 28 cohort studies revealed that while STN-DBS with appropriate patient selection is a safe therapy in terms of cognitive function, a mild decline in executive function and verbal learning was observed along with a relatively marked decline in semantic and phonemic verbal fluency.

Many studies examining declining cognitive function have noted that a decline in verbal fluency is prominent and that attention should be paid to deteriorating language skills (Okun et al. 2009; Gironell et al. 2003; Smeding et al. 2006). Unfortunately, studies on cognitive function have concluded that it is difficult to distinguish a decline in cognitive function caused by STN-DBS from that caused by PD progression, making randomized controlled trials difficult. Witt et al. allocated patients either to STN-DBS ($n=60$) or drug therapy alone ($n=63$) and tested cognitive function after 6 months. While overall cognitive function scores did not decrease, scores for verbal fluency, the Stroop test, and executive function decreased after STN-DBS. More importantly, QOL improved in patients who experienced a decline in executive function after STN-DBS, which mitigated any clinical decrease in ADL after treatment (Witt et al. 2008). Subscores for elderly individuals, high doses of levodopa, and axial symptoms with high UPDRS scores are risk factors for deterioration in executive function after STN-DBS. However, these preoperative risk factors may reflect the degree of disease progression. Other factors, including surgical procedure, correct electrode placement, and postoperative management may also be involved in the deterioration of executive function after STN-DBS.

In order to examine whether the electrode trajectory affects changes in cognitive function, Witt et al. (2013) divided patients into an STN-DBS group ($n=31$) and a drug therapy alone group ($n=31$) and examined the association between changes in cognitive function and electrode entry point, region transected, and site of active contact within the STN. An electrode trajectory passing through the head of the caudate nucleus caused an overall cognitive decline as well as a decline in working memory. A site of active contact that deviated from within the STN resulted in a decline in semantic verbal fluency. Therefore, the electrode path should avoid the head of the caudate nucleus and the electrode should be placed correctly within the STN; together, this can decrease the risk of cognitive decline following STN-DBS.

Depression after STN-DBS is thought to occur in approximately 20–25% patients. However, in a review of 22 articles, Takeshita et al. (2005) found the incidence of postoperative depression to be 2–33.3 % and that of mania to be 4.2–8.1 %, with STN-DBS having an antidepressant effect in 16.7–76 % patients. Overall, they concluded that the depression scores remained unchanged. In two randomized controlled trials, the STN-DBS group experienced a slight antidepressant effect at 6 months compared with the drug therapy alone group. Postoperative risk factors for depression were identified to be an excessive tapering of dopaminergic medication and a history of depression (Weaver et al. 2009; Witt et al. 2008).

Some reports on suicides by patients who underwent STN-DBS have been published (Burkhard et al. 2004; Soulas et al. 2008). A review of 5,311 patients at 75 facilities by Voon et al. found the rate of successful suicide to be 0.45% and the rate of unsuccessful suicide to be 0.90 %. The incidence in the first year after surgery was significantly high and correlated with postoperative depression (Voon et al. 2008). Rodrigues et al. (2010) retrospectively examined suicide cases and reported levodopa dose tapering to be a significant factor.

Mood and impulsiveness are also thought to be involved in the limbic part of the STN, and stimulation of this region by STN-DBS may result in changes in mood and behavior. During the initial stage of STN-DBS, dopaminergic medication and stimulus adjustment are often difficult to balance and may increase mood-related complications. Therefore, excessive dose tapering in the early postoperative period is a significant risk factor, and drug and DBS adjustments must be appropriate, tolerable, and monitored.

7.8 Comparison of DBS Targets

DBS targeting the STN or GPi is a common treatment for motor fluctuations and dyskinesia associated with advanced PD. Several recent reports have seen little difference in the effectiveness of STN-DBS and GPi-DBS in ameliorating motor symptoms (Okun et al. 2009; Rodriguez-Oroz et al. 2005; Moro et al. 2010; Anderson et al. 2005; Follett et al. 2010). Weaver et al. (2005) conducted a meta-analysis of 31 papers on STN-DBS and 14 papers on GPi-DBS and concluded that motor function improvement

(UPDRS-III) after 6 months was 54 % with STN-DBS and 40 % with GPi-DBS, indicating no significant difference between groups. ADL also improved by 40 % in both groups, although no significant difference was observed. While GPi-DBS ameliorated both the on-period and off-period symptoms, STN-DBS only ameliorated the off-period symptoms. In contrast, the drug dosage was tapered by 52 % with STN-DBS, whereas no tapering was possible with GPi-DBS. In a number of randomized controlled trials, improvements in motor function and ADL were comparable. However, adverse effects such as cognitive and mental dysfunction occurred more commonly with STN-DBS and rarely with GPi-DBS. Drug tapering was possible in these trials with STN-DBS, but not with GPi-DBS (Okun et al. 2009; Rodriguez-Oroz et al. 2005; Moro et al. 2010; Anderson et al. 2005; Follett et al. 2010).

The randomized controlled COMPARE trial compared the effectiveness of STN-DBS and GPi-DBS in ameliorating nonmotor symptoms and revealed a significant decline in verbal fluency and mental function (such as mood and cognitive function) in the STN-DBS group compared with that in the GPi-DBS group (Okun et al. 2009). Follett et al. (2010) allocated 299 patients to either an STN-DBS group ($n = 147$) or a GPi-DBS group ($n = 152$) and examined UPDRS-III score, self-reported function, QOL, neurocognitive function, and adverse events after 2 years. No difference in UPDRS-III score was observed between the two groups. Drug dosage was significantly tapered in the STN-DBS group compared with that in the GPi-DBS group; however, a decline in visuomotor processing speed was observed in the former group. Furthermore, depression was ameliorated in the GPi-DBS group but exacerbated in the STN-DBS group, and serious adverse effects were generally the same in both groups. Motor symptoms were also ameliorated by both STN-DBS and GPi-DBS, with individual differences in nonmotor function. Till date, the overall improvement rates for motor symptoms in randomized controlled trials have been 26–48 % with STN-DBS and 16.9–37 % with GPi-DBS. Therefore, the rate of amelioration of motor symptoms after STN-DBS tended to be lower in these trials.

In the recent Netherlands Subthalamic and Pallidal Stimulation (NSTAPS) study, patients were allocated either to an STN-DBS group ($n = 63$) or a GPi-DBS group ($n = 65$), and the weighted Academic Medical Center Linear Disability Scale (ALDS), cognitive function, mood, effects on behavior, UPDRS III score, QOL, adverse effects, and drug usage were examined after 1 year. No difference in weighted ALDS score was observed between the two groups. However, the off-period symptom improvement rate was 45.7 % in the STN-DBS group compared with 26 % in the GPi-DBS group, indicating a significant improvement. Compared with that in the GPi-DBS group, a significant tapering of drug dosage was possible in the STN-DBS group, resulting in significant amelioration of off-period symptoms as per ALDS scores and posture and gait as per UPDRS scores. In addition, there were no differences in cognitive, mood, and behavioral adverse effects between groups (Odekerken et al. 2013). Tapering of drug dosage was again possible in the STN-DBS group, which led to amelioration of levodopa-induced dyskinesia. In contrast, dose tapering was not possible in the GPi-DBS group, although a direct inhibitory effect on levodopa-induced dyskinesia was observed.

Stimulation of the ventral intermediate nucleus of the thalamus (Vim) has no effect on motor fluctuation and dyskinesia in patients with advanced PD, but it has a strong inhibitory effect on drug therapy-resistant tremors (Schuurman et al. 2000, 2008). Individualized target selection based on these differences in clinical efficacy is necessary.

Conclusions

DBS is indicated for advanced PD patients with motor fluctuations and dyskinesia whose symptoms are difficult to control with drugs or who suffer from drug therapy-resistant tremors. Further improvements in the safety and adjustability of DBS can be expected from future advances in DBS devices. Several crucial factors need to be considered to achieve favorable treatment outcomes: careful patient selection, optimally timed treatment initiation, technically correct surgical procedures, careful management of postoperative drugs, and controlled adjustment of DBS.

References

Alexander GE, DeLong MR, Strick PL (1986) Parallel organization of functionally segregated circuits linking basal ganglia and cortex. Annu Rev Neurosci 9:357–381

Anderson VC, Burchiel KJ, Hogarth P et al (2005) Pallidal vs subthalamic nucleus deep brain stimulation in Parkinson disease. Arch Neurol 62(4):554–560

Andrade-Souza YM, Schwalb JM, Hamani C et al (2005) Comparison of three methods of targeting the subthalamic nucleus for chronic stimulation in Parkinson's disease. Neurosurgery 56(2 Suppl):360–368

Benabid AL, Pollak P, Louveau A et al (1987) Combined (thalamotomy and stimulation) stereotactic surgery of the VIM thalamic nucleus for bilateral Parkinson disease. Appl Neurophysiol 50(1–6):344–346

Benabid AL, Pollak P, Gross C et al (1994) Acute and long-term effects of subthalamic nucleus stimulation in Parkinson's disease. Stereotact Funct Neurosurg 62(1–4):76–84

Benarroch EE (2008) Subthalamic nucleus and its connections: anatomic substrate for the network effects of deep brain stimulation. Neurology 70(21):1991–1995

Benazzouz A, Breit S, Koudsie A et al (2002) Intraoperative microrecordings of the subthalamic nucleus in Parkinson's disease. Mov Disord 17(Suppl 3): S145–S149

Bronstein JM, Tagliati M, Alterman RL et al (2011) Deep brain stimulation for Parkinson disease: an expert consensus and review of key issues. Arch Neurol 68(2):165–171

Burchiel KJ, Anderson VC, Favre J et al (1999) Comparison of pallidal and subthalamic nucleus deep brain stimulation for advanced Parkinson's disease: results of a randomized, blinded pilot study. Neurosurgery 45(6):1375–1382

Burkhard PR, Vingerhoets FJ, Berney A et al (2004) Suicide after successful deep brain stimulation for movement disorders. Neurology 63(11):2170–2172

Castrioto A, Lozano AM, Poon YY et al (2011) Ten-year outcome of subthalamic stimulation in Parkinson disease: a blinded evaluation. Arch Neurol 68(12):1550–1556

Charles PD, Van Blercom N, Krack P et al (2002) Predictors of effective bilateral subthalamic nucleus stimulation for PD. Neurology 59(6):932–934

Czernecki V, Schüpbach M, Yaici S et al (2008) Apathy following subthalamic stimulation in Parkinson disease: a dopamine responsive symptom. Mov Disord 23(7):964–969

Davis JT, Lyons KE, Pahwa R (2006) Freezing of gait after bilateral subthalamic nucleus stimulation for Parkinson's disease. Clin Neurol Neurosurg 108(5):461–464

Deep-Brain Stimulation for Parkinson's Disease Study Group (2001) Deep-brain stimulation of the subthalamic nucleus or the pars interna of the globus pallidus in Parkinson's disease. N Engl J Med 345(13): 956–963

Defer GL, Widner H, Marié RM et al (1999) Core assessment program for surgical interventional therapies in Parkinson's disease (CAPSIT-PD). Mov Disord 14(4):572–584

Deuschl G, Schade-Brittinger C, Krack P et al (2006) A randomized trial of deep-brain stimulation for Parkinson's disease. N Engl J Med 355(9):896–908

Espay AJ, Vaughan JE, Marras C et al (2010) Early versus delayed bilateral subthalamic deep brain stimulation for Parkinson's disease: a decision analysis. Mov Disord 25(10):1456–1463

Fasano A, Romito LM, Daniele A et al (2010) Motor and cognitive outcome in patients with Parkinson's disease 8 years after subthalamic implants. Brain 133(9): 2664–2676

Follett KA, Weaver FM, Stern M et al (2010) Pallidal versus subthalamic deep-brain stimulation for Parkinson's disease. N Engl J Med 362(22):2077–2091

Funkiewiez A, Ardouin C, Caputo E et al (2004) Long term effects of bilateral subthalamic nucleus stimulation on cognitive function, mood, and behaviour in Parkinson's disease. J Neurol Neurosurg Psychiatry 75(6):834–839

Gironell A, Kulisevsky J, Rami L et al (2003) Effects of pallidotomy and bilateral subthalamic stimulation on cognitive function in Parkinson disease. A controlled comparative study. J Neurol 250(8):917–923

Gross RE, Krack P, Rodriguez-Oroz MC et al (2006) Electrophysiological mapping for the implantation of deep brain stimulators for Parkinson's disease and tremor. Mov Disord 21(Suppl 14):S259–S283

Herzog J, Volkmann J, Krack P et al (2003) Two-year follow-up of subthalamic deep brain stimulation in Parkinson's disease. Mov Disord 18(11):1332–1337

Houeto JL, Damier P, Bejjani PB et al (2000) Subthalamic stimulation in Parkinson disease: a multidisciplinary approach. Arch Neurol 57(4):461–465

Katayama Y, Kasai M, Oshima H et al (2001) Subthalamic nucleus stimulation for Parkinson disease: benefits observed in levodopa-intolerant patients. J Neurosurg 95(2):213–221

Katayama Y, Oshima H, Kano T et al (2006) Direct effect of subthalamic nucleus stimulation on levodopa-induced peak-dose dyskinesia in patients with Parkinson's disease. Stereotact Funct Neurosurg 84(4):176–179

Kleiner-Fisman G, Fisman DN, Sime E et al (2003) Long-term follow up of bilateral deep brain stimulation of the subthalamic nucleus in patients with advanced Parkinson disease. J Neurosurg 99(3):489–495

Kleiner-Fisman G, Herzog J, Fisman DN et al (2006) Subthalamic nucleus deep brain stimulation: summary and meta-analysis of outcomes. Mov Disord 21(Suppl 14):S290–S304

Krack P, Batir A, Van Blercom N et al (2003) Five-year follow-up of bilateral stimulation of the subthalamic nucleus in advanced Parkinson's disease. N Engl J Med 349(20):1925–1934

Kumar R, Lozano AM, Kim YJ et al (1998) Double-blind evaluation of subthalamic nucleus deep brain stimulation in advanced Parkinson's disease. Neurology 51(3): 850–855

Kumar R, Lozano AM, Sime E et al (1999) Comparative effects of unilateral and bilateral subthalamic nucleus deep brain stimulation. Neurology 53(3):561–566

Lang AE, Widner H (2002) Deep brain stimulation for Parkinson's disease: patient selection and evaluation. Mov Disord 17(Suppl 3):S94–S101

Limousin P, Krack P, Pollak P et al (1998) Electrical stimulation of the subthalamic nucleus in advanced Parkinson's disease. N Engl J Med 339(16):1105–1111

López-Flores G, Miguel-Morales J, Teijeiro-Amador J et al (2003) Anatomic and neurophysiological methods for the targeting and lesioning of the subthalamic nucleus: Cuban experience and review. Neurosurgery 52(4): 817–830

Lopiano L, Rizzone M, Bergamasco B et al (2002) Deep brain stimulation of the subthalamic nucleus in PD: an analysis of the exclusion causes. J Neurol Sci 195(2): 167–170

Minguez-Castellanos A, Escamilla-Sevilla F, Katati MJ et al (2005) Different patterns of medication change after subthalamic or pallidal stimulation for Parkinson's disease: target related effect or selection bias? J Neurol Neurosurg Psychiatry 76(1):34–39

Molinuevo JL, Valldeoriola F, Tolosa E et al (2000) Levodopa withdrawal after bilateral subthalamic nucleus stimulation in advanced Parkinson disease. Arch Neurol 57(7):983–988

Morrison CE, Borod JC, Perrine K et al (2004) Neuropsychological functioning following bilateral subthalamic nucleus stimulation in Parkinson's disease. Arch Clin Neuropsychol 19(2):165–181

Moro E, Scerrati M, Romito LM et al (1999) Chronic subthalamic nucleus stimulation reduces medication requirements in Parkinson's disease. Neurology 53(1):85–90

Moro E, Lozano AM, Pollak P et al (2010) Long-term results of a multicenter study on subthalamic and pallidal stimulation in Parkinson's disease. Mov Disord 25(5):578–586

Muniz AS, Liu W, Liu H et al (2010) Gait initiation evaluation after deep brain stimulation for Parkinson's disease: a 7-year follow-up. Conf Proc IEEE Eng Med Biol Soc 2010:3650–3653

Odekerken VJ, van Laar T, Staal MJ et al (2013) Subthalamic nucleus versus globus pallidus bilateral deep brain stimulation for advanced Parkinson's disease (NSTAPS study): a randomised controlled trial. Lancet Neurol 12(1):37–44

Okun MS, Fernandez HH, Wu SS et al (2009) Cognition and mood in Parkinson's disease in subthalamic nucleus versus globus pallidus interna deep brain stimulation: the COMPARE trial. Ann Neurol 65(5): 586–595

Okun MS, Gallo BV, Mandybur G et al (2012) Subthalamic deep brain stimulation with a constant-current device in Parkinson's disease: an open-label randomised controlled trial. Lancet Neurol 11(2):140–149

Ory-Magne F, Brefel-Courbon C, Simonetta-Moreau M et al (2007) Does ageing influence deep brain stimulation outcomes in Parkinson's disease? Mov Disord 22(10):1457–1463

Østergaard K, Aa Sunde N (2006) Evolution of Parkinson's disease during 4 years of bilateral deep brain stimulation of the subthalamic nucleus. Mov Disord 21(5):624–631

Parsons TD, Rogers SA, Braaten AJ et al (2006) Cognitive sequelae of subthalamic nucleus deep brain stimulation in Parkinson's disease: a meta-analysis. Lancet Neurol 5(7):578–588

Patel NK, Khan S, Gill SS (2008) Comparison of atlas- and magnetic-resonance-imaging-based stereotactic targeting of the subthalamic nucleus in the surgical treatment of Parkinson's disease. Stereotact Funct Neurosurg 86(3):153–161

Piboolnurak P, Lang AE, Lozano AM et al (2007) Levodopa response in long-term bilateral subthalamic stimulation for Parkinson's disease. Mov Disord 22(7):990–997

Pillon B, Ardouin C, Damier P et al (2000) Neuropsychological changes between "off" and "on" STN or GPi stimulation in Parkinson's disease. Neurology 55(3):411–418

Pinter MM, Alesch F, Murg M et al (1999) Deep brain stimulation of the subthalamic nucleus for control of extrapyramidal features in advanced idiopathic Parkinson's disease: one year follow-up. J Neural Transm 106(7–8): 693–709

Pollak P, Krack P, Fraix V et al (2002) Intraoperative micro- and macrostimulation of the subthalamic nucleus in Parkinson's disease. Mov Disord 17(Suppl 3):S155–S161

Rodriguez-Oroz MC, Zamarbide I, Guridi J et al (2004) Efficacy of deep brain stimulation of the subthalamic nucleus in Parkinson's disease 4 years after surgery: double blind and open label evaluation. J Neurol Neurosurg Psychiatry 75(10):1382–1385

Rodriguez-Oroz MC, Obeso JA, Lang AE et al (2005) Bilateral deep brain stimulation in Parkinson's disease: a multicentre study with 4 years follow-up. Brain 128(Pt 10):2240–2249

Rodrigues AM, Rosas MJ, Gago MF et al (2010) Suicide attempts after subthalamic nucleus stimulation for Parkinson's disease. Eur Neurol 63(3):176–179

Saint-Cyr JA, Trépanier LL, Kumar R et al (2000) Neuropsychological consequences of chronic bilateral stimulation of the subthalamic nucleus in Parkinson's disease. Brain 123(Pt 10):2091–2108

Sansur CA, Frysinger RC, Pouratian N et al (2007) Incidence of symptomatic hemorrhage after stereotactic electrode placement. J Neurosurg 107(5): 998–1003

Schüpbach WM, Chastan N, Welter ML et al (2005) Stimulation of the subthalamic nucleus in Parkinson's disease: a 5 year follow up. J Neurol Neurosurg Psychiatry 76(12):1640–1644

Schüpbach WM, Maltête D, Houeto JL et al (2007) Neurosurgery at an earlier stage of Parkinson disease: a randomized, controlled trial. Neurology 68(4): 267–271

Schuepbach WM, Rau J, Knudsen K et al (2013) Neurostimulation for Parkinson's disease with early motor complications. N Engl J Med 368(7):610–622

Schuurman PR, Bosch DA, Bossuyt PM et al (2000) A comparison of continuous thalamic stimulation and thalamotomy for suppression of severe tremor. N Engl J Med 342(7):461–468

Schuurman PR, Bosch DA, Merkus MP et al (2008) Long-term follow-up of thalamic stimulation versus thalamotomy for tremor suppression. Mov Disord 23(8):1146–1153

Scotto di Luzio AE, Ammannati F, Marini P et al (2001) Which target for DBS in Parkinson's disease? Subthalamic nucleus versus globus pallidus internus. Neurol Sci 22(1):87–88

Shih LC, Tarsy D (2007) Deep brain stimulation for the treatment of atypical parkinsonism. Mov Disord 22(15):2149–2155

Shin M, Lefaucheur JP, Penholate MF et al (2007) Subthalamic nucleus stimulation in Parkinson's disease: postoperative CT-MRI fusion images confirm accuracy of electrode placement using intraoperative multi-unit recording. Neurophysiol Clin 37(6): 457–466

Simuni T, Jaggi JL, Mulholland H et al (2002) Bilateral stimulation of the subthalamic nucleus in patients with Parkinson disease: a study of efficacy and safety. J Neurosurg 96(4):666–672

Smeding HM, Speelman JD, Koning-Haanstra M et al (2006) Neuropsychological effects of bilateral STN stimulation in Parkinson disease: a controlled study. Neurology 66(12):1830–1836

Smeding HM, Speelman JD, Huizenga HM et al (2011) Predictors of cognitive and psychosocial outcome after STN DBS in Parkinson's disease. J Neurol Neurosurg Psychiatry 82(7):754–760

Soulas T, Gurruchaga JM, Palfi S et al (2008) Attempted and completed suicides after subthalamic nucleus stimulation for Parkinson's disease. J Neurol Neurosurg Psychiatry 79(8):952–954

Starr PA, Theodosopoulos PV, Turner R (2003) Surgery of the subthalamic nucleus: use of movement-related neuronal activity for surgical navigation. Neurosurgery 53(5):1146–1149

St George RJ, Nutt JG, Burchiel KJ et al (2010) A meta-regression of the long-term effects of deep brain stimulation on balance and gait in PD. Neurology 75(14):1292–1299

Takeshita S, Kurisu K, Trop L et al (2005) Effect of subthalamic stimulation on mood state in Parkinson's disease: evaluation of previous facts and problems. Neurosurg Rev 28(3):179–186

Tarsy D, Apetauerova D, Ryan P et al (2003) Adverse effects of subthalamic nucleus DBS in a patient with multiple system atrophy. Neurology 61(2):247–249

Tavella A, Bergamasco B, Bosticco E et al (2002) Deep brain stimulation of the subthalamic nucleus in Parkinson's disease: long-term follow-up. Neurol Sci 23(Suppl 2):S111–S112

Temel Y, Kessels A, Tan S et al (2006) Behavioural changes after bilateral subthalamic stimulation in advanced Parkinson disease: a systematic review. Parkinsonism Relat Disord 12(5):265–272

Thobois S, Mertens P, Guenot M et al (2002) Subthalamic nucleus stimulation in Parkinson's disease: clinical evaluation of 18 patients. J Neurol 249(5):529–534

Thobois S, Ardouin C, Lhommée E et al (2010) Non-motor dopamine withdrawal syndrome after surgery for Parkinson's disease: predictors and underlying mesolimbic denervation. Brain 133(Pt 4):1111–1127

Toda H, Sawamoto N, Hanakawa T et al (2009) A novel composite targeting method using high-field magnetic resonance imaging for subthalamic nucleus deep brain stimulation. J Neurosurg 111(4):737–745

Tsai ST, Lin SH, Chou YC et al (2009) Prognostic factors of subthalamic stimulation in Parkinson's disease: a comparative study between short- and long-term effects. Stereotact Funct Neurosurg 87(4):241–248

Valldeoriola F, Pilleri M, Tolosa E et al (2002) Bilateral subthalamic stimulation monotherapy in advanced Parkinson's disease: long-term follow-up of patients. Mov Disord 17(1):125–132

Vingerhoets FJ, Villemure JG, Temperli P et al (2002) Subthalamic DBS replaces levodopa in Parkinson's disease: two-year follow-up. Neurology 58(3):396–401

Volkmann J, Allert N, Voges J et al (2001) Safety and efficacy of pallidal or subthalamic nucleus stimulation in advanced PD. Neurology 56(4):548–551

Volkmann J, Moro E, Pahwa R (2006) Basic algorithms for the programming of deep brain stimulation in Parkinson's disease. Mov Disord 21(Suppl 14): S284–S289

Volkmann J, Albanese A, Kulisevsky J et al (2009) Long-term effects of pallidal or subthalamic deep brain stimulation on quality of life in Parkinson's disease. Mov Disord 24(8):1154–1161

Voon V, Krack P, Lang AE et al (2008) A multicentre study on suicide outcomes following subthalamic stimulation for Parkinson's disease. Brain 131(Pt 10): 2720–2728

Weaver F, Follett K, Hur K et al (2005) Deep brain stimulation in Parkinson disease: a metaanalysis of patient outcomes. J Neurosurg 103(6):956–967

Weaver FM, Follett K, Stern M et al (2009) Bilateral deep brain stimulation vs best medical therapy for patients with advanced Parkinson disease: a randomized controlled trial. JAMA 301(1):63–73

Welter ML, Houeto JL, Tezenas du Montcel S et al (2002) Clinical predictive factors of subthalamic stimulation in Parkinson's disease. Brain 125(Pt 3):575–583

Williams A, Gill S, Varma T et al (2010) Deep brain stimulation plus best medical therapy versus best medical

therapy alone for advanced Parkinson's disease (PD SURG trial): a randomised, open-label trial. Lancet Neurol 9(6):581–591
Witt K, Daniels C, Herzog J et al (2006) Differential effects of L-dopa and subthalamic stimulation on depressive symptoms and hedonic tone in Parkinson's disease. J Neuropsychiatry Clin Neurosci 18(3):397–401
Witt K, Daniels C, Reiff J et al (2008) Neuropsychological and psychiatric changes after deep brain stimulation for Parkinson's disease: a randomised, multicentre study. Lancet Neurol 7(7):605–614
Witt K, Granert O, Daniels C et al (2013) Relation of lead trajectory and electrode position to neuropsychological outcomes of subthalamic neurostimulation in Parkinson's disease: results from a randomized trial. Brain 136(Pt 7):2109–2119
Woods SP, Fields JA, Tröster AI (2002) Neuropsychological sequelae of subthalamic nucleus deep brain stimulation in Parkinson's disease: a critical review. Neuropsychol Rev 12(2):111–126

Stimulation of Globus Pallidus

8

Mitsuhiro Ogura

8.1 Introduction

Choosing which nucleus to target with deep brain stimulation (DBS) for the treatment of Parkinson's disease (PD)—the subthalamic nucleus (STN) or globus pallidus internus (GPi)—is a subject of debate (Anderson et al. 2005; Follett et al. 2010; Group TD-BSfPsDS 2001; Peppe et al. 2004). Currently, the STN is chosen more frequently than the GPi.

Recent comparative studies between STN-DBS and GPi-DBS have revealed that the improvement of motor function was not significantly different between the two targets (Follett et al. 2010; Anderson et al. 2005; Zahodne et al. 2009; Okun et al. 2009; Nakamura et al. 2007; Moro et al. 2010; Rodriguez-Oroz et al. 2005; Volkmann et al. 2009; Sauleau et al. 2009). Although STN-DBS can reduce levodopa dosages after surgery (Machado et al. 2006), it is also more frequently associated with cognitive impairments and psychogenic complications. However, while GPi-DBS rarely reduces medication dosage, it carries a lower risk of neuropsychological complications. Moreover, GPi-DBS strongly inhibits PD-related involuntary movements, such as drug-induced dyskinesia and painful dystonia. Camptocormia is also reduced by GPi-DBS.

M. Ogura, MD, PhD
Department of Neurological Surgery,
Wakayama Medical University, Wakayama, Japan
e-mail: ogura@wakayama-med.ac.jp

Because there are unique characteristics associated with the stimulation of the STN or GPi, target selection should depend on the clinical features of each patient. For instance, GPi-DBS should be chosen for those patients in whom the thresholds of levodopa-induced dyskinesia and psychological abnormalities are low.

The most important step of DBS surgery is accurate electrode placement. This requires identifying the optimal target and introducing the electrode lead to the target appropriately. Here, the surgical procedures of GPi-DBS for PD are reviewed.

8.2 History of Pallidal Surgery

The world's first stereotactic operation was a pallidotomy performed in 1947 on a patient with Huntington's chorea by using a stereotactic instrument developed by Spiegel and Wycis (Spiegel et al. 1947). The dawn rose on stereotactic operations in 1954 when a pallidoansotomy was performed on a patient with PD (Spiegel and Wycis 1954), while Hassler et al. conducted a ventral lateral thalamotomy. At the same time, Narabayashi et al. performed a pallidotomy by injecting procaine oil into patients with PD. Leksell improved pallidotomies by targeting the posterior ventral region of the globus pallidus, which is the region of origin for the ansa lenticularis. The long-term effects of such operations

T. Itakura (ed.), *Deep Brain Stimulation for Neurological Disorders: Theoretical Background and Clinical Application*, DOI 10.1007/978-3-319-08476-3_8,

were reported by Svennilson et al. (1960), and showed that pallidotomies are effective at reducing rigidity and tremor, in addition to akinesia.

However, stereotactic surgeons in the latter half of the 1950s became more interested in ventral lateral and ventral intermediate thalamotomies, while the pallidotomy proposed by Hassler et al. was all but forgotten and Leksell's pallidotomy was no longer in demand. The temporary decrease in the number of stereotactic operations was concomitant with the popularization of levodopa therapy. As the limitations of levodopa therapy became clear, however, there was renewed interest in stereotactic operations. In 1992, Laitinen et al. reinvigorated Leksell's pallidotomy, and the posterior ventral pallidotomy was widely received for its ability to relieve rigidity and akinesia in contrast to thalamotomies, which were effective only at reducing tremors. Benabid et al. (1987) reported on thalamic ventral intermediate nucleus stimulation therapy for tremors. Assessments of its safety and regulation led to the application of DBS in bilateral operations, which resulted in a high frequency of side effects in an ablation surgery. Siegfried and Lippitz (1994) performed GPi-DBS, thus popularizing DBS.

8.3 Anatomy and Physiology of the Globus Pallidus

The GPi forms a banana shape, with the globus pallidus externus (GPe) located dorsolaterally, the internal capsule located caudally, and the optic tract (OT) located ventrally. The volume of the GPi in humans is approximately 500 mm^3, which is three times larger than the STN (150 mm^3) (Guridi et al. 2000); however, the optimal stimulation site is not large. Thus, a better anatomical understanding of the GPi is needed.

The GPi is an output nucleus that projects information integrated in the basal ganglia to the thalamus (Albin et al. 1989; Alexander and Crutcher 1990; Smith et al. 1998). The projection fiber is comprised of the ansa lenticularis and the lenticular fasciculus (Forel's H2 field), and projects to the lateral ventral nucleus of the thalamus. The corpus striatum, which acts as the input nucleus for the basal ganglia, receives projections from the cerebral cortex, and sends inhibitory projections to the GPe, GPi, and substantia nigra pars reticulata (SNr) (Fig. 8.1). The direct pathway is responsible for the direct projection from the corpus striatum to the GPi/SNr, while the indirect pathway goes through the GPe or the STN to the GPi/SNr. The output nucleus of the basal ganglia, the GPi/SNr, projects to the thalamus; information from the thalamus is sent back to the cerebral cortex or corpus striatum. Dopaminergic cells in the substantia nigra pars compacta (SNc) send projections to the corpus striatum that have excitatory effects on neurons of the direct pathway and inhibitory effects on neurons of the indirect pathway (Levy et al. 1997).

The optimal stimulatory site for GPi-DBS in the treatment of PD is the sensorimotor region located in the posterior ventrolateral region of the GPi. The association system loop projects dorsally to the GPi. Moreover, the rostromedial part of the GPi contains projections from the limbic system. The sensorimotor region of the GPi is somatotopically organized, with the face and upper and lower limbs arranged in order from the ventral to dorsal side.

As previously stated, the GPi is a larger nucleus compared to the STN. However, accurate targeting in the sensorimotor region reduces the transport of stimulatory effects to the limbic system, and reduces the risk of neuropsychological side effects.

8.4 Surgical Methods

8.4.1 Patient Selection

Patient selection is a critical step for obtaining optimal benefits and decreasing morbidity. Several factors should be considered when determining if a patient is a suitable candidate for GPi-DBS. The most important point is to confirm that a patient has been diagnosed with idiopathic PD prior to surgery (Bronte-Stewart 2003). Patients with other Parkinson syndromes, such as

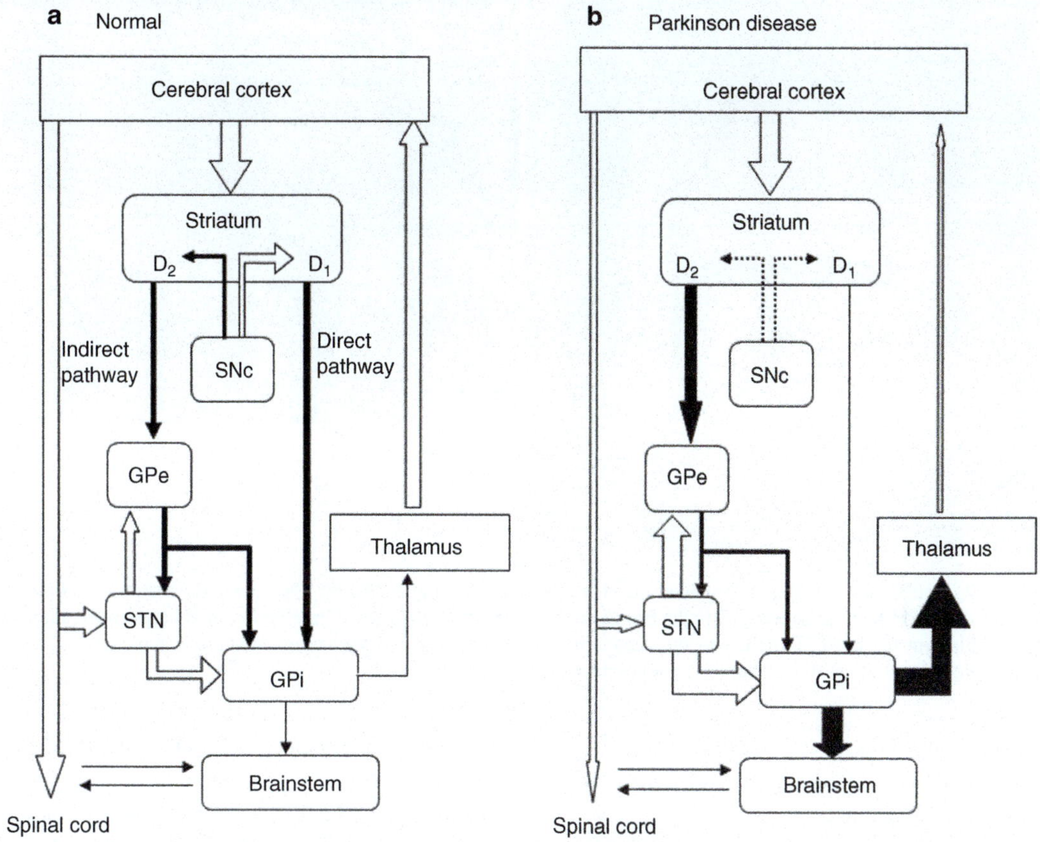

Fig. 8.1 Schematic diagram of the basal ganglia–thalamocortical circuitry under normal conditions (**a**) and in Parkinson's disease (**b**). In Parkinson's disease, decreased excitatory inputs from the substantia nigra compacta (*SNc*) to striatal D1 neurons lead to the disinhibition of globus pallidus internus (*GPi*) neurons and increase the inhibitory output to the thalamus (direct pathway). Decreased inhibitory projection from the SNc leads to the disinhibition of striatal D2 neurons, and inhibition of globus pallidus externus (*GPe*) neurons. Decreased GPe activity induces overactivation of the subthalamic nucleus (*STN*) and consequently of the GPi (indirect pathway). *Black arrows* inhibitory projections, *white arrows* excitatory projections

progressive supranuclear palsy (PSP) and multiple system atrophy (MSA), will not benefit from DBS surgery. Therefore, a patient's response to levodopa is the best indicator of suitability for GPi-DBS. Severe drug-induced dyskinesia and motor fluctuations, such as wearing-off and on-off phenomena, impair the abilities of daily living despite appropriate medication therapy. The long-term problems associated with levodopa therapy may occur anywhere from 3 to 10 years after treatment initiation, but GPi-DBS can improve these symptoms. Tremor is also fairly suppressed by GPi-DBS as well as thalamic (Vim) stimulation. Nevertheless, it is not advisable to use either STN-DBS or GPi-DBS in elderly patients with brain atrophy and those with dementia.

8.4.2 Preoperative Preparation

Preoperative assessment is essential for evaluating a patient's suitability for surgery and their risk of poor postoperative outcome and complications. Videotaped recordings of the patient's behaviors are useful for comparing pre- and postoperative statuses. The Unified Parkinson's Disease Rating Score (UPDRS) is a widely used rating scale for following the course and symptoms of PD, and patients should be assessed both on and off

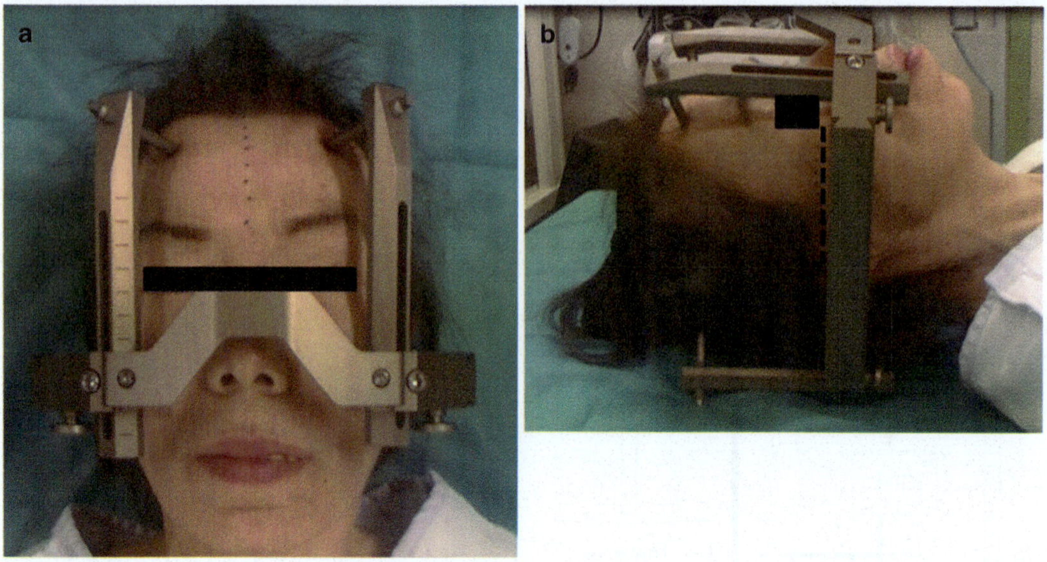

Fig. 8.2 Application of the stereotactic head frame (Leksell). (*Left*) The head is centered in the frame, so that the midline on the head is aligned to the center of the frame. Note the midline of the head is parallel to the posts of the frame. (*Right*) The lateral view shows the base of the frame is placed parallel to a line between the inferior orbital rim and the external auditory canal

medication. Neuropsychological testing is also necessary to evaluate patients for dementia and cognitive disturbance.

The night prior to surgery, antiparkinsonian medications are usually stopped to permit the pronouncement of PD symptoms during surgery. Any anticoagulant and platelet aggregation medications should be discontinued at least 7–10 days preoperatively to avoid intracerebral hemorrhage, which is the most serious complication associated with stereotactic surgery.

8.4.3 Stereotactic Frame Application

Stereotactic surgery is performed under local anesthesia; a mixture of lidocaine, marcaine, and epinephrine are injected into the frame pin site. An appropriate dose of propofol can be given prior to pin insertion to minimize suffering when placing the frame. During surgery, care should be taken to maintain blood pressure within a normal range to avoid intracerebral hemorrhage.

A variety of stereotactic head frames are available, such as Leksell, CRW, and Riechert–Mundinger. Surgical procedure details differ between institutes, and stereotactic surgeons should master the use of their institution's apparatus. During frame placement, it is important to place the frame with its axes orthogonal to the standard anatomical planes of the brain (Machado et al. 2006; Starr 2002) (Fig. 8.2). Earplugs may be used to facilitate straight frame placement while applying the pins. Moreover, the base of the frame should be applied parallel to a line between the inferior orbital rim and the external auditory canal, which is approximately parallel to the anterior commissure–posterior commissure (AC–PC) line. When indirect targeting is used, it is important to lay axial targeting image planes coplanar to the AC–PC plane, as the placement will be less accurate if deviations are present between both planes.

Once the frame is in place, preoperative imaging, such as computed tomography (CT), magnetic resonance imaging (MRI), and ventriculography, is performed to construct the stereotactic images required for DBS surgery. Several image-guided software systems are available to integrate data sets from multiple imaging methods. We use a StealthStation Framelink

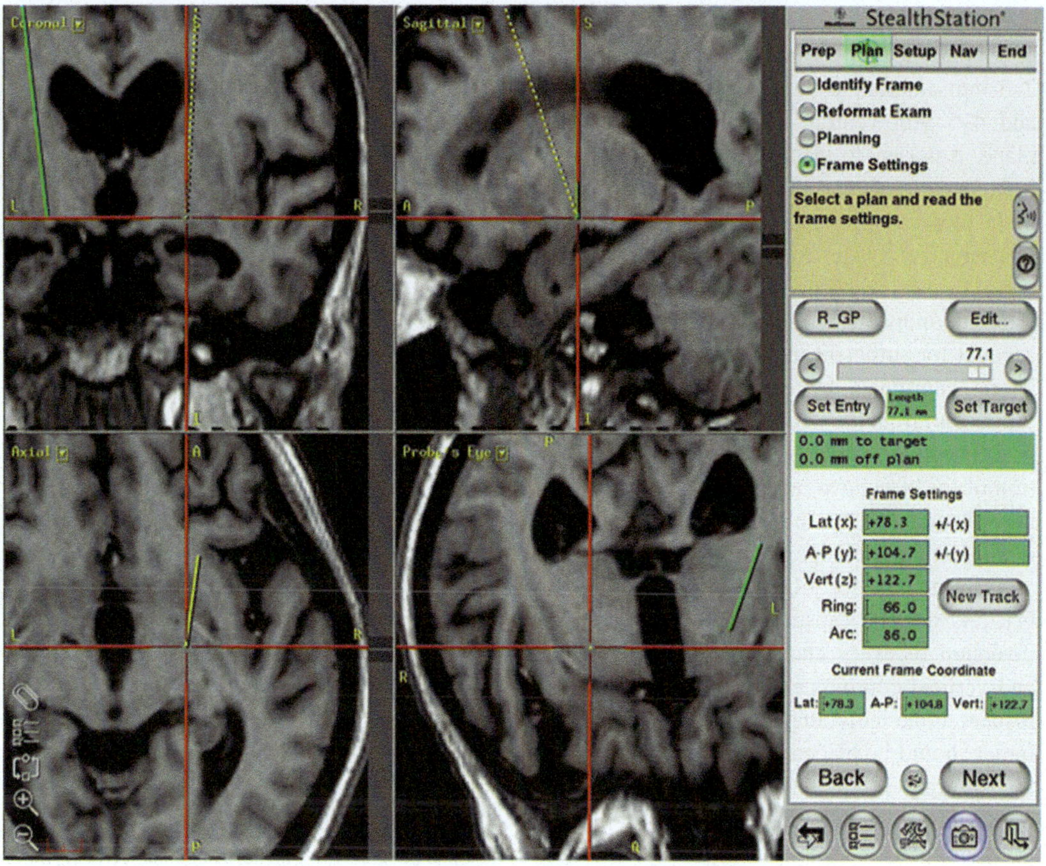

Fig. 8.3 Determining the target and planning the trajectory by using the T1-magnetization-prepared rapid gradient-echo (MPRage) sequence on the software StealthStation Framelink. The trajectory avoids the lateral ventricle while targeting the globus pallidus internus (GPi)

package (Medtronic navigation, Louisville, CO) to generate integrated images by fusing MR images obtained preoperatively without the frame, with CT images obtained immediately after frame placement (Fig. 8.3). The CT images are always used as the main reference during surgery.

8.4.4 Operative Procedures

The most important step of GPi-DBS surgery is accurate electrode placement into the optimal portion of the GPi. To do this, it is important to perform each of the three steps in the operative procedure appropriately, including target setting, microelectrode recordings (MERs), and macrostimulations.

8.4.5 Target Setting

There are two methods for defining the initial anatomical target in GPi: direct and indirect targeting. Indirect targeting is based on a standardized stereotactic atlas established on AC and PC landmarks. Direct targeting is based on the imaging data set of an individual's own anatomy (Lemaire et al. 1999). Direct targeting seems to have obvious benefits over the indirect method; however, both of these techniques have disadvantages. We employ a hybrid of these two methods to define the initial target.

Indirect targeting has been the traditional method employed in stereotactic neurosurgery. It is based on a standardized stereotactic atlas, and uses fixed distances from the midcommissural point (Pallavaram et al. 2008). The typical GPi coordinates are 19–21 mm lateral to the midline, 2–3 mm anterior to the midcommissural point, and 4–5 mm ventral to the intercommissural plane. It is easy to identify the commissures on MRI, and target coordinates are readily available in the literature. However, a disadvantage of indirect targeting is the existence of discrete variations in the anatomy of the brain between different individuals. Care should be taken to account for sufficient individual variation in the lateral coordinate by expanding the range to 16–23 mm from the midline.

Direct targeting is based on MRI visualization of the structures, and it is helpful for making fine adjustments to the indirect coordinates in an attempt to compensate for individual variation in nuclear location. As the GPi, adjacent OT, and internal capsule can be visualized via inversion recovery and T2 images, the lateral and vertical coordinates are then checked with respect to the individual's nuclear anatomy. The target should be placed in the posterior third of the ventral GPi directly over the OT, which passes just ventral to the motor territory of the GPi, and can be used as a targeting landmark. When the borders of the GPi are not perfectly visualized, the vertical and lateral coordinates can be checked to ensure that they correspond to the dorsal border of the OT on a coronal T1-MR image in 3D mode, just traversing the mamillary bodies (Fig. 8.4).

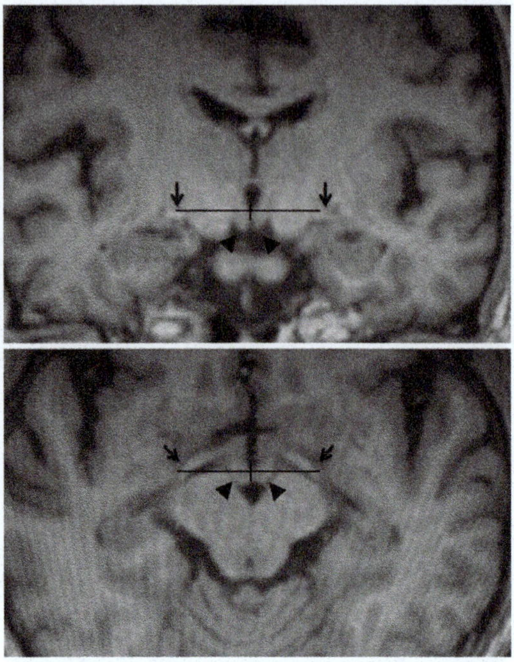

Fig. 8.4 Stereotactic targeting of the globus pallidus internus (GPi) on the reformatted T1-magnetization-prepared rapid gradient-echo (MPRage) images. (*Upper*) Coronal image at 3 mm anterior to the midcommissural point, which usually traverses the mamillary bodies. (*Lower*) Axial image passing through the dorsal border of the optic tracts (OTs). The horizontal and vertical coordinates are determined from the dorsal border of the OT. *Arrowheads* mamillary body, *arrows* optic tracts

8.4.6 Patient Position and Opening

The head frame is secured to the operating table by using the Mayfield with an adaptor. The patient is positioned supine on the operating table, with the knees flexed and the head of the table elevated to about 30°. This position avoids cerebrospinal fluid (CSF) leakage and prevents excessive intraoperative brain shift (Fig. 8.5).

The entry point and final trajectory are established using T1-MRI in 3D mode with the aid of planning software to avoid the ventricles, sulci, and vessels along the electrode trajectory. We usually place the burr hole 1–2 cm anterior to the coronal suture and 2.5–3 cm from the midline. The planned burr hole sites are anesthetized, and the scalp is incised in a semicircular fashion (Fig. 8.6).

8.4.7 MERs

Several factors may prevent targeting accuracy when only preoperative image sets are used; therefore, image-guided anatomical targeting alone is not sufficient for optimally placing a DBS lead (Guridi et al. 2000; Starr 2002).

The accuracy of targeting is limited by the mechanical properties of the stereotactic system itself. Moreover, anatomic targeting precision can be decreased by MRI slice thickness and distortion effects, brain shift due to CSF leakage during surgery, and imperfect visualization of the

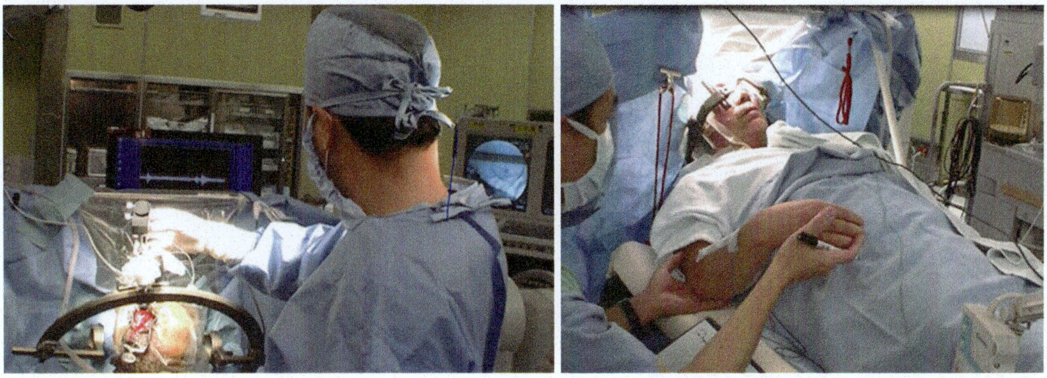

Fig. 8.5 Operative setup and patient positioning. (*Left*) The sterile area is located at the top of the patient's head. The C-arm is draped. The monitors displaying the microelectrode recordings and fluoroscopic image are placed over the operating table, such that the surgeon can easily view the monitors during the procedures. (*Right*) The patient is positioned supine with the head of the table elevated. The sterile transparent drape acts as a barrier between the sterile head area and the nonsterile area where the examiner stands, while providing good visualization of the patient's face during the surgery

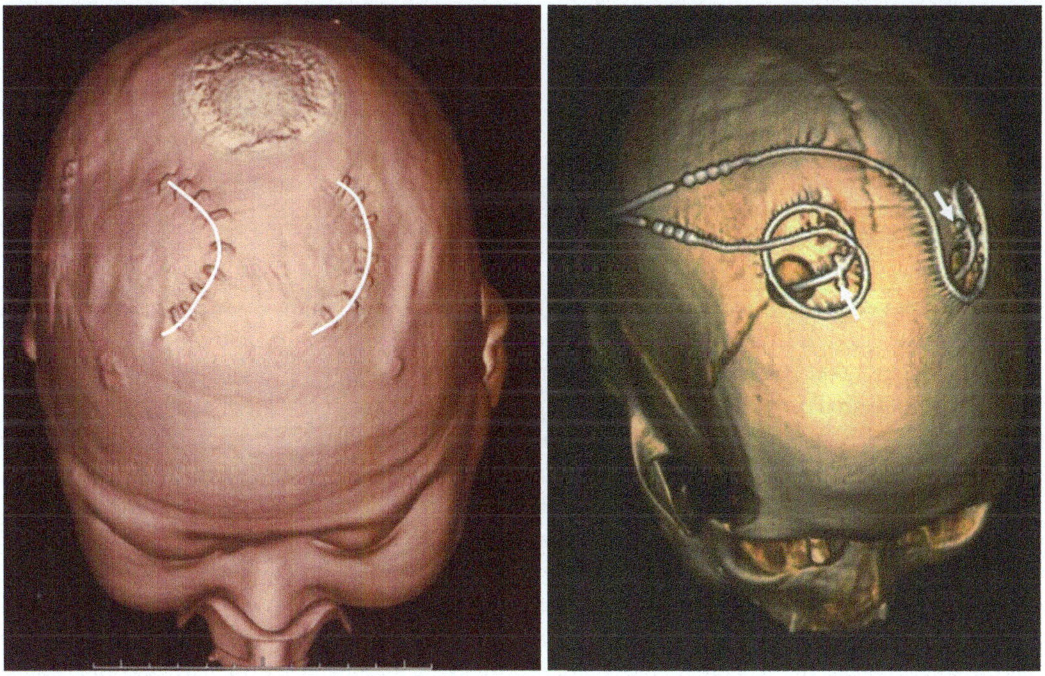

Fig. 8.6 Postoperative 3D-computed tomography (CT) images showing the location of the skin incisions (*left, semicircular lines*) and burr holes (*right*). The deep brain stimulation (DBS) leads were fixed using titanium miniplates (*right, arrows*)

GPi. Hence, physiological studies are important for confirming or adjusting final placement.

Using MER, the structures surrounding the GPi that will be traversed by the electrode can be identified on the basis of their characteristic firing patterns. Furthermore, efficacy and side effects are assessed by macrostimulation. As the electrode passes in close proximity to neurons, the unit activity from the neurons is transmitted through the microelectrode and displayed on a computer monitor.

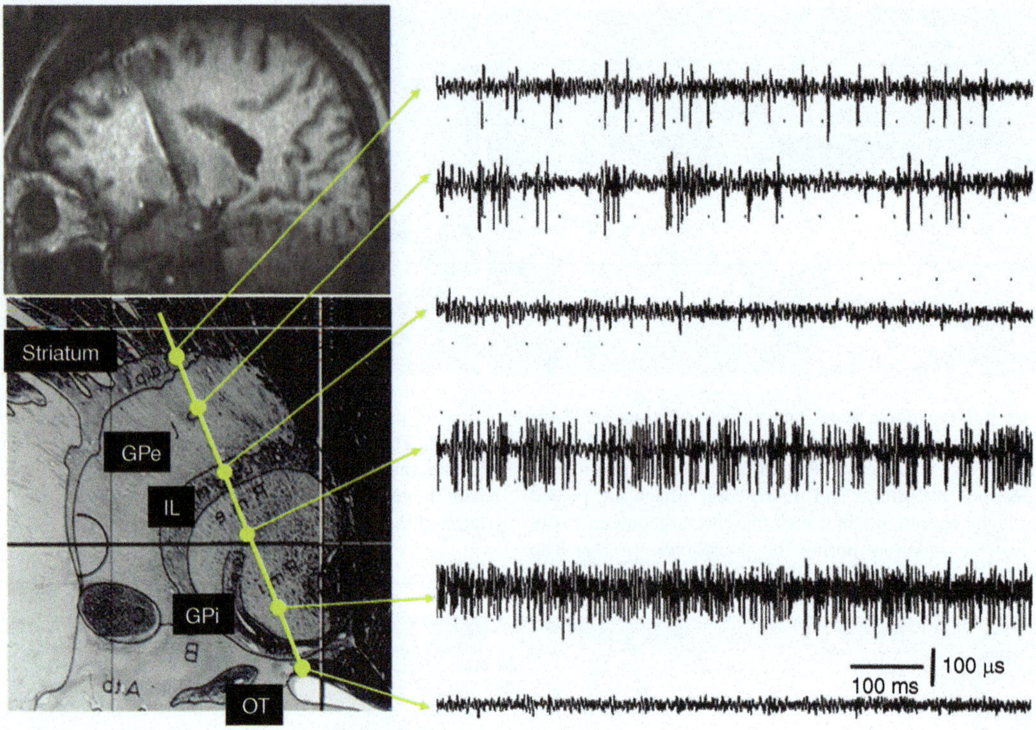

Fig. 8.7 Chart showing the characteristic neuronal activity of a typical track targeting the globus pallidus internus (*GPi*). The microelectrode passes through the striatum, globus pallidus externus (*GPe*), and internal laminae (*IL*), and finally enters the GPi, where a high-frequency tonic neuronal activity is recorded. Note the ventral position of the optic tract (*OT*)

Usually, single-unit extracellular action potentials are recorded using high-impedance (0.1–1.0 MΩ at 1,000 Hz) tungsten or platinum-iridium microelectrodes, with a 15- to 25-μm tip diameter. The impedance of larger electrode tips is too low to make single-unit discriminations from neuronal activity recorded near the tip. The impedance of smaller-sized electrode tips is higher; thus, only single cells with lower background recordings are achieved. The MERs are started from 20 mm above to 4 mm below the potential target, depending on individual anatomical findings. The neuronal activity in each brain structure has a characteristic pattern (Fig. 8.7). The major structures identified by MER are the striatum, GPe and GPi, internal and external medullary laminae, nucleus basalis, OT, and internal capsule (Vitek et al. 1998).

8.4.7.1 Striatum

The microelectrode typically first encounters striatal cells, and then GPe cells prior to reaching the GPi. The striatum is separated from the GPe by the external laminae. Striatal neurons mainly have low spontaneous discharge rates (lower than 10 Hz) with a tonic pattern and have a relatively long duration with high-amplitude action potentials.

8.4.7.2 GPe

In the GPe, two distinct patterns of spontaneous activity are recorded. Most GPe neurons fire in a regular fashion with high-frequency discharges of 30–60 Hz separated irregularly by brief pauses. Approximately 10–20 % of GPe neurons fire at a low frequency (around 10 Hz) with high-frequency, short-duration bursts.

8.4.7.3 GPi

The GPi is separated from the GPe by an approximately 1-mm-thick internal laminae of white matter that can be identified by the lack of cellular activity and the frequent presence of border cells.

After passing the internal laminae, the entrance to the GPi is easily recognized by a sharp, distinct increase in activity. In the GPi, neurons generally have a tonic discharge pattern with a high frequency (higher than 70 Hz in PD), but without the distinct pauses observed in the GPe. In addition, some neurons fire synchronously with the patient's tremor (tremor-related cells).

The location of the sensorimotor region of the GPi is found predominantly in the structures' posterolateral portions. A substantial number of neurons in the motor region modulate their firing rate in response to passive manipulations and active movement of the extremities and orofacial structures on the contralateral side of the body. The anteromedial region of the GPi is related to nonmotor associative functions; this finding is consistent with those of animal experiments. There is a general somatotopic organization in the motor region of the GPi. Cells representing the leg tend to be more dorsal and medial to those representing the arm and face. The base of the GPi can be identified by an abrupt diminution in neuronal activity as the microelectrode exits the GPi, at which point border cells may be encountered.

Approximately 1–2 mm below the inferior margin of the GPi is the OT. There is usually no spontaneous activity within the OT, and although monophasic spikes are sometimes recorded, they can be identified as OT by light-evoked fiber activity. Microstimulation evokes visual sensations at currents less than 20 μA.

During typical penetration through the longer central extent of the GPi, the neuronal activity in a 6-mm-long segment of the GPi is recorded, and the OT is identified 2 mm below the GPi base. If the region of GPi neuronal activity is shorter than 6 mm and the OT cannot be identified, it is possible that the track was not optimal, and a second track should be considered.

Subsequent tracks should be at least 2 mm away from the first track. The second track is made either anterior or posterior to the initial track to confirm the posterior border, depending on the apparent location of the first track within the GPi. Additional tracks are made either laterally or medially to delineate the lateral border of the GPi.

8.4.8 Macrostimulation

Prior to internalizing the lead, we perform a final location check by testing it intraoperatively with macrostimulation, which can elicit visual, motor, or cutaneous sensory responses by affecting structures near the probe. Rigidity; finger tap; opening and closing of hand; heeltap; and observations of tremor, voice, and vision are recorded during test stimulation. Owing to the proximity of the internal capsule and OT, it is important to determine the threshold of stimulation-induced phenomena. The corticobulbar tract (CBT) and corticospinal tract (CST) in the internal capsule are identified by evoking muscle contractions. If dysarthria, conjugate eye movement, or tonic facial contraction is elicited at low stimulation thresholds, the lead is too close to the CBT and should be moved posterolaterally. If muscle contractions of the contralateral hand and leg are evoked at low stimulation thresholds, the lead is too close to the CST and should be moved anterolaterally. If CBT- or CST-related responses are not observed at high intensity stimulation, it indicates electrode failure or poor positioning (too anterior, lateral, or superior) (Fig. 8.8).

As the typical thresholds of CBT/CST responses evoked by Lead Point electrodes (Medtronic, Louisville, CO) are within a range of 3–5 mA, a trajectory with a threshold of <2.5 or >5 mA is not optimal. Because the OT passes beneath the motor region of the GPi, if an optimal track inferior to the GPi is stimulated, most patients report transient visual flashes. Although intraoperative test stimulation is not used for assessing therapeutic benefits, if a tremor is present, it is immediately reduced during test stimulation. Other symptoms besides tremor do not respond intraoperatively.

Motor symptoms in PD may be either partially or completely suppressed by mechanical insertion of the electrode itself without electrical stimulation. Observation of this so-called microlesion effect is evidence that the electrode is positioned appropriately within the motor region of the GPi, even though failure to observe a microlesion effect does not necessarily predict a poor chronic stimulation outcome.

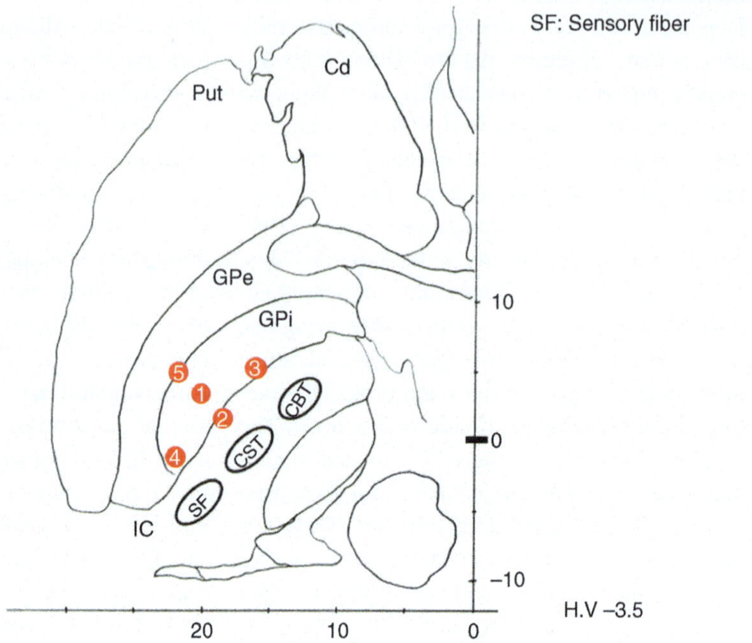

Fig. 8.8 Macrostimulation-induced phenomena and possible electrode locations. ① Optimum location: usually, tremor and dyskinesia disappear. Rigidity also diminishes. ② Medial shift: muscle contractions of the contralateral hand and leg are evoked at a low stimulation threshold because of the activation of the corticospinal tract (*CST*). ③ Anteromedial shift: dysarthria, conjugate eye movement, or tonic facial contraction is elicited because of the activation of the corticobulbar tract (*CBT*). ④ Posterior shift: numbness is evoked on the contralateral face and hand because of the activation of the sensory fiber (*SF*). ⑤ Lateral shift: no evoked responses are shown during a high-intensity stimulation

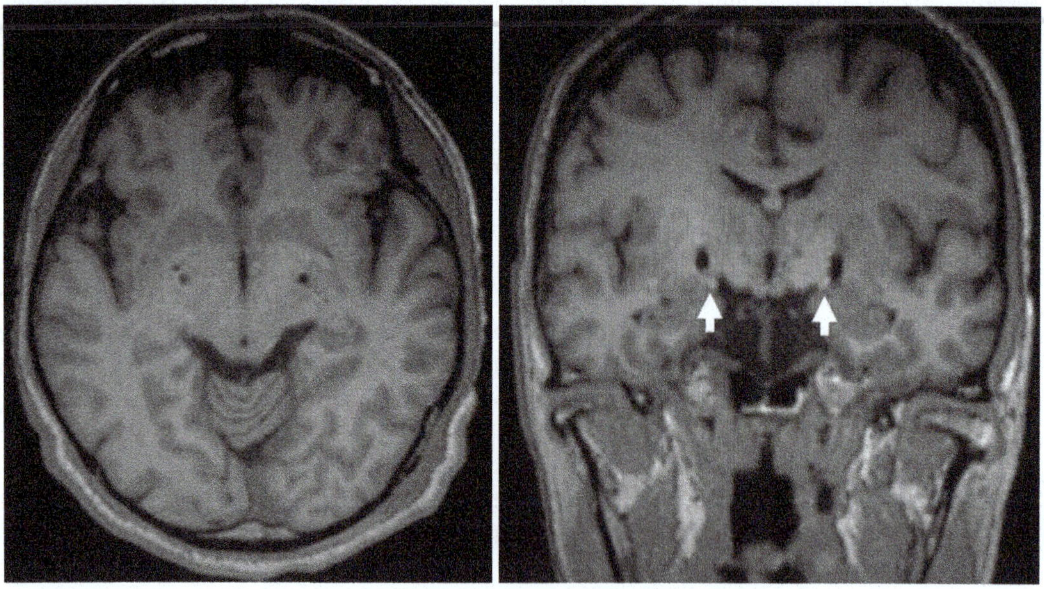

Fig. 8.9 Axial (*left*) and coronal (*right*) T1-weighted postoperative magnetic resonance (MR) images showing the electrodes in the globus pallidus. Note the location of the electrode tips dorsolateral to the optic tracts (*arrows*)

8.4.9 Electrode Placement

Once the optimal track for electrode implantation has been determined using MERs and macrostimulations, the microelectrode is replaced with the DBS (Fig. 8.9) lead under fluoroscopic monitoring. Additional test stimulation, especially for side effects, is also commonly performed using the DBS lead. Usually, bipolar stimulation with a pulse width of 90 μs and a rate of 130 Hz is performed at contact 0 (the most ventral contact of the lead) as cathodes with the extracranial end are attached to the Medtronic model 3625 hand-held pulse generator. If corticospinal activation, dysarthria, and conjugate eye deviation occur below 3 V, the surgeon should consider moving the lead.

8.4.10 Implantation of the Pulse Generator

After the final confirmation of appropriate track position and depth, the cannula is withdrawn over the DBS electrode under fluoroscopic monitoring. The stylet is removed from the DBS lead and the electrode is attached to the cranium by using titanium microplates. Implantation of the implantable pulse generator (IPG) is performed under general anesthesia; the patient is positioned supine with the head turned away from the side of implant, similar to a ventriculoperitoneal shunt procedure. Because the IPG should be placed in a location that minimizes pressure and trauma to the unit, the most common location for IPG implantation is the infraclavicular area. The generator should be placed at least 2 cm below the clavicle or 3 cm away from the shoulder joint so that the IPG does not rub against either structure, which may cause pain. If the IPG is placed in an area other than the infraclavicular area, it should be positioned away from any bony prominence, such as the rib or the iliac crest.

An infraclavicular incision several centimeters long is made parallel to the clavicle, and a subcutaneous pocket is dissected between the pectoralis muscle and its fascia. Care should be taken to place the generator at a depth of no more than 2 cm from the skin surface, as greater depths may impede the programmer's ability to communicate with the generator. From a small parietal incision to the infraclavicular pocket, a tunnel is made using the tunneling device and the extension wire is pulled up from the chest. The extension wire is then connected with the DBS lead proximally and the IPG distally.

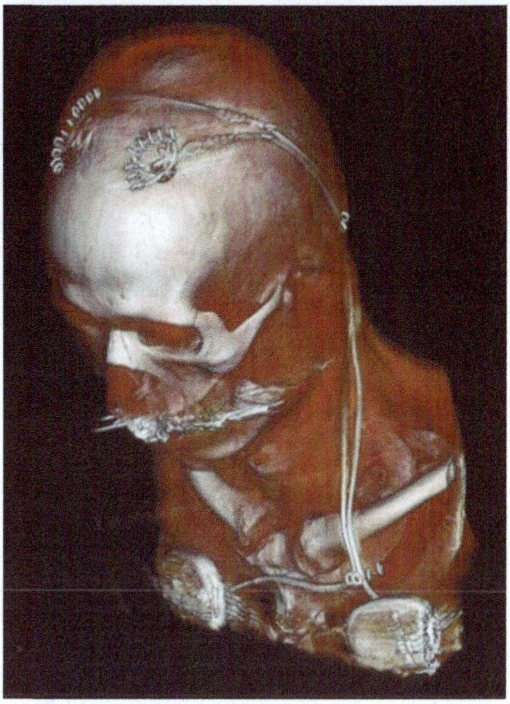

Fig. 8.10 Postoperative 3D-computed tomography (CT) image showing the subcutaneous course of the extension wires and infraclavicular placement of the implantable pulse generators (IPGs)

The connector on the lead extender should be placed at the upper part of the temporal muscle, 2–4 cm posterior to the auricle. If the connector is placed near the ear, it can cause erosion and discomfort while wearing glasses. If it is located too posteriorly, it may cause pain during sleep by contacting the greater occipital nerves when in a supine position. If it is placed in the neck below the mastoid, mobility at the lead-connector junction can cause hardware failure. Once the appropriate position has been established, the generator is placed in its pocket and the excess extension lead is coiled behind the generator. Finally, the skin is closed after sufficient irrigation of the wounds (Fig. 8.10).

8.5 Postoperative Management

Immediately after surgery, it is important to maintain arterial blood pressure in the normal range to prevent cerebral hemorrhage.

Postoperative CT or MRI is performed to evaluate electrode location and intracranial status. Plain radiography of the head and chest are also performed to assess the location and geometry of the leads, extension wire, and IPG. Side effects and efficacy are systematically evaluated under each stimulation condition, including active contacts, intensity, frequency, and pulse duration. The most effective contact for the patient is then selected for chronic stimulation.

8.6 Surgical Results

GPi-DBS is a well-established treatment option for the motor fluctuations and dyskinesia of advanced PD (Ghika et al. 1998; Gross et al. 1997; Kumar et al. 2000; Volkmann et al. 1998). A number of randomized controlled trials have been conducted in clinical investigations of GPi-DBS. In a comparative study of 121 DBS-treated patients (61 GPi-DBS and 60 STN-DBS) and 134 patients receiving best medical therapy, off-period motor function improved significantly in the DBS group at the 6-month time point (Weaver et al. 2009). Furthermore, prolongation of on time without troubling dyskinesia was observed. Additionally, GPi-DBS improves off-period UPDRS part-III scores by approximately 40 %, whereas improvement during the on-period was less (20–30 %). Short-term effects measured 1 year postoperatively demonstrated improvements in all subscores (tremor, rigidity, akinesia, gait, instability, and speech).

The most beneficial characteristic of GPi-DBS is its ability to suppress levodopa-induced dyskinesia. In a number of reports, postoperative dyskinesia scores improved by 70–80 % compared to preoperative scores (Andrade et al. 2009; Rodrigues et al. 2007a; Rouaud et al. 2010; Weaver et al. 2005; Rodriguez-Oroz et al. 2005; Ogura et al. 2004). Levodopa reductions do not occur with GPi-DBS; therefore, the suppressive effects of dyskinesia have been thought to be a direct effect of the stimulation. Thus, the wearing-off can be reduced by improving motor function during the off-period and improving dyskinesia during the on-period.

In studies comparing the clinical effects of different GPi stimulation sites (Krack et al. 1998; Bejjani et al. 1997), posterior ventral stimulation of the GPi improved muscular rigidity and dyskinesia dramatically in the on-state; however, gait disturbance and akinesia can worsen in the off-state. In contrast, stimulation of the dorsal part of the GPi led to improvements in gait disturbance, akinesia, and muscle rigidity; however, increasing the stimulation intensity can induce dyskinesia. Central stimulation is thought to have a combined improvement effect on both posterior ventral and dorsal stimulation. These findings need to be taken into consideration when determining the optimal target for surgical treatment of PD.

After GPi-DBS, the improvement of motor function in the off-period can be maintained for about 4–5 years; however, the effects in the on-period gradually decrease over time. Worsening axial signs, such as instability and speech, are notable; however, the suppressive effects on dyskinesia are maintained in the long term. In 152 GPi-DBS patients assessed 2 years after surgery, the UPDRS motor score did not change compared to the 6-month motor score (Follett et al. 2010), indicating a maintained stimulatory effect. Moreover, in a multicenter study investigating the long-term effects at 3–4 and 5–6 years after surgery (Moro et al. 2010; Rodriguez-Oroz et al. 2005), the off-period UPDRS part-III scores maintained a 35.6 % improvement at 5–6 years postoperatively. All motor subscores improved 3–4 years postoperatively, except postural instability and speech scores, whereas only tremors, muscle rigidity, and activities of daily living (ADL) improved significantly 5–6 years postoperatively. However, during the on-period, motor UPDRS improvement was not observed 5–6 years postoperatively, and it worsened compared to the 3–4 year mark. Analysis of each motor subscore revealed a 75 % improvement of dyskinesia that was maintained. A reduction in improvement was not observed after 5–6 years; however, all other criteria worsened, most notably speech. In addition, in a meta-analysis (St George et al. 2010) of the long-term effects of DBS on gait and postural instability, the improvement effect of

GPi-DBS was maintained over 5 years for the primary symptoms, such as tremor, muscle rigidity, and akinesia. However, gait and postural instability worsened during the on-period.

8.7 Comparison of the Effects of STN-DBS and GPi-DBS

Through studies comparing STN-DBS and GPi-DBS, the characteristics of GPi-DBS have become clear. For instance, in a meta-analysis (Weaver et al. 2005) of 31 STN-DBS and 14 GPi-DBS studies, no significant differences in the improvements of the UPDRS part-III scores at 6 months after operation were detected between STN-DBS (54 %) and GPi-DBS (40 %). Similarly, both STN-DBS and GPi-DBS demonstrated a 40 % improvement in ADL; however, GPi-DBS showed improvement during both the on- and off-periods, whereas STN-DBS showed improvement only during the off-period. Randomized comparative studies (Follett et al. 2010; Anderson et al. 2005; Zahodne et al. 2009; Okun et al. 2009; Nakamura et al. 2007) and nonrandomized comparative studies (Moro et al. 2010; Rodriguez-Oroz et al. 2005; Volkmann et al. 2009; Sauleau et al. 2009; Group TD-BSfPsDS 2001) have both shown that motor function and ADL improvement were equal between STN-DBS and GPi-DBS; however, adverse events, such as cognitive and neuropsychological disorders, occurred more frequently with STN-DBS.

Interestingly, a clear difference was observed with regard to levodopa dosage reduction. Levodopa dosages decreased 52 % with STN-DBS, whereas no such decrease was observed with GPi-DBS. Both comparative and noncomparative studies have confirmed that the medication dosages were not reduced in patients who had undergone GPi-DBS.

The Cognition and Mood in Parkinson's disease in STN versus GPi-DBS (COMPARE) trial was a randomized study that compared the nonmotor effects of both STN-DBS and GPi-DBS (Zahodne et al. 2009; Okun et al. 2009; Taba et al. 2010). The results from this trial have shown that there were no significant differences in the co-primary outcome measures (mood and cognition) between STN and GPi in the optimal DBS state. A worsening of letter verbal fluency was seen in STN-DBS. Additionally, the trial also measured weight gain over time and found that in 70 % of the patients with GPi-DBS, the average weight gain was 10.65 ± 6.98 lbs, which was comparable to that with STN-DBS (Locke et al. 2011; Sauleau et al. 2009).

Although significant differences were not observed with respect to motor function improvement after either GPi-DBS or STN-DBS, differences were apparent in nonmotor symptoms. Therefore, nonmotor factors may be considered when selecting a surgical target for DBS (Follett et al. 2010; Rodrigues et al. 2007b). GPi-DBS is more suitable in certain patients, such as those with a low levodopa-induced threshold for dyskinesia (Minguez-Castellanos et al. 2005) and those with a high risk for neurological disorders (Rouaud et al. 2010).

8.8 Complications

Complications of GPi-DBS include intracranial bleeding, infection, skin erosion, and lead breakage. Combined with minor troubles, complications occur at a rate of 10–20 %. A major complication during surgery is cerebral hemorrhage due to vascular injury during insertion of the leads (Hariz et al. 2008). The frequency of cerebral hemorrhage is about 1–2 %. Since an increased number of microelectrode insertions can increase the risk of intracranial bleeding, caution must be taken. Neuropsychological complications, including cognitive impairment, hallucinations/delusions, depression/apathy/anxiety, and disturbed consciousness, can arise through GPi-DBS. However, the frequency of these complications is relatively low with GPi-DBS compared to STN-DBS. Adverse symptoms induced by electrical stimulation include headache, nausea, scintillation, muscle contraction of the face and limbs, numbness, and abnormal eye movements. However, many of those symptoms are temporary, occurring only within several seconds to several minutes after the start of the stimulations.

Conclusion

The most important step of GPi-DBS surgery is the accurate placement of the electrode within the optimal target region. To do so, care must be taken in each step of the surgery. First, the stereotactic head frame should be attached with its axes orthogonal to the standard anatomical planes of the brain. A hybrid of direct and indirect targeting is then employed for initial anatomical target localization. To compensate for individual anatomical variation of the nucleus, direct visualization helps to make fine adjustments to the indirect targeting. Image-guided stereotactic targeting alone is not sufficient to place a DBS lead accurately. Therefore, physiological studies are important to confirm or adjust electrode placement. Using MERs, the motor region of the target can be determined from characteristic patterns of spontaneous discharge, and by mapping movement-related neurons during passive movement examination. Furthermore, the ventral boundaries of the GPi can be identified in real time. Based on MER, macrostimulation is performed at the level of the selected target to determine the threshold for the internal capsule response.

Both the GPi and STN are viable DBS targets for the treatment of motor symptoms, and the therapeutic benefits are similar for both surgical targets. The advantages and disadvantages of STN-DBS or GPi-DBS should be recognized conclusively. Cognitive or behavioral side effects were less frequently encountered in patients treated with GPi-DBS, while a significant reduction in the daily dose of levodopa was achieved in patients with STN-DBS. Therefore, the selection of a DBS target may be tailored on the basis of each patient's therapeutic need and nonmotor symptom risk profiles. If cognitive or behavioral issues are of concern, GPi-DBS should be considered.

References

Albin RL, Young AB, Penney JB (1989) The functional anatomy of basal ganglia disorders. Trends Neurosci 12(10):366–375

Alexander GE, Crutcher MD (1990) Functional architecture of basal ganglia circuits: neural substrates of parallel processing. Trends Neurosci 13(7):266–271

Anderson VC, Burchiel KJ, Hogarth P et al (2005) Pallidal vs subthalamic nucleus deep brain stimulation in Parkinson disease. Arch Neurol 62(4):554–560. doi:10.1001/archneur.62.4.554

Andrade P, Carrillo-Ruiz JD, Jimenez F (2009) A systematic review of the efficacy of globus pallidus stimulation in the treatment of Parkinson's disease. J Clin Neurosci 16(7):877–881. doi:10.1016/j.jocn.2008.11.006

Bejjani B, Damier P, Arnulf I et al (1997) Pallidal stimulation for Parkinson's disease. Two targets? Neurology 49(6):1564–1569

Benabid AL, Pollak P, Louveau A et al (1987) Combined (thalamotomy and stimulation) stereotactic surgery of the VIM thalamic nucleus for bilateral Parkinson disease. Appl Neurophysiol 50(1–6):344–346

Bronte-Stewart H (2003) Parkinson's disease: surgical options. Curr Treat Options Neurol 5(2):131–147

Follett KA, Weaver FM, Stern M et al (2010) Pallidal versus subthalamic deep-brain stimulation for Parkinson's disease. N Engl J Med 362(22):2077–2091. doi:10.1056/NEJMoa0907083

Ghika J, Villemure JG, Fankhauser H et al (1998) Efficiency and safety of bilateral contemporaneous pallidal stimulation (deep brain stimulation) in levodopa-responsive patients with Parkinson's disease with severe motor fluctuations: a 2-year follow-up review. J Neurosurg 89(5):713–718. doi:10.3171/jns.1998.89.5.0713

Gross C, Rougier A, Guehl D et al (1997) High-frequency stimulation of the globus pallidus internalis in Parkinson's disease: a study of seven cases. J Neurosurg 87(4):491–498. doi:10.3171/jns.1997.87.4.0491

Group TD-BSfPsDS (2001) Deep-brain stimulation of the subthalamic nucleus or the pars interna of the globus pallidus in Parkinson's disease. N Engl J Med 345(13):956–963. doi:10.1056/NEJMoa000827

Guridi J, Rodriguez-Oroz MC, Lozano AM et al (2000) Targeting the basal ganglia for deep brain stimulation in Parkinson's disease. Neurology 55(12 Suppl 6): S21–S28

Hariz MI, Rehncrona S, Quinn NP et al (2008) Multicenter study on deep brain stimulation in Parkinson's disease: an independent assessment of reported adverse events at 4 years. Mov Disord 23(3):416–421. doi:10.1002/mds.21888

Krack P, Pollak P, Limousin P et al (1998) Opposite motor effects of pallidal stimulation in Parkinson's disease. Ann Neurol 43(2):180–192. doi:10.1002/ana.410430208

Kumar R, Lang AE, Rodriguez-Oroz MC et al (2000) Deep brain stimulation of the globus pallidus pars interna in advanced Parkinson's disease. Neurology 55(12 Suppl 6):S34–S39

Lemaire JJ, Durif F, Boire JY et al (1999) Direct stereotactic MRI location in the globus pallidus for chronic stimulation in Parkinson's disease. Acta Neurochir 141(7):759–765; discussion 766

Levy R, Hazrati LN, Herrero MT et al (1997) Re-evaluation of the functional anatomy of the basal ganglia in normal and Parkinsonian states. Neuroscience 76(2):335–343

Locke MC, Wu SS, Foote KD et al (2011) Weight changes in subthalamic nucleus vs globus pallidus internus deep brain stimulation: results from the COMPARE Parkinson disease deep brain stimulation cohort. Neurosurgery 68(5):1233–1237. doi:10.1227/NEU.0b013e31820b52c5; discussion 1237–1238

Machado A, Rezai AR, Kopell BH et al (2006) Deep brain stimulation for Parkinson's disease: surgical technique and perioperative management. Mov Disord 21(Suppl 14):S247–S258. doi:10.1002/mds.20959

Minguez-Castellanos A, Escamilla-Sevilla F, Katati MJ et al (2005) Different patterns of medication change after subthalamic or pallidal stimulation for Parkinson's disease: target related effect or selection bias? J Neurol Neurosurg Psychiatry 76(1):34–39. doi:10.1136/jnnp.2003.032623

Moro E, Lozano AM, Pollak P et al (2010) Long-term results of a multicenter study on subthalamic and pallidal stimulation in Parkinson's disease. Mov Disord 25(5):578–586. doi:10.1002/mds.22735

Nakamura K, Christine CW, Starr PA et al (2007) Effects of unilateral subthalamic and pallidal deep brain stimulation on fine motor functions in Parkinson's disease. Mov Disord 22(5):619–626. doi:10.1002/mds.21300

Ogura M, Nakao N, Nakai E et al (2004) The mechanism and effect of chronic electrical stimulation of the globus pallidus for treatment of Parkinson disease. J Neurosurg 100(6):997–1001. doi:10.3171/jns.2004.100.6.0997

Okun MS, Fernandez HH, Wu SS et al (2009) Cognition and mood in Parkinson's disease in subthalamic nucleus versus globus pallidus interna deep brain stimulation: the COMPARE trial. Ann Neurol 65(5):586–595. doi:10.1002/ana.21596

Pallavaram S, Yu H, Spooner J et al (2008) Intersurgeon variability in the selection of anterior and posterior commissures and its potential effects on target localization. Stereotact Funct Neurosurg 86(2):113–119. doi:10.1159/000116215

Peppe A, Pierantozzi M, Bassi A et al (2004) Stimulation of the subthalamic nucleus compared with the globus pallidus internus in patients with Parkinson disease. J Neurosurg 101(2):195–200. doi:10.3171/jns.2004.101.2.0195

Rodriguez-Oroz MC, Obeso JA, Lang AE et al (2005) Bilateral deep brain stimulation in Parkinson's disease: a multicentre study with 4 years follow-up. Brain 128(Pt 10):2240–2249. doi:10.1093/brain/awh571

Rodrigues JP, Walters SE, Watson P et al (2007a) Globus pallidus stimulation in advanced Parkinson's disease. J Clin Neurosci 14(3):208–215. doi:10.1016/j.jocn.2005.11.023

Rodrigues JP, Walters SE, Watson P et al (2007b) Globus pallidus stimulation improves both motor and nonmotor aspects of quality of life in advanced Parkinson's disease. Mov Disord 22(13):1866–1870. doi:10.1002/mds.21427

Rouaud T, Dondaine T, Drapier S et al (2010) Pallidal stimulation in advanced Parkinson's patients with contraindications for subthalamic stimulation. Mov Disord 25(12):1839–1846. doi:10.1002/mds.23171

Sauleau P, Leray E, Rouaud T et al (2009) Comparison of weight gain and energy intake after subthalamic versus pallidal stimulation in Parkinson's disease. Mov Disord 24(14):2149–2155. doi:10.1002/mds.22765

Siegfried J, Lippitz B (1994) Chronic electrical stimulation of the VL-VPL complex and of the pallidum in the treatment of movement disorders: personal experience since 1982. Stereotact Funct Neurosurg 62(1–4):71–75

Smith Y, Bevan MD, Shink E et al (1998) Microcircuitry of the direct and indirect pathways of the basal ganglia. Neuroscience 86(2):353–387

Spiegel EA, Wycis HT, Marks M et al (1947) Stereotaxic apparatus for operations on the human brain. Science 106(2754):349–350. doi:10.1126/science.106.2754.349

Spiegel EA, Wycis HT (1954) Ansotomy in paralysis agitans. AMA Arch Neurol Psychiatry 71(5):598–614

Starr PA (2002) Placement of deep brain stimulators into the subthalamic nucleus or Globus pallidus internus: technical approach. Stereotact Funct Neurosurg 79(3–4):118–145. doi:10.1159/000070828

St George RJ, Nutt JG, Burchiel KJ et al (2010) A meta-regression of the long-term effects of deep brain stimulation on balance and gait in PD. Neurology 75(14):1292–1299. doi:10.1212/WNL.0b013e3181f61329

Svennilson E, Torvik A, Lowe R et al (1960) Treatment of parkinsonism by stereotatic thermolesions in the pallidal region. A clinical evaluation of 81 cases. Acta Psychiatr Scand 35:358–377

Taba HA, Wu SS, Foote KD et al (2010) A closer look at unilateral versus bilateral deep brain stimulation: results of the National Institutes of Health COMPARE cohort. J Neurosurg 113(6):1224–1229. doi:10.3171/2010.8.JNS10312

Vitek JL, Bakay RA, Hashimoto T et al (1998) Microelectrode-guided pallidotomy: technical approach and its application in medically intractable Parkinson's disease. J Neurosurg 88(6):1027–1043. doi:10.3171/jns.1998.88.6.1027

Volkmann J, Sturm V, Weiss P et al (1998) Bilateral high-frequency stimulation of the internal globus pallidus in advanced Parkinson's disease. Ann Neurol 44(6):953–961. doi:10.1002/ana.410440615

Volkmann J, Albanese A, Kulisevsky J et al (2009) Long-term effects of pallidal or subthalamic deep brain stimulation on quality of life in Parkinson's disease. Mov Disord 24(8):1154–1161. doi:10.1002/mds.22496

Weaver F, Follett K, Hur K et al (2005) Deep brain stimulation in Parkinson disease: a metaanalysis of patient outcomes. J Neurosurg 103(6):956–967. doi:10.3171/jns.2005.103.6.0956

Weaver FM, Follett K, Stern M et al (2009) Bilateral deep brain stimulation vs best medical therapy for patients with advanced Parkinson disease: a randomized controlled trial. JAMA 301(1):63–73. doi:10.1001/jama.2008.929

Zahodne LB, Okun MS, Foote KD et al (2009) Greater improvement in quality of life following unilateral deep brain stimulation surgery in the globus pallidus as compared to the subthalamic nucleus. J Neurol 256(8):1321–1329. doi:10.1007/s00415-009-5121-7

9 Thalamic Stimulation for Parkinson's Disease: Clinical Studies on DBS

Yasushi Miyagi

9.1 Tremor of Parkinson's Disease

Parkinson's disease (PD) is clinically characterized by several major motor symptoms: rest tremor, muscle rigidity, akinesia and, in the later stage, postural instability. The primary pathology of PD is the degeneration of dopaminergic cells within the substantia nigra pars compacta and the subsequent dopamine depletion in the striatum. Although a majority of parkinsonian patients exhibit rest tremor as an initial motor sign, a clinical evaluation of the severity of the tremor is not correlated with the disease progression, and the tremor-dominant variant has a better prognosis in disease progression than those with the akinesia/rigid variant (Louis et al. 1999). The medial substantia nigra, especially the retrorubral area A8, is more severely affected by dopaminergic cell degeneration in the tremor-dominant variant in contrast to more severe damage of the lateral substantia nigra (A9) in the akinesia/rigid variant (Hirsch et al. 1992; Jellinger 1999). This indicates that the tremor is associated with cell loss of the retrorubral substantia nigra (Deuschl et al. 2000). Although dopamine replacement therapy alleviates most of the motor symptoms, some tremors are quite resistant to dopamine replacement therapy. Clinicians frequently prescribe excessive doses of dopaminergic medication for tremor-dominant patients without any akinesia/rigid symptoms. Parkinsonian tremor, if the amplitude is small enough or not associated with postural/kinetic tremor, is not disabling by itself, but most patients are disabled by akinesia, rigidity and postural instability. Therefore, a complete cessation of tremor cannot be a therapeutic target of pharmacotherapy for the tremor-dominant PD, and the difference in symptomatic progression between two variants should be taken into account when deciding on a surgical strategy for intractable tremors of PD.

9.2 Surgical Treatment of Parkinsonian Tremor

Various preliminary surgical interventions, such as removing parts of the motor cortex or lesioning of the internal capsule, were performed in the early 1900s, and the first established surgical treatment was thalamotomy by a stereotactic technique developed in the 1950s. Although the development and widespread use of levodopa therapy of the early 1960s led to a decrease in surgical treatments (Tasker et al. 1983), 50 % of parkinsonian tremors still responded poorly to medical treatment (Koller 1986). Stereotactic thalamotomy survived among a few institutes as a surgical option for medically intractable

Y. Miyagi, MD, PhD
Department of Stereotactic and Functional Neurosurgery, Kaizuka Hospital, Fukuoka, Japan
e-mail: miyagi@kaizuka-hosp.or.jp

T. Itakura (ed.), *Deep Brain Stimulation for Neurological Disorders: Theoretical Background and Clinical Application*, DOI 10.1007/978-3-319-08476-3_9,

tremors, as well as other movement disorders exhibiting tremor, such as essential tremor, post-stroke tremor, multiple sclerosis and so on. In association with the refinement of the microrecording technique in thalamotomy, high frequency electrical stimulation was developed for the intraoperative physiological identification of the optimal point for thalamotomy (Ohye and Narabayashi 1979; Lenz et al. 1988). Such surgical experiences as reversible functional ablation have been applied to deep brain stimulation (DBS) of thalamus to date, and the most promising surgical target for intractable tremor of PD is the nucleus ventro-intermedius (Vim) of the thalamus.

9.3 Anatomy and Functional Connectivity of Thalamic Nuclei

The most currently established stereotactic targets of deep brain stimulation for Parkinson's disease are subthalamic nucleus (STN), globus pallidus internus (GPi), and Vim (Pollak et al. 2002). These nuclei are the important elements in the motor circuit among the cortex, thalamus, and basal ganglia. They involve the cells that respond to the movement of contralateral skeletal muscle or joints ("movement-related" or "kinesthetic" neurons) and play an important role in the physiological regulation of muscle tone, voluntary movement and also the pathological development of involuntary movement. Microrecording techniques during stereotactic neurosurgery have detected movement-related neurons located in the posterolateral part of GPi (Vitek et al. 1998) and dorsolateral part of STN (Rodriguez-Oroz et al. 2001); therefore they are known as the sensorimotor area of each structure. As for the thalamus, movement-related neurons are located in its ventrolateral part. There are four types of cells, the activities of which are related to active voluntary movement (voluntary cells), somatosensory stimulation (somatosensory cells), both active movement and somatosensory stimulation (combined cells), and neither active movement nor somatosensory stimulation (no-response cell) (Lenz et al. 1990). Identifying the firing activities of these cells, the ventrolateral part of the thalamus can be segmented into four nuclei from anterior to posterior; the nucleus ventro-oralis anterior and posterior (Voa/Vop), Vim and ventro-caudalis (Vc), according to the terminology by Hassler and Riechert (1954). These nuclei correspond to VLa, VLp and VPL/VPM, respectively according to the parcellation of human thalamus by Hirai and Jones (1989). Voa/Vop receives the input from GPi (pallidal receiving area) (Ohye 1997), and projects to the premotor cortex (Hirai and Jones 1989; Krack et al. 2002). Vim primarily receives the input from the cerebellum and projects to the primary motor cortex (Krack et al. 2002; Macchi and Jones 1997). Vc receives the input from lemniscus medialis (Hirai and Jones 1989) and projects to area 3a and 2 of the primary somatosensory cortex. In electrophysiological mapping with the microrecording technique, the neurons of Voa/Vop can be identified by the presence of voluntary cells which increase firing rates in response to active movement of contralateral joints while those of Vim are identified by the kinesthetic response to passive movements of contralateral joints (Lenz et al. 1990; Molnar et al. 2005). The activity of somatosensory cells lagged behind the tremor while activity of combined cells often led the tremor; therefore, both activities of the somatosensory and combined cell types may be related to the generation of the tremor by different mechanisms (Lenz et al. 1994). Parkinsonian tremor can result from the oscillation of two anatomically segregated loops; the basal ganglia loop including Voa/Vop and the cerebellar loop including Vim. In addition to the oscillation of the basal ganglia loop, the cerebellar loop may indirectly contribute to the expression of parkinsonian tremor through the rhythmic neuronal activity of Vim proprioceptive cells. The oscillation of both the cerebellar and the basal ganglia loops could also result from interconnections between the cerebellar and basal ganglia thalamic nuclei through the thalamic reticular nucleus or thalamo-cortico-thalamic loops (Krack et al. 1998). The beneficial effect of the thalamotomy or Vim-DBS must be due to an interaction between the basal ganglia-thalamo-cortical and the cerebello-thalamo-cortical projection (Deuschl et al. 2000). DBS of the center median nucleus/parafascicular complex (CM/PF) is under investigation as a therapeutic target of PD (Peppe et al. 2008). In a retrospective study, a possible involvement of the CM/PF is suggested to explain the efficacy of thalamic Vim-DBS on levodopa-induced dyskinesia in PD (Caparros-Lefebvre et al. 1999).

9.4 Experiences in Thalamotomy

The stereotactic lesioning technique has been applied to the thalamus for alleviation of various kinds of tremors or movement disorders (Hassler and Riechert 1954; Cooper and Bravo 1958). Although the number of stereotactic thalamotomy decreased markedly when levodopa therapy emerged in the 1960s, some parkinsonian tremors were resistant to levodopa or other dopamine replacement therapies (Koller 1986). The surgery survived for only severe parkinsonian tremors that were resistant to medical treatment (Siegfried 1980; Matsumoto et al. 1984; Narabayashi 1989). Thalamotomy was effective in 70–90 % of intractable tremors of PD (Matsumoto et al. 1984; Fox et al. 1991; Jankovic et al. 1995; Cardoso et al. 1995). Ohye (1997) reported that only a small lesion (40 mm^3) is effective to attenuate a tremor in the area of Vim involving the kinesthetic neurons that respond to contralateral joint movement. Lenz et al. (1995) reported that a lesion volume of 60 mm^3 has long-term tremor relief if it was put within 2 mm from the center of kinesthetic neurons, but a lesion more than 2 mm from the center of kinesthetic neurons has no long-lasting effect. However, no correlation between thalamotomy lesion size and clinical outcome was reported (Hariz and Hirabayashi 1997). Optimal target localization for thalamotomy requires topographical consideration about the distributions of tremor neurons within Vim and the body part that has an intractable tremor. Post-stroke or post-traumatic tremor is characterized by coarse and irregular oscillation involving proximal muscles, requiring a relatively larger coagulative lesion for relief of the tremor. In contrast, parkinsonian and essential tremors are usually of low amplitude, regular and distal in distribution. For the relief of such a tremor, the lesion could be very small; if aided by electrophysiological methods to identify Vim neurons, the minimal effective volume of the lesion was estimated to be about 40 mm^3 and restricted to Vim (Hirai et al. 1983). The kinesthetic neurons within Vim appear to be arranged primarily in a dorsolateral to ventromedial direction corresponding to a lower limb-upper limb-face sequence (Ohye and Narabayashi 1979; Hirai et al. 1983). In many cases, a hand tremor is the most disabling for tremor-dominant PD that directly affects the patients' daily activity. It also affects the patients' appearances and brings the mental stresses. Neurons responding to the hand are topographically arranged in the relatively ventrolateral part of Vim. Therefore, pursuing hand area in Vim associates with the risk of getting close to internal capsule. Thalamotomy was considered to be effective also for rigidity and levodopa-induced dyskinesia if the lesion was placed extensively, anterior enough to involve Voa/Vop (Narabayashi et al. 1984).

9.5 Vim-DBS for Parkinson's Disease

Deep brain stimulation at Vim (Vim-DBS) was initially proposed as an additional treatment for patients who had already undergone thalamotomy on the contralateral side (Benabid et al. 1987). Since Vim-DBS has been shown to be effective for intractable tremors in the short term (Benabid et al. 1987, 1996; Alesch et al. 1995; Koller et al. 1997; Limousin et al. 1999) and in the long term (Benabid et al. 1991; Blond et al. 1992; Lyons et al. 2001; Rehncrona et al. 2003; Putzke et al. 2003; Pahwa et al. 2006), Vim-DBS has replaced thalamotomy in the treatment of parkinsonian tremor, essential tremor and other various types of tremor in the past 20 years because of its safety, reversibility and adaptability. Vim-DBS actually improved the majority of PD disabling tremors and the quality of life in tremor-dominant cases (Limousin-Dowsey 2002); however, its effect on other motor symptoms has been equivocal. Ventrolateral thalamotomy attenuated levodopa-induced dyskinesia (Hughes et al. 1971; Narabayashi et al. 1984; Jankovic et al. 1995); Vim-DBS alleviated only 18 % of dyskinesia (Benabid et al. 1993) and only peak-dose but not diphasic dyskinesia (Caparros-Lefebvre et al. 1993). Contralateral limb akinesia/rigidity was mildly alleviated but ipsilateral akinesia/rigidity and axial symptoms, such as dysarthria, postural instability and gait disturbance were not changed by unilateral or bilateral surgery (Limousin et al. 1999). In another study, Vim-DBS itself had no therapeutic effect on the other PD symptoms, such as akinesia, motor fluctuation, postural instability, and gait disturbance (Koller et al. 1997; Hariz et al. 1998; Benabid et al. 1996; Ondo et al. 1998; Lyons et al. 2001; Putzke et al. 2003). Stimulation involving Voa/Vop is thought to generate a significant therapeutic effect on levodopa-induced dyskinesia because hyperkinetic involuntary movements such as dystonia and dyskinesia are alleviated if the Voa/Vop are involved in the thalamotomy (Narabayashi et al. 1984; Blond et al. 1992). The effect of Vim-DBS on PD symptoms other than tremor is also very mild. Even though long-term Vim-DBS remained effective on tremors, the improvement in the patients' ability to cope with daily living was variable (Hariz et al. 1998; Schuurman et al. 2000). STN and GPi are the more appropriate DBS targets for non-tremor symptoms of advanced parkinsonian patients who had previously undergone thalamic DBS for treatment of tremors (Fraix et al. 2005). Therefore, Vim-DBS is now targeted in uncommon and much selected circumstances, such as cases in which a tremor is apparently the only clinical feature (Walter and Vitek 2004; Moro and Lang 2006; Pahwa et al. 2006) or if the tremor is dominant with a clinically unfavorable background, such as cases of elderly patients, presence of psychosis, and/or other surgical risks (Hariz et al. 2008).

9.6 Surgical Procedure of Vim-DBS

The first key point of Vim-DBS surgery is the anatomical targeting of Vim. Recent advances in imaging technology have enabled the direct anatomical localization of Vim, such as 3-T MRI (Spiegelmann et al. 2006), diffusion tensor imaging (Ziyan et al. 2006; Yamada et al. 2010), and 1.5-T white matter-attenuated inversion recovery (Vassal et al. 2012) although these technologies are not yet widely available. In general, an indirect targeting method based on the midline between anterior and posterior commissures (AC and PC) is used with a physiological mapping technique. In Kaizuka Hospital, for example, the *Y*-coordinate of Vim is placed 5–6 mm (or 25 % of AC–PC distance) anterior to PC, just on the AC–PC line (Z-coordinate = 0 mm) and the laterality (*X*-coordinate) is 11 mm from the lateral wall of the third ventricle. In the ventriculography era, the *X*-coordinates were based on the distance from the anatomical midline (Blond et al. 1992; Benabid et al. 1996). Because the patients that required Vim-DBS are often elderly, brain atrophy and enlargement of third ventricle are frequently an issue and the laterality of the tentative target is subject to the width of the third ventricle. Proper determination of the laterality is very important in order to localize the hand area of Vim and to avoid the current spread to the internal capsule; however, ordinary MR imaging cannot visualize a clear boundary between the thalamus and the internal capsule. Therefore, the distance from the lateral wall of the third ventricle seems to be more reliable than that from the anatomical midline.

Generally, the burr hole and entry point are placed around the coronal suture, which makes the trajectory angled 60–70° to the AC–PC line, penetrating the caudate, and the thalamus from dorsal to ventral Voa/Vop and Vim (Fig. 9.1). To supplement the accuracy of the target, microelectrode recording is used to refine the physiological mapping of Vim in almost half of DBS centers (Gross et al. 2006). In this trajectory, many spontaneous tremor-related discharges are easily encountered about 2–4 mm before reaching the

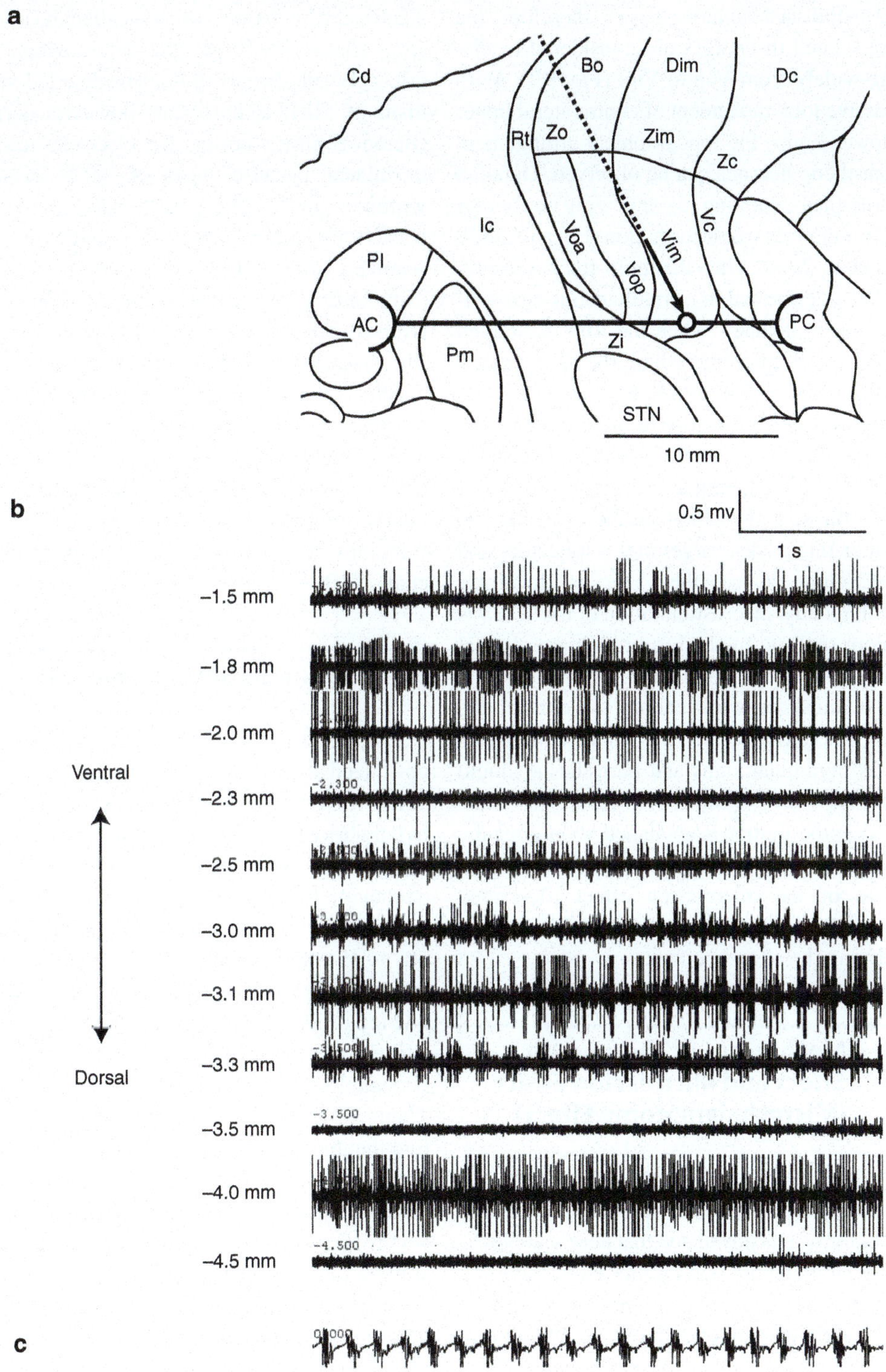

Fig. 9.1 Microelectrode recording of Vim and electromyogram of tremor in 60-year-old male with tremor-dominant Parkinson's disease. (**a**) Schematic presentation of trajectory to Vim in Schaltenbrand–Wahren atlas (1977) at 12 mm lateral to midline. Circle on the AC–PC line indicates tentative target at 25 % distance anterior to PC. The trajectory makes an approximately 60° angle from the AC–PC line, passing through the interface of Vop/Vim and the most ventral part of Vim. (**b**) Microelectrode recording on the trajectory to Vim. The grouping discharges, which were mildly to strongly related to the tremor activity, were observed at various depths to the tentative target. (**c**) Tremor activity (5 Hz) on the surface electromyogram on the right biceps muscle

above-mentioned tentative target; therefore, the tremor-related discharges are considered to distribute widely from Vop to Vim (Fig. 9.1). With the passive joint movement of contralateral upper and lower limbs, the topographical arrangement of kinesthetic neurons can be observed. Detailed physiological mapping of the Vim/Vc border may provide valuable information (Lozano 2000; Gross et al. 2006) when the multi-track microrecording is performed in a simultaneous or a serially repeated manner. When the Vim is targeted by single-track microrecording, the absence of a somatosensory response to light touch should be monitored in this trajectory in order not to enter Vc, especially at the ventral portion close to the AC–PC level. A stereotactic X-ray is useful to confirm the spatial relationship between the site of tremor-related discharges in this trajectory and AC–PC line. Once the Vim is localized physiologically, macrostimulation or trial DBS is the more realistic method to predict the clinical efficacy of chronic stimulation. The therapeutic window must be wide enough to control the tremor, whereas the thresholds for adverse effects such as pyramidal signs and paresthesia should be as high as possible. However, in some instances, the tremor is abolished soon after the DBS lead or macroelectrode passes through Vim because of the microlesion effect (described later), and macrostimulation is helpful only in identifying the adverse effect.

9.7 Mechanism of Therapeutic Effect and Microlesion Effect (Microthalamotomy Effect)

The mechanism underlying Vim-DBS is unknown. Since Vim-DBS acts as a reversible thalamotomy, it is postulated that neuronal blocking and jamming are possibilities (Benabid et al. 1996), but the activation of inhibitory mechanisms should also be considered (Strafella et al. 1997). Many tremors tend to be transiently alleviated soon after microelectrode recording or insertion of DBS leads even without lesioning or electrical stimulation, which is called the microlesion effect (MLE) or the microthalamotomy effect (Benabid et al. 1996). The detailed mechanism of MLE is not clear; however, perifocal edema or gliosis around the electrode track are postulated because most of MLE disappear within a few weeks postoperatively (Benabid et al. 1996; Tasker 1998). A few studies showed a relatively long MLE lasting up to 6 months (Sitburana et al. 2010) or more than 1 year (Kondziolka and Lee 2004; Blond et al. 1992). The duration of MLE may depend on the extent of gliosis or tissue reaction (Blond et al. 1992) or the focal metabolism in the cerebello-thalamocortical network (Mure et al. 2011). The existence of MLE did not predict the tremor outcome but the stimulation parameters remained lower at 6 months in the marked MLE group (Sitburana et al. 2010).

9.8 Stimulation Parameters

Detailed settings for Vim-DBS can be usually optimized after the MLE disappears. The contact at the ventral Vim is initially selected as a negative polarity (cathode) of unipolar configuration. Typically, a pulse width of 60 μsec and a frequency of 130 Hz are selected. The pulse width required for tremor inhibition was as short as 50 μs (Strafella et al. 1997). The therapeutic effect of Vim-DBS can be obtained at the frequency of 100–1,000 Hz, and the frequency of 130 Hz is generally used for stable tremor relief (Benabid et al. 1996; Limousin-Dowsey 2002). Then the voltage is progressively increased to find the threshold for tremor cessation of the target limb (Limousin-Dowsey 2002). In PD patients, some tolerance and rebound effect can occur. Possible stimulation tolerance during stimulation and tremor rebound at terminating stimulation should be made clear to the candidates for Vim-DBS. Blond et al. (1992) reported the reappearance of tremor in three out of ten PD patients during a mean follow-up period of 19.4 months. There was a significant increase in voltage at 3 months compared to 1 week after surgery and at 6 months compared to 3 months Hariz et al. 1999). Rebound tremor was observed by several studies (Blond et al. 1992; Benabid et al. 1996; Albanese et al. 1999; Kumar et al. 1999). In order to avoid tolerance development, we instruct patients to turn on Vim-DBS when getting up in the morning and terminate it before sleep. If the rebound tremor returns as soon as the DBS is turned off, producing a tremor-induced insomnia, a family member is advised to turn off DBS after the patient falls asleep. On the other hand, a patient with STN-DBS is told to keep DBS on all day long even during sleep, because nocturnal awakening is a frequent problem when DBS is turned off during sleep. Vim-DBS, unlike thalamotomy, selectively reduces tremors without altering sleep or sleep spindles (Arnulf et al. 2000a). STN-DBS showed both subjective and polysomnographic evidence of improvement of sleep (Arnulf et al. 2000b; Hjort et al. 2004). In an empirical observation, the recurrence of tremor in both upper and lower extremities after Vim-DBS can be alleviated by STN-DBS (Fraix et al. 2005), while no patient with STN-DBS has needed to be secondarily implanted in the Vim because of lack or loss of effect, so far.

9.9 Complications

Complications are usually related to incorrectly placed lesions or unnecessarily large lesions (Fox et al. 1991; Jankovic et al. 1995), Vim borders the posterior limb of the internal capsule laterally and the Vc posteriorly. Even within Vim, too laterally placed lesions lead to contralateral hemiparesis and too posteriorly placed lesions lead to paresthesia or numbness of the contralateral fingers and lip corner. Also lateropulsion is frequently but transiently seen in the immediate postoperative period, which may be related to the interruption of cerebellar afferents. Similarly, the lateral current spread from Vim-DBS may result in contralateral muscle rigidity and the posterior current spread may result in dysesthesia. Benabid et al. (1991) recorded paresthesia (9.4 %), dystonia (6.3 %), gait disorders (12.5 %), and dysarthria (21.9 %) in 32 Vim-DBS cases. The side effects related to Vim-DBS were generally mild and well tolerated and acceptable if the DBS significantly alleviated the tremor (Hariz et al. 1999). Because bilateral thalamotomy inevitably results in persistent dysarthria as a complication (Matsumoto et al. 1984), irrespective of staged or contemporaneous surgery, a bilateral Vim-DBS or a combination of unilateral Vim-DBS and contralateral thalamotomy should be recommended for tremor cases of bilateral limbs, head or jaw (Koller et al. 1997; Schuurman et al. 2000). In 44 % of the patients who had a previous thalamotomy, DBS on the contralateral Vim provoked some dysarthria when the stimulation was activated (Hariz et al. 1999). The DBS effect itself is reversible in nature, and the stimulation intensities or parameters should be explored within the extent that does not produce adverse effects. With the recent advancement of a neurostimulator (Activa SC, Medtronic), patients can adjust the stimulation intensity of one or both sides by themselves to find an optimal intensity.

9.10 Vim-DBS Versus Thalamotomy; The Surgical Results in Kaizuka Hospital

In a comparison study by Schuurman et al. (2000, 2008) between the efficacy of unilateral thalamotomy and that of unilateral or bilateral Vim-DBS for a drug-resistant tremor in 45 parkinsonian patients, 93 % of thalamotomy and 88 % of Vim-DBS patients still experienced satisfactory tremor suppression at 5 years. Adverse effects, such as cognitive decline, dysarthria, and gait and balance disturbance were more often seen after thalamotomy (Schuurman et al. 2000), while some DBS-treated patients had hardware-related complications requiring additional surgery (Pollak et al. 2002). Vim-DBS is safer than

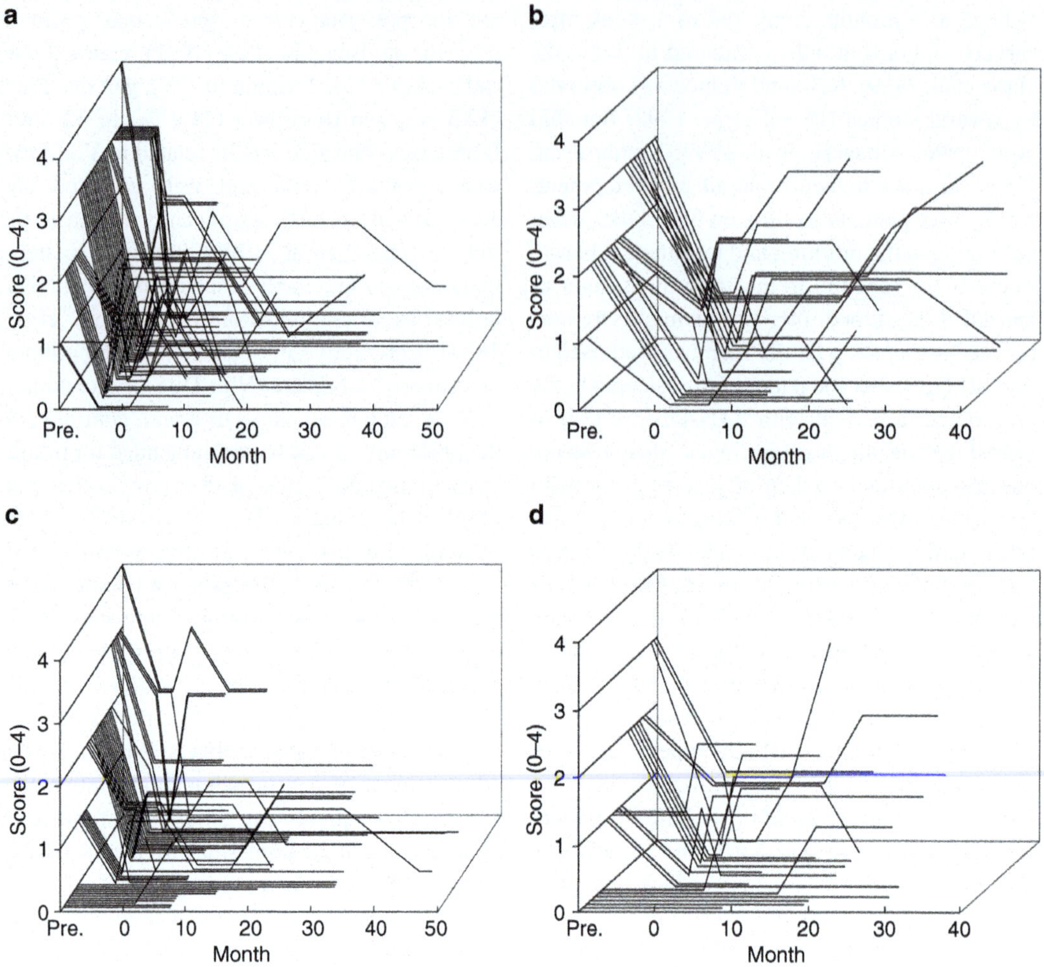

Fig. 9.2 Postoperative change in individual tremor severity in parkinsonian patients. (**a, b**) Rest tremor, item 20 of UPDRS part 2, (**c, d**) action or postural tremor, item 21 of UPDRS part 2. (**a, c**) Vim-DBS ($n = 51$), (**b, d**) thalamotomy ($n = 22$)

thalamotomy and can be carried out bilaterally in either one or two stages (Benabid et al. 1991). In Kaizuka Hospital, 35 thalamotomies and 54 Vim-DBS procedures were performed in tremor-dominant Parkinson's disease cases between April 1993 and February 2004. In this period, thalamotomy was gradually replaced by Vim-DBS because of the nature of safety, reversibility and adjustability in Vim-DBS although the targeting method of Vim-DBS was the same as the method used in thalamotomy. The tentative target coordinates for Vim was determined by an indirect method based on the AC–PC line on MRI findings: 5.5 mm (or 25 % of AC–PC distance) anterior to the PC (*Y*), 11 mm lateral to the lateral wall of the third ventricle (*X*) and 0 mm above AC–PC line (*Z*). The target determination was supplemented by the guidance of microelectrode recording and electromyogram (Fig. 9.1); the tremor neurons were identified by discharges synchronized with tremor activity on electromyogram. The scores of rest tremor in the medical records were available for 22 thalamotomies and 51 Vim-DBS procedures, and the longest follow-up visits were 36 and 48 months, respectively (Fig. 9.2). At the first month postoperatively, excellent results with complete tremor disappearance or decreased tremor score over two points were observed in 15 out of 22 thalamotomies (68.2 %) and 36 out of 51 Vim-DBS (70.6 %). The tremor evaluation after each surgery was terminated when additional surgery was needed due to tremor recurrence or other parkinsonian symptoms. Thalamotomy brought an immediate tremor cessation, but one-third of patients presented the tremor recurrence, most of which were apparent within 1 year. Vim-DBS also produced an immediate and powerful therapeutic effect, and most tremor recurrence in the acute phase was seen within 1 month postoperatively as well (Fig. 9.2), suggesting the resolution of the microlesion (microthalamotomy) effect; however, all of the recurred tremors were attenuated to a level lower than their preoperative tremor score by adjustment of stimulation parameters. In Fig. 9.3, the postoperative courses of tremor severity for 2 years were compared between 14 thalamotomies and 16 Vim-DBS. The therapeutic effect of Vim-DBS was stable for 2 years, while that of thalamotomy were stabilized after 1 year. When tremor recurrence was defined as the deterioration over one point of score from the peak benefit after surgery, the cumulative recurrences of thalamotomy were 18 % at 3 months and 19 % at 1 year postoperatively, while those of Vim-DBS were 6 % at 3 months and 18 % at 1 year (Fig. 9.3c).

9.11 Stimulation Parameters and Stimulation Site of Vim-DBS

Most of the adjustment was the increase in voltage, pulse width, and frequency. Some of the adjustment included the change in polarity (bipolar to unipolar configuration) and multiple cathode contacts. There was a significant increase in voltage at 3 months compared to 1 week after surgery and at 6 months compared to 3 months as also observed by another study (Hariz et al. 1999). The surgical procedure for targeting Vim is the same for thalamotomy and Vim-DBS. Contrary to the immediate surgical results in thalamotomy, in Vim-DBS, the stimulation parameters are inevitably increased from the initial setting in order to attenuate any possible tremor recurrence because the actual intensities required for tremor relief are usually masked by the microlesion effect immediately after the implantation. The spatial relationship between the effective sites of thalamotomy lesion and effective active contact for Vim-DBS is unclear. We have investigated this problem by focusing on the positive results of 6 thalamotomy and 22 Vim-DBS. To determine the *Y*- and *Z*-coordinates, the center of the thalamotomy lesion and the active contact for the effective cathode were localized using postoperative MR imaging (Miyagi et al. 2007; Yoshida et al. 2008). As shown in Fig. 9.4, the sagittal sections parallel to the mid-plane, including the AC–PC line and DBS contacts and thalamotomy lesion, were overlaid. The *X*-coordinates were measured from the lateral wall of the third ventricle on the horizontal section. Both the centers of lesion and effective cathode were located around 12 mm to the lateral wall of the third ventricle, corresponding to the external portion of Vim (Fig. 9.4c) which is adjacent to the pyramidal tract in the posterior limb of the internal capsule. Although the lateral distribution showed no significant difference between lesion center and effective cathode, the centers of effective cathode distributed more posteriorly than the centers of effective lesion. The adjusted energy use (AEU) of the implantable pulse generator at the 2-year follow up showed two peaks in the histogram (Fig. 9.5a): under 20 (low AEU group) and over 20 (high AEU group). The low AEU group was distributed more posteriorly than the centers of lesion ($p=0.003$, Fig. 9.5b), while the high AEU group showed the same distribution as effective lesion (Fig. 9.5c). The battery longevities estimated for high and low AEU groups were 5 and 10 years, respectively (Table 9.1). Therefore, when the lower intensity with minimal active contact is assumed to indicate the more favorable results, the effective cathode must locate as posteriorly as adjacent to Vc and as ventrally as close to AC–PC line. This observation is similar to

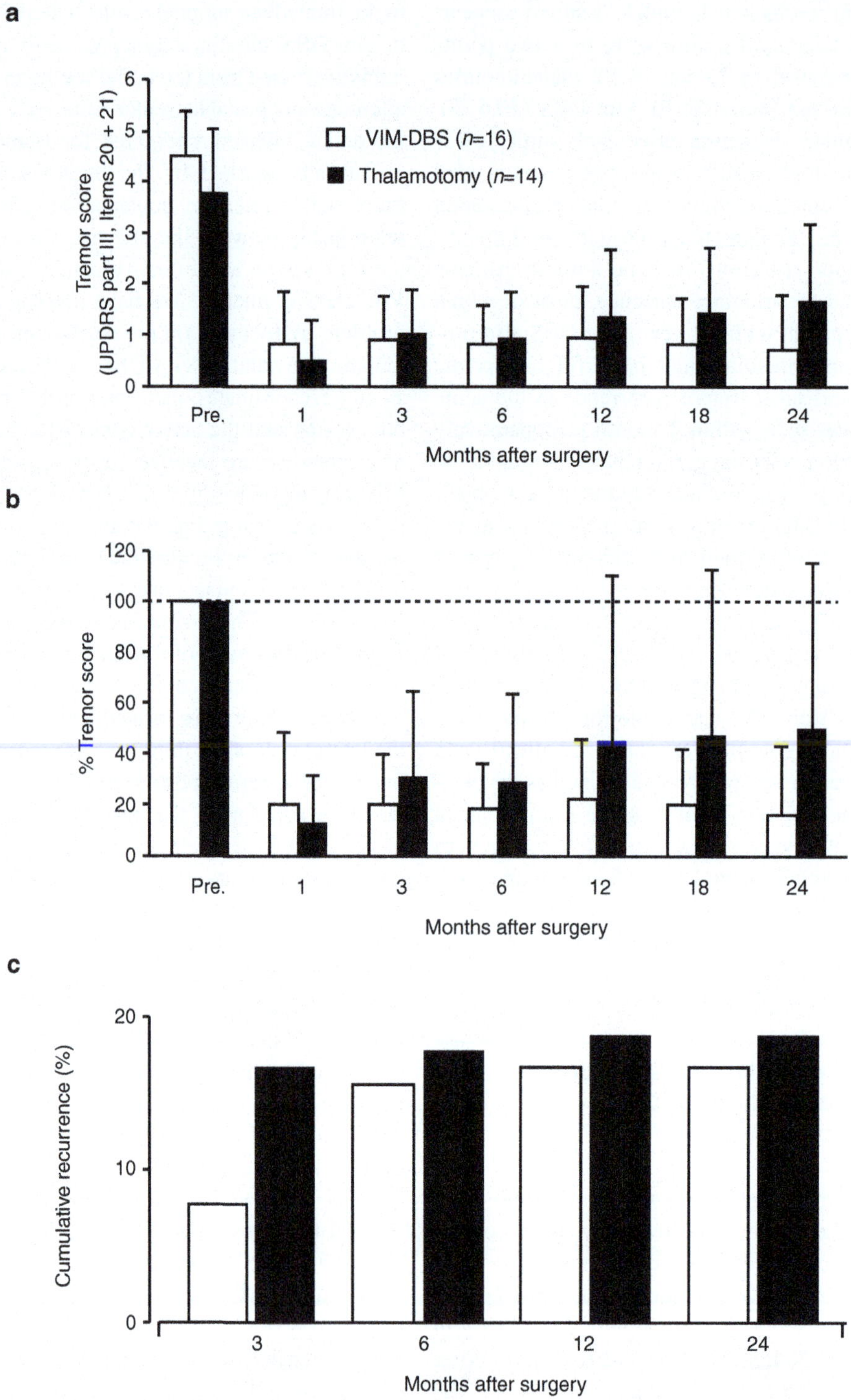

Fig. 9.3 Summary of surgical results of Vim-DBS (*open column*, $n = 16$) and thalamotomy (*closed column*, $n = 14$). *Bars* indicate standard deviation. (**a**) Postoperative changes in tremor score (items 20 and 21 of UPDRS part 2). (**b**) Percent tremor score show the relative changes when the preoperative value was assumed to be 100 %. (**c**) Cumulative recurrence rate of tremor

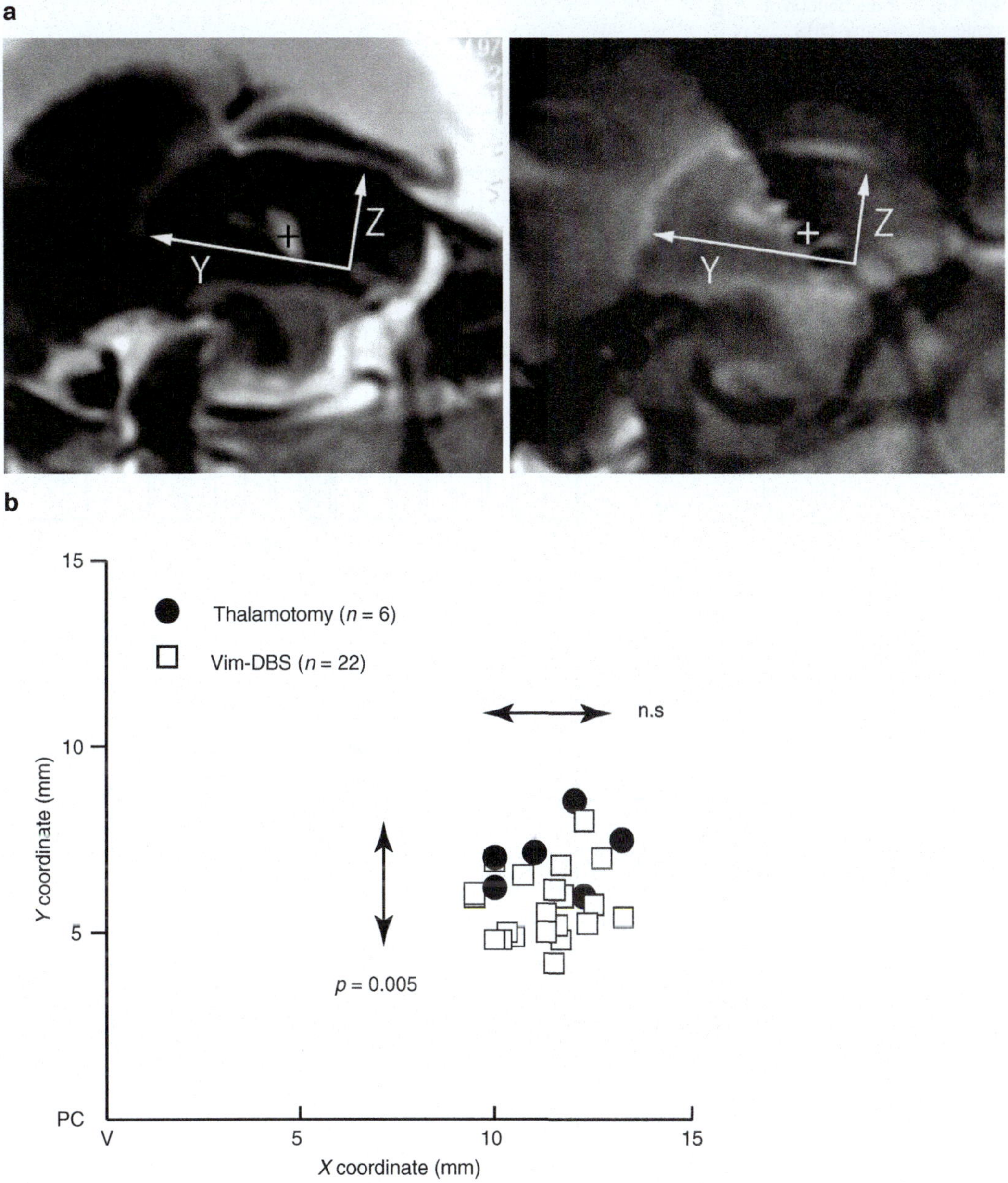

Fig. 9.4 Distribution of centers of effective lesion and effective cathode. (**a**) Method of measurement of lesion center (*left*) and DBS cathode (*right*) by magnetic resonance imaging. The sagittal sections parallel to the midplane, including AC–PC line and DBS contacts and thalamotomy lesion, were overlaid (Miyagi et al. 2007; Yoshida et al. 2008). The *X*-coordinates were measured from the lateral wall of the third ventricle on the horizontal section. The center was measured assuming AC–PC line as *Y* axis and anterior edge of PC as the origin of a three-dimensional axis. (**b**) *X*–*Y* distribution of centers of effective lesion and effective cathode of the cases showing excellent tremor control. *X* coordinate was the distance from the lateral wall of the third ventricle (*V*). *Closed circle* thalamotomy, *open square* Vim-DBS. Mann–Whitney *U*-test detected the significantly posterior distribution of effective cathodes of Vim-DBS ($n = 0.005$)

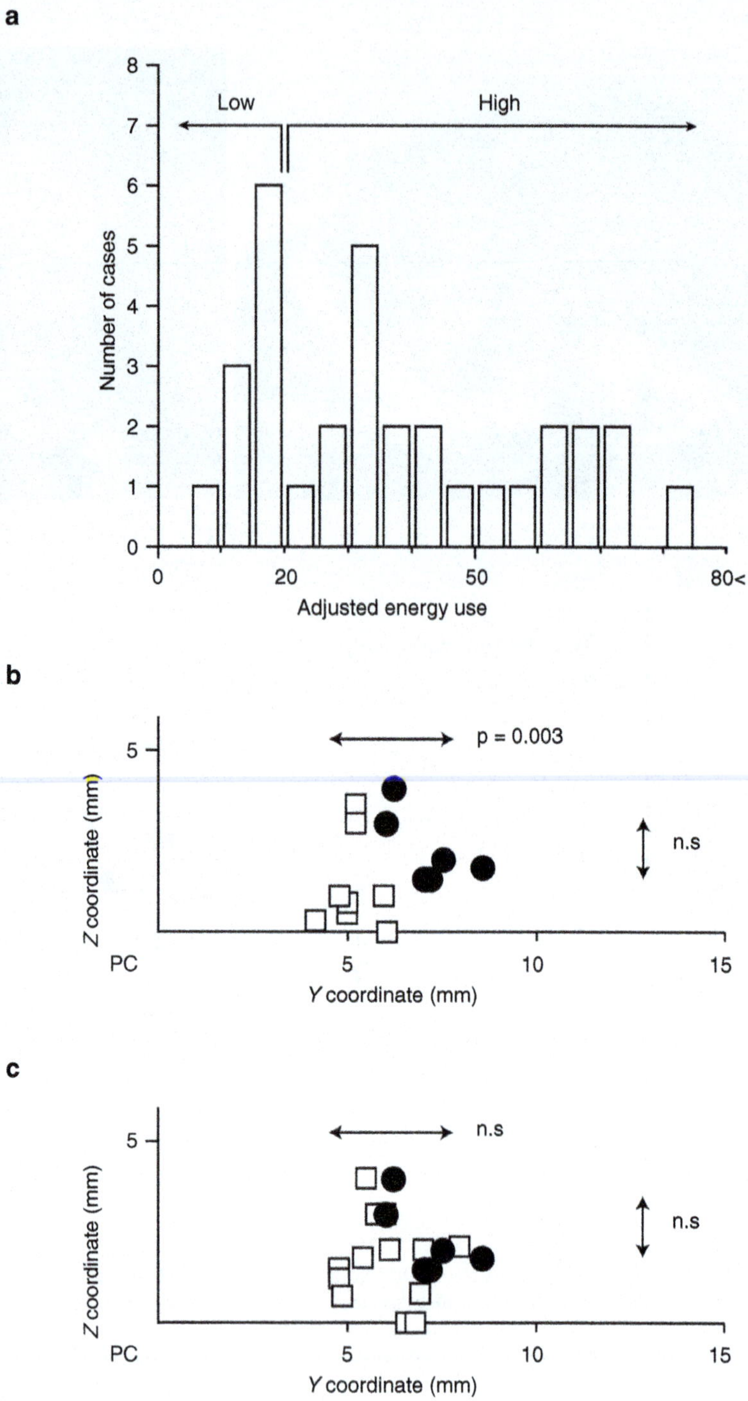

Fig. 9.5 *Y–Z* distribution of centers of effective DBS cathodes and the relationship with adjusted energy use. (**a**) Histogram of adjusted energy use of Vim-DBS with excellent outcomes. (**b**, **c**) *X–Y* distribution of centers of effective lesion ($n=6$) and effective cathode of the cases showing excellent tremor control with low AEU (**b**, $n=8$) and high AEU (**c**, $n=22$). *Closed circle* thalamotomy, *open square* Vim-DBS. Mann–Whitney *U*-test detected the significantly posterior distribution of effective cathodes of Vim-DBS of low AEU group ($n=0.003$) but not high AEU group

Table 9.1 Summary of DBS parameters

Adjusted energy use		High, ≥20 (41.4±14.1)	Low, <20 (15.3±3.3)
Case number		14	8
Follow up (month)		40.5±17.8	40.8±22.9
Parameter			
Pulse width (μsec)		146.3±63.0	78.8±22.3
Frequency (Hz)		149.4±24.4	151.9±18.3
Amplitude (volt)		2.4±0.5	1.7±0.5
Impedance (ohm)		1218.8±339.7	1679.8±301.8
Current (mA)		2.1±0.3	1.1±0.4
Polarity configuration			
Bipolar	1 cathode	6 (42.9 %)	7 (87.5 %)
	2 cathodes	4 (28.6 %)	0 (0 %)
Unipolar	1 cathode	3 (21.4 %)	1 (12.5 %)
	2 cathodes	1 (7.1 %)	0 (0 %)
Estimated IPG longevity (years)		5.1±1.1	10.0±1.3

Cases of excellent surgical outcome ($n=22$) were divided into two groups by adjusted energy use to estimate the longevity of internal pulse generator (IPG); high AEU equal or more than 20 and low AEU less than 20

another study of thalamotomy (Atkinson et al. 2002), which found that the lesion including the interface of the Vim with the anterior Vc is necessary for inclusion of proprioceptive thalamus to get an excellent outcome. However, the posteriorly located the thalamotomy lesion, the higher risk for paresthesia is anticipated. On the other hand, the active contacts used for chronic Vim-DBS were significantly anterior and dorsal to the ideal thalamotomy target (Kiss et al. 2003), which may reflect the advantage of adjustability in Vim-DBS. In contrast to thalamotomy lesions, electrodes for Vim-DBS can be arranged in such a way that wide areas can be stimulated (Katayama et al. 2005).

9.12 Vim-DBS or STN DBS?

Tremor-dominant PD is known to exhibit slower disease progression than the akinesia/rigid type of tremor (Zetusky et al. 1985; Vu et al. 2012). On the other hand, it is empirically known that some tremors decrease its severity in exchange for the progression of akinesia or rigidity in the advanced stage of PD. Vim-DBS may have a significant role in improving the quality of life threatened by disabling tremors; however, in PD patients whose tremor was successfully controlled after unilateral and bilateral Vim-DBS over 3 years, 65 % of them had disability due to akinetic-rigid symptoms and levodopa-induced dyskinesias (Pollak et al. 1997, 2002), making the long-term follow up limited to only 15 %. Progression of PD is still inevitable after Vim-DBS, and there was significant increase in dopamine replacement therapy in a long-term follow up (Tarsy et al. 2005). From our operative series, the typical course of disease progression of the PD patient who had unilateral Vim-DBS followed by bilateral STN-DBS was presented in Fig. 9.6. In this case, the activity of daily living (ADL) gradually deteriorated during Vim-DBS because of the progression of akinesia and rigidity although tremor control was stable for over 8 years. Switching to bilateral STN-DBS, the

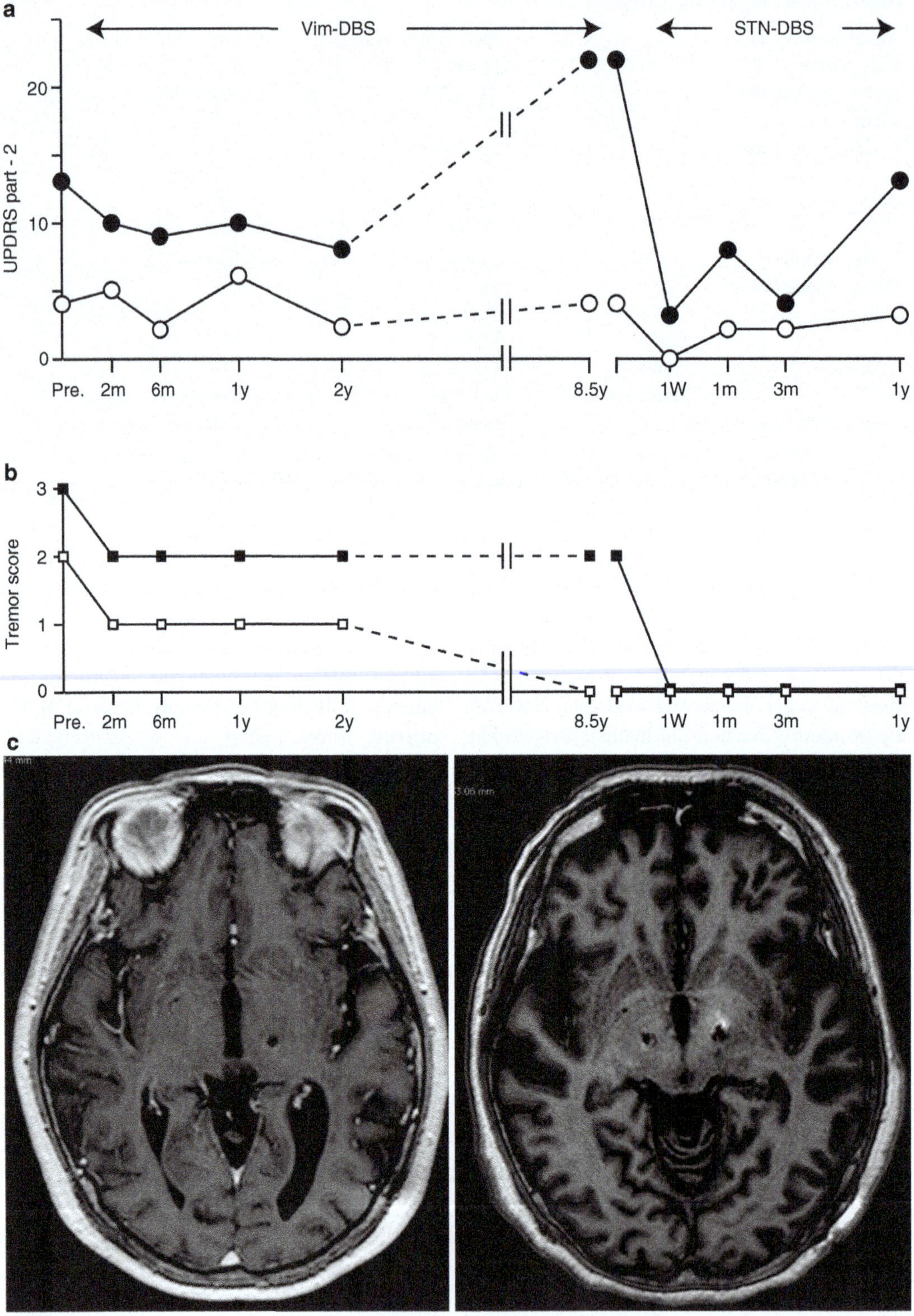
a
Vim-DBS
STN-DBS
UPDRS part - 2
20
10
0
Pre. 2m 6m 1y 2y 8.5y 1W 1m 3m 1y
b
Tremor score
3
2
1
0
Pre. 2m 6m 1y 2y 8.5y 1W 1m 3m 1y
c

Fig. 9.6 Typical clinical course of tremor-dominant PD. A 64-year-old female developed rest tremor at the age of 54. She was diagnosed as PD and was treated with dopamine replacement therapy and also took anticholinergics. Although the parkinsonism showed some alleviation, the large amplitude tremor at rest was not alleviated at all but associated with adverse effect of nausea. At the age of 55, she underwent Vim-DBS and her rest tremor was successfully treated by bipolar stimulation of contact 1 as cathode, 120 μs pulse width, 130 Hz frequency and 2.4 V amplitude (82 μA). Until the 8-year follow up, her akinesia had gradually advanced irrespective of dopamine replacement therapy and associated with a wearing off and marked motor fluctuation. She suffered from peak-dose dyskinesia of the trunk and, during off phase, she suffered from severe muscle rigidity, tremor, dysarthria, end-dose toe dystonia, tingling pain of bilateral leg, cold sensation of the left leg and hallucination. (**a**) Unified Parkinson's disease rating scale (*UPDRS*), part 2 (ADL) showing the development of wearing off and motor fluctuation. *Closed circle*, med-off phase, *open circle* med-on phase. (**b**) Tremor score (UPDRS, part 3), *Closed square*, item 20 (rest tremor); *open circle* item 21 (action tremor). (**c**) Postoperative MR imaging of Vim-DBS (*left*) and STN-DBS (*right*)

ADL during the off period was significantly improved. Furthermore, tremors completely ceased, which could not be achieved by Vim-DBS. Even if tremor amplitude is very large, the therapeutic targets (Vim, STN and GPi) should be carefully selected in the light of disease progression. For advanced PD patients, STN and GPi are more appropriate targets of DBS to relieve intractable tremors, while also alleviating tremors (Volkmann et al. 1998; Pollak et al. 2002; Krack et al. 2003; Hariz et al. 2008). The effect of STN DBS on rest and postural tremor has been reported to be stable over time (Krack et al. 1998; Rodriguez et al. 1998). STN-DBS affects the network metabolism of cerebello-thalamo-cortical pathways more widely than Vim-DBS (Mure et al. 2011). On the contrary, Vim-DBS could be an appropriate treatment of intractable tremors of PD when the cognitive decline is worried about. Preexisting mild cognitive dysfunction in PD patients was not worsened after Vim-DBS as evaluated by neuropsychological testing (Caparros-Lefebvre et al. 1992), but Vim-DBS exhibited significant improvement on measures of conceptualization, verbal memory, emotional adjustment, and QOL at 1-year follow up (Woods et al. 2001). Tröster et al. (1998) found that Vim-DBS subtly improved semantic verbal fluency but interfered with immediate recall of word lists. It should be argued that Vim-DBS remains a reasonable option for parkinsonian patients with long-standing, non-progressive tremor-dominant variant, especially in the elderly or cognitively impaired cases.

References

Albanese A, Nordera GP, Caraceni T et al (1999) Long-term ventralis intermedius thalamic stimulation for parkinsonian tremor. Italian Registry for Neuromodulation in Movement Disorders. Adv Neurol 80:631–634

Alesch F, Pinter MM, Helscher RJ et al (1995) Stimulation of the ventral intermediate thalamic nucleus in tremor dominated Parkinson's disease and essential tremor. Acta Neurochir (Wien) 136(1–2):75–81

Arnulf I, Bejjani BP, Garma L et al (2000a) Effect of low and high frequency thalamic stimulation on sleep in patients with Parkinson's disease and essential tremor. J Sleep Res 9(1):55–62

Arnulf I, Bejjani BP, Garma L et al (2000b) Improvement of sleep architecture in PD with subthalamic nucleus stimulation. Neurology 55(11):1732–1734

Atkinson JD, Collins DL, Bertrand G et al (2002) Optimal location of thalamotomy lesions for tremor associated with Parkinson disease: a probabilistic analysis based on postoperative magnetic resonance imaging and an integrated digital atlas. J Neurosurg 96(5):854–866

Benabid AL, Pollak P, Louveau A et al (1987) Combined (thalamotomy and stimulation) stereotactic surgery of the VIM thalamic nucleus for bilateral Parkinson disease. Appl Neurophysiol 50(1–6):344–346

Benabid AL, Pollak P, Gervason C et al (1991) Long-term suppression of tremor by chronic stimulation of the ventral intermediate thalamic nucleus. Lancet 337(8738):403–406

Benabid AL, Pollak P, Seigneuret E et al (1993) Chronic VIM thalamic stimulation in Parkinson's disease, essential tremor and extra-pyramidal dyskinesias. Acta Neurochir Suppl (Wien) 58:39–44

Benabid AL, Pollak P, Gao D et al (1996) Chronic electrical stimulation of the ventralis intermedius nucleus of the thalamus as a treatment of movement disorders. J Neurosurg 84(2):203–214

Blond S, Caparros-Lefebvre D, Parker F et al (1992) Control of tremor and involuntary movement disorders by chronic stereotactic stimulation of the ventral intermediate thalamic nucleus. J Neurosurg 77(1): 62–68

Caparros-Lefebvre D, Blond S, Pecheux N et al (1992) Neuropsychological evaluation before and after thalamic stimulation in 9 patients with Parkinson disease. Rev Neurol (Paris) 148(2):117–122

Caparros-Lefebvre D, Blond S, Vermersch P et al (1993) Chronic thalamic stimulation improves tremor and levodopa induced dyskinesias in Parkinson's disease. J Neurol Neurosurg Psychiatry 56(3):268–273

Caparros-Lefebvre D, Blond S, Feltin MP et al (1999) Improvement of levodopa induced dyskinesias by thalamic deep brain stimulation is related to slight variation in electrode placement: possible involvement of the centre median and parafascicularis complex. J Neurol Neurosurg Psychiatry 67(3):308–314

Cardoso F, Jankovic J, Grossman RG et al (1995) Outcome after stereotactic thalamotomy for dystonia and hemiballismus. Neurosurgery 36(3):501–507; discussion 507–508

Cooper IS, Bravo G (1958) Chemopallidectomy and chemothalamectomy. J Neurosurg 15(3):244–250

Deuschl G, Raethjen J, Baron R et al (2000) The pathophysiology of parkinsonian tremor: a review. J Neurol 247(Suppl 5):V33–V48

Fox MW, Ahlskog JE, Kelly PJ (1991) Stereotactic ventrolateralis thalamotomy for medically refractory tremor in post-levodopa era Parkinson's disease patients. J Neurosurg 75(5):723–730

Fraix V, Pollak P, Moro E et al (2005) Subthalamic nucleus stimulation in tremor dominant parkinsonian patients with previous thalamic surgery. J Neurol Neurosurg Psychiatry 76(2):246–248

Gross RE, Krack P, Rodriguez-Oroz MC et al (2006) Electrophysiological mapping for the implantation of deep brain stimulators for Parkinson's disease and tremor. Mov Disord 21(Suppl 14):S259–S283

Hariz MI, Hirabayashi H (1997) Is there a relationship between size and site of the stereotactic lesion and symptomatic results of pallidotomy and thalamotomy? Stereotact Funct Neurosurg 69(1–4 Pt 2):28–45

Hariz GM, Bergenheim AT, Hariz MI et al (1998) Assessment of ability/disability in patients treated with chronic thalamic stimulation for tremor. Mov Disord 13(1):78–83

Hariz MI, Shamsgovara P, Johansson F et al (1999) Tolerance and tremor rebound following long-term chronic thalamic stimulation for Parkinsonian and essential tremor. Stereotact Funct Neurosurg 72(2–4): 208–218

Hariz MI, Krack P, Alesch F et al (2008) Multicentre European study of thalamic stimulation for parkinsonian tremor: a 6 year follow-up. J Neurol Neurosurg Psychiatry 79(6):694–699

Hassler R, Riechert T (1954) Indikationen und Lokalisations – methode der gezilten Hirnoperationen. Nervenarzt 25(11):441–447

Hirai T, Jones EG (1989) A new parcellation of the human thalamus on the basis of histochemical staining. Brain Res Brain Res Rev 14(1):1–34

Hirai T, Miyazaki M, Nakajima H et al (1983) The correlation between tremor characteristics and the predicted volume of effective lesions in stereotaxic nucleus ventralis intermedius thalamotomy. Brain 106(Pt 4): 1001–1018

Hirsch EC, Mouatt A, Faucheux B et al (1992) Dopamine, tremor, and Parkinson's disease. Lancet 340(8811): 125–126

Hjort N, Ostergaard K, Dupont E (2004) Improvement of sleep quality in patients with advanced Parkinson's disease treated with deep brain stimulation of the subthalamic nucleus. Mov Disord 19(2):196–199

Hughes RC, Polgar JG, Weightman D et al (1971) L-dopa in Parkinsonism and the influence of previous thalamotomy. Br Med J 1(5739):7–13

Jankovic J, Cardoso F, Grossman RG et al (1995) Outcome after stereotactic thalamotomy for parkinsonian, essential, and other types of tremor. Neurosurgery 37(4):680–686; discussion 686–687

Jellinger KA (1999) Post mortem studies in Parkinson's disease–is it possible to detect brain areas for specific symptoms? J Neural Transm Suppl 56:1–29

Katayama Y, Kano T, Kobayashi K et al (2005) Difference in surgical strategies between thalamotomy and thalamic deep brain stimulation for tremor control. J Neurol 252(Suppl 4):IV17–IV22

Kiss ZH, Wilkinson M, Krcek J et al (2003) Is the target for thalamic deep brain stimulation the same as for thalamotomy? Mov Disord 18(10): 1169–1175

Koller WC (1986) Pharmacologic treatment of parkinsonian tremor. Arch Neurol 43(2):126–127

Koller W, Pahwa R, Busenbark K et al (1997) High-frequency unilateral thalamic stimulation in the treatment of essential and parkinsonian tremor. Ann Neurol 42(3):292–299

Kondziolka D, Lee JY (2004) Long-lasting microthalamotomy effect after temporary placement of a thalamic stimulating electrode. Stereotact Funct Neurosurg 82(2–3):127–130

Krack P, Benazzouz A, Pollak P et al (1998) Treatment of tremor in Parkinson's disease by subthalamic nucleus stimulation. Mov Disord 13(6):907–914

Krack P, Dostrovsky J, Ilinsky I et al (2002) Surgery of the motor thalamus: problems with the present nomenclatures. Mov Disord 17(Suppl 3):S2–S8

Krack P, Batir A, Van Blercom N et al (2003) Five-year follow-up of bilateral stimulation of the subthalamic nucleus in advanced Parkinson's disease. N Engl J Med 349(20):1925–1934

Kumar K, Kelly M, Toth C (1999) Deep brain stimulation of the ventral intermediate nucleus of the thalamus for control of tremors in Parkinson's disease and essential tremor. Stereotact Funct Neurosurg 72(1):47–61

Lenz FA, Dostrovsky JO, Kwan HC et al (1988) Methods for microstimulation and recording of single neurons and evoked potentials in the human central nervous system. J Neurosurg 68(4):630–634

Lenz FA, Kwan HC, Dostrovsky JO et al (1990) Single unit analysis of the human ventral thalamic nuclear group. Activity correlated with movement. Brain 113(Pt 6): 1795–1821

Lenz FA, Kwan HC, Martin RL et al (1994) Single unit analysis of the human ventral thalamic nuclear group. Tremor-related activity in functionally identified cells. Brain 117(Pt 3):531–543

Lenz FA, Normand SL, Kwan HC et al (1995) Statistical prediction of the optimal site for thalamotomy in parkinsonian tremor. Mov Disord 10(3):318–328

Limousin P, Speelman JD, Gielen F et al (1999) Multicentre European study of thalamic stimulation in parkinsonian and essential tremor. J Neurol Neurosurg Psychiatry 66(3):289–296

Limousin-Dowsey P (2002) Postoperative management of Vim DBS for tremor. Mov Disord 17(Suppl 3): S208–S211

Louis ED, Tang MX, Cote L et al (1999) Progression of parkinsonian signs in Parkinson disease. Arch Neurol 56(3):334–337

Lozano AM (2000) Vim thalamic stimulation for tremor. Arch Med Res 31(3):266–269

Lyons KE, Koller WC, Wilkinson SB et al (2001) Long term safety and efficacy of unilateral deep brain stimulation of the thalamus for parkinsonian tremor. J Neurol Neurosurg Psychiatry 71(5):682–684

Macchi G, Jones EG (1997) Toward an agreement on terminology of nuclear and subnuclear divisions of the motor thalamus. J Neurosurg 86(4):670–685

Matsumoto K, Shichijo F, Fukami T (1984) Long-term follow-up review of cases of Parkinson's disease after unilateral or bilateral thalamotomy. J Neurosurg 60(5): 1033–1044

Miyagi Y, Shima F, Sasaki T (2007) Brain shift: an error factor during implantation of deep brain stimulation electrodes. J Neurosurg 107(5):989–997

Molnar GF, Pilliar A, Lozano AM et al (2005) Differences in neuronal firing rates in pallidal and cerebellar receiving areas of thalamus in patients with Parkinson's disease, essential tremor, and pain. J Neurophysiol 93(6):3094–3101

Moro E, Lang AE (2006) Criteria for deep-brain stimulation in Parkinson's disease: review and analysis. Expert Rev Neurother 6(11):1695–1705

Mure H, Hirano S, Tang CC et al (2011) Parkinson's disease tremor-related metabolic network: characterization, progression, and treatment effects. Neuroimage 54(2):1244–1253

Narabayashi H (1989) Stereotaxic Vim thalamotomy for treatment of tremor. Eur Neurol 29(Suppl 1):29–32

Narabayashi H, Yokochi F, Nakajima Y (1984) Levodopa-induced dyskinesia and thalamotomy. J Neurol Neurosurg Psychiatry 47(8):831–839

Ohye C (1997) Functional organization of the human thalamus. In: Steriade M, Jones EG, McComick DA (eds) Thalamus, vol II. Elsevier, Amsterdam, pp 517–542

Ohye C, Narabayashi H (1979) Physiological study of presumed ventralis intermedius neurons in the human thalamus. J Neurosurg 50(3):290–297

Ondo W, Jankovic J, Schwartz K et al (1998) Unilateral thalamic deep brain stimulation for refractory essential tremor and Parkinson's disease tremor. Neurology 51(4):1063–1069

Pahwa R, Lyons KE, Wilkinson SB et al (2006) Long-term evaluation of deep brain stimulation of the thalamus. J Neurosurg 104(4):506–512

Peppe A, Gasbarra A, Stefani A et al (2008) Deep brain stimulation of CM/PF of thalamus could be the new elective target for tremor in advanced Parkinson's Disease? Parkinsonism Relat Disord 14(6):501–504

Pollak P, Benabid AL, Limousin P et al (1997) Chronic intracerebral stimulation in Parkinson's disease. Adv Neurol 74:213–220

Pollak P, Fraix V, Krack P et al (2002) Treatment results: Parkinson's disease. Mov Disord 17(Suppl 3): S75–S83

Putzke JD, Wharen RE Jr, Wszolek ZK et al (2003) Thalamic deep brain stimulation for tremor-predominant Parkinson's disease. Parkinsonism Relat Disord 10(2):81–88

Rehncrona S, Johnels B, Widner H et al (2003) Long-term efficacy of thalamic deep brain stimulation for tremor: double-blind assessments. Mov Disord 18(2): 163–170

Rodriguez MC, Guridi OJ, Alvarez L et al (1998) The subthalamic nucleus and tremor in Parkinson's disease. Mov Disord 13(Suppl 3):111–118

Rodriguez-Oroz MC, Rodriguez M, Guridi J et al (2001) The subthalamic nucleus in Parkinson's disease: somatotopic organization and physiological characteristics. Brain 124(Pt 9):1777–1790

Schaltenbrand G, Wahren W (1977) Atlas for stereotaxy of the human brain. Georg Thieme, Stuttgart

Schuurman PR, Bosch DA, Bossuyt PM et al (2000) A comparison of continuous thalamic stimulation and thalamotomy for suppression of severe tremor. N Engl J Med 342(7):461–468

Schuurman PR, Bosch DA, Merkus MP et al (2008) Long-term follow-up of thalamic stimulation versus thalamotomy for tremor suppression. Mov Disord 23(8):1146–1153

Siegfried J (1980) Neurosurgical treatment of Parkinson's disease. Present indications and value. In: Rinne UK, Klinger M, Stamm G (eds) Parkinson's disease. Current progress, problems and management. Elsevier, Amsterdam, pp 369–376

Sitburana O, Almaguer M, Ondo WG (2010) A pilot study: microlesion effects and tremor outcome in the ventrointermediate deep brain stimulation (VIM-DBS). Clin Neurol Neurosurg 112(2):106–109

Spiegelmann R, Nissim O, Daniels D et al (2006) Stereotactic targeting of the ventrointermediate nucleus of the thalamus by direct visualization with high-field MRI. Stereotact Funct Neurosurg 84(1): 19–23

Strafella A, Ashby P, Munz M et al (1997) Inhibition of voluntary activity by thalamic stimulation in humans: relevance for the control of tremor. Mov Disord 12(5):727–737

Tarsy D, Scollins L, Corapi K et al (2005) Progression of Parkinson's disease following thalamic deep brain stimulation for tremor. Stereotact Funct Neurosurg 83(5–6):222–227

Tasker RR (1998) Deep brain stimulation is preferable to thalamotomy for tremor suppression. Surg Neurol 49(2):145–153; discussion 153–144

Tasker RR, Siqueira J, Hawrylyshyn P et al (1983) What happened to VIM thalamotomy for Parkinson's disease? Appl Neurophysiol 46(1–4):68–83

Troster AI, Wilkinson SB, Fields JA et al (1998) Chronic electrical stimulation of the left ventrointermediate (Vim) thalamic nucleus for the treatment of pharmacotherapy-resistant Parkinson's disease: a differential impact on access to semantic and episodic memory? Brain Cogn 38(2):125–149

Vassal F, Coste J, Derost P et al (2012) Direct stereotactic targeting of the ventrointermediate nucleus of the thalamus based on anatomic 1.5-T MRI mapping with a white matter attenuated inversion recovery (WAIR) sequence. Brain Stimul 5(4):625–633

Vitek JL, Bakay RA, Hashimoto T et al (1998) Microelectrode-guided pallidotomy: technical approach and its application in medically intractable Parkinson's disease. J Neurosurg 88(6):1027–1043

Volkmann J, Sturm V, Weiss P et al (1998) Bilateral high-frequency stimulation of the internal globus pallidus in advanced Parkinson's disease. Ann Neurol 44(6): 953–961

Vu TC, Nutt JG, Holford NH (2012) Progression of motor and nonmotor features of Parkinson's disease and their response to treatment. Br J Clin Pharmacol 74(2): 267–283

Walter BL, Vitek JL (2004) Surgical treatment for Parkinson's disease. Lancet Neurol 3(12):719–728

Woods SP, Fields JA, Lyons KE et al (2001) Neuropsychological and quality of life changes following unilateral thalamic deep brain stimulation in Parkinson's disease: a one-year follow-up. Acta Neurochir (Wien) 143(12):1273–1277; discussion 1278

Yamada K, Akazawa K, Yuen S et al (2010) MR imaging of ventral thalamic nuclei. AJNR Am J Neuroradiol 31(4):732–735

Yoshida F, Miyagi Y, Morioka T et al (2008) Assessment of contact location in subthalamic stimulation for Parkinson's disease by co-registration of computed tomography images. Stereotact Funct Neurosurg 86(3):162–166

Zetusky WJ, Jankovic J, Pirozzolo FJ (1985) The heterogeneity of Parkinson's disease: clinical and prognostic implications. Neurology 35(4):522–526

Ziyan U, Tuch D, Westin CF (2006) Segmentation of thalamic nuclei from DTI using spectral clustering. Med Image Comput Comput Assist Interv 9(Pt 2):807–814

Deep Brain Stimulation for Dystonia

10

Takaomi Taira

10.1 Introduction

Dystonia is a neurological movement disorder, in which sustained muscle contractions cause twisting and repetitive movements or abnormal postures (Fahn et al. 1998). The disorder may be hereditary or caused by other factors such as birth-related or other physical trauma, infection, or reaction to pharmaceutical drugs, particularly neuroleptics. Although pathophysiology of dystonia is not clear, it is agreed that abnormal functional disorganization is present in the thalamo-cortical-basal ganglia neural loop (Albanese and Lalli 2012). Recently, involvement of cerebellar and brainstem mechanisms is postulated in animal studies (Filip et al. 2013; Hisatsune et al. 2013). In the past, dystonia was often regarded as psychogenic origin, and even today many patients with dystonia are misdiagnosed. A story of such typical dilemma was well described by Cooper (1976).

Treatment is difficult and has been limited to minimizing the symptoms of the disorder (Delnooz and van de Warrenburg 2012). Ablative stereotactic surgeries such as pallidotomy and thalamotomies were used to control dystonia in 1960s–1970s with various intracerebral targets. The most subjects were dystonia musculorum deformans which is known as DYT-1-positive young onset hereditary generalized dystonia. The results of surgery were not uniform with high incidence of complications, especially due to bilateral procedures. Surprisingly, some neurosurgeons have already tried deep brain stimulation before 1980, and had suggested the usefulness of DBS for movement disorders (Cooper et al. 1980; Mundinger 1977; Andy 1983; Hariz et al. 2010).

In early 1990s, Laitinen et al. (1992a, b) reported effectiveness of postero-ventro-lateral pallidotomy for Parkinson disease (PD), and it was dramatically effective for rigidity, dyskinesia, and frozen gait. Because dyskinesia and dystonia seen in PD are symptomatically similar to idiopathic generalized dystonia, Iacono et al. (1996) started such new pallidotomy for patients with generalized dystonia with favorable results. Many reports (Yoshor et al. 2001; Lin et al. 1999; Islekel et al. 1999; Vitek et al. 1998; Ondo et al. 1998; Vitek and Bakay 1997; Bhatia et al. 1998; Lai et al. 1999) on pallidotomy for generalized dystonia in late 1990s, around that time deep brain stimulation (DBS) of the thalamic Vim nucleus and subthalamic nucleus had been established for control of parkinsonian symptoms. Superiority of DBS over pallidotomy or thalamotomy had been shown in Parkinson disease and tremor, not because of effectiveness of controlling symptoms, but because of adjustability and reversibility of DBS that resulted in lower

T. Taira, MD, PhD
Department of Neurosurgery,
Tokyo Women's Medical University, Tokyo, Japan
e-mail: ttaira@nij.twmu.ac.jp

T. Itakura (ed.), *Deep Brain Stimulation for Neurological Disorders: Theoretical Background and Clinical Application*, DOI 10.1007/978-3-319-08476-3_10,

incidence of complications. Since then DBS has become a standard surgical treatment of PD and various types of tremor. However, it is interesting that there are no studies on randomized comparison of DBS and pallidotomy for dystonias. Pallidal DBS was adapted since late 1990s (Tronnier and Fogel 2000) without scientific evidence of superiority over pallidotomy with assumption that DBS should be better. Over the past 15 years, pallidal DBS has become a standard established treatment of generalized dystonia (Tagliati et al. 2011; Moro et al. 2013; Reese et al. 2011). Stable long-term effect of pallidal DBS has been reported (Mehrkens et al. 2009). However, there are still many issues to be solved.

10.2 Classification of Dystonias and Diagnosis

Dystonia is not a single disease. When neurosurgeons say "DBS for dystonia," the term "dystonia" generally mean "primary generalized dystonia" or "young-onset DYT-1-positive dystonia." However, there are many other types and etiologies in dystonia as shown in Table 10.1. Dystonia can be classified by the age of onset, body distribution, and etiology (Table 10.2). DBS is usually indicated for primary generalized dystonias, while incidence of adult-onset "focal" dystonia such as cervical dystonia and blephalospasm is much higher. Among secondary dystonias, cerebral palsy (CP) and tardive dystonia induced by anti-psychotic medications are most common. Genes and loci of hereditary dystonias have been found, and more than 20 types are listed as DTY dystonia (Table 10.3), and this indicates that dystonia is a clinically and genetically heterogeneous disorder (Kline 2009).

The diagnosis of dystonia is based mainly upon clinical features, although gene analysis can provide supportive evidence. Observation and examination of the patient with detailed clinical history are most important in diagnosis of dystonia. Patients with typical DYT-1 dystonia have normal milestones of development during early childhood, and then symptom starts from a leg or an arm. In the early stage of dystonia, sensory trick phenomenon (simple touching of a certain part of the body improves the symptoms) and morning benefit (symptoms are better immediately after waking up in the morning) are observed. The symptoms are always the same and stereotype. If these three manifestations are confirmed, diagnosis is not difficult. For further details, please refer to the UpToDate (Comella 2013).

10.3 Surgical Indication

It is well established that young-onset DYT-1-positive generalized dystonia is the best indication of pallidal DBS (Panov et al. 2013; Haridas et al. 2011; Isaias et al. 2009), while other non-hereditary adult-onset primary generalized dystonia respond to pallidal DBS as well. It has been shown that younger onset and shorter duration of the disease are the favorable factors of DBS treatment (Yamada et al. 2013; Lumsden et al. 2013). Symptoms of the trunk and proximal parts of extremities seem to respond better than the neck or the distal part of the extremities. This means that patients may have persistent difficulty of writing due to focal hand dystonia even after well controlled other symptoms. Tonic neck dystonia may be a residual symptom after DBS, and peripheral surgical procedure or botulinum toxin injections may be necessary. Speech difficulty may be refractory to DBS.

Patients with phasic or complex type cervical dystonia or orofacial dystonia (Meige syndrome) can be good candidates of pallidal DBS, if the symptoms are refractory to botulinum toxin injections (Kim et al. 2012; Ostrem et al. 2011; Morgan and Sethi 2008; Krauss 2007; Lyons et al. 2010; Witt et al. 2013; Walsh et al. 2013). It is often said that secondary dystonia does not respond well to pallidal DBS as compared with primary dystonia. Although this may be generally true, tardive dystonia due to anti-psychotic medications can be as well controlled as primary dystonias (Eltahawy et al. 2004; Franzini et al. 2005; Cohen et al. 2007; Sako et al. 2008; Gruber et al. 2009; Chang et al. 2010; Trinh et al. 2014). Functional or social outcome of tardive dystonia after DBS depends on the psychiatric state, and therefore medications necessary for their psychiatric symptoms should not be

Table 10.1 Classification of dystonia by etiology

Primary dystonia	
Typically early-onset: generalized	
DYT1 generalized dystonia	
Non-DYT1 generalized dystonia	
Paroxysmal dystonia and dyskinesias	
Dopa-responsive dystonia	
Myoclonic dystonia	
Rapid-onset dystonia-parkinsonism	
X-linked dystonia-parkinsonism	
Typically adult-onset: focal	
Blephalospasm	
Cervical dystonia	
Writer's cramp	
Embouchure dystonia	
Oromandibular dystonia	
Laryngeal dystonia	
Secondary dystonia	
Medications, trauma, toxins, infections, or stroke.	Pelizaeus-Merzbacher disease
Perinatal cerebral injury	Dystonia-deafness syndrome
Viral encephalitis	MERRF
SSPE	MELAS Leber's disease
AIDS	Leigh's syndrome
Creutzfeldt-Jakob disease	Neuroacanthocytosis
Kernicterus	Intranuclear inclusion disease
Huntington's disease	Hemochromatosis
Parkinson's disease	Progressive supranuclear palsy
Spinocerebellar ataxias	Multiple system atrophy
HARP syndrome	Corticobasal degeneration
Familial frontotemporal dementias	Dentatorubropalidoluysian atrophy
Familial basal ganglia calcifications	Glutaric academia
Wilson's disease	Methylmalonic academia
Juvenile parkinsonism	Homocystinuria
Ataxia-telangiectasia	Metachromatic leukodystrophy
Triosephosphate isomerase def	Neuronal ceroid lipofuscinosis
Vitamin E deficiency	Primary antiphospholipid antibody
Biopterin deficiency	Gangliosidoses
Sphingolipidoses	Hallervorden-Spatz disease
Niemann-Pick disease	Multiple sclerosis
Ceroid lipofuscinosis	Atlantoaxial sublaxation
Homocystinuria	Syringomyelia
Hartnup disease	Arnold-Chiari malformation
Methylmalonic aciduria	Congenital Klippel-Feil syndrome
Tyrosinemia	
Lesch-Nyhan syndrome	
Rett's syndrome	

stopped and close follow-up by psychiatrists is mandatory (Mentzel et al. 2012; Jahanshahi et al. 2011). There are few reports on DBS for dystonias of cerebral palsy origin (Katsakiori et al. 2009; Koy et al. 2013; Marks et al. 2013). Because of heterogeneity of the symptoms of cerebral palsy such as mixture of dystonia, spasticity, and athetosis, the effect of pallidal DBS in CP seems modest.

Table 10.2 Classification of dystonia by age and distribution

Classification by age of onset
Early onset (childhood and young adulthood, generally <26 years old)
Late onset (generally ≥26 years old)
Classification by anatomic distribution
Focal (involving a single body area)
Segmental (involving two or more contiguous body areas)
Generalized (involving at least one leg, the trunk, and another body area)
Multifocal (involving two or more noncontiguous body areas)
Hemidystonia (involving one side of the body)

However, even with such modest improvement of dystonia, patients may often feel great improvement probably because lifelong motor impairment had been so severe. A few patients with mild CP may develop severe generalized dystonia, and such patients can be good candidates of pallidal DBS.

Many congenital metabolic disorders can induce dystonias. Among them, dystonia in Lesch-Nyhan syndrome (Taira and Hori 2003; Deon et al. 2012; Cif et al. 2007) and Hallervorden-Spatz disease (Umemura et al. 2004; Timmermann et al. 2010; Ge et al. 2011) is considered to be an indication of DBS.

Table 10.3 List of hereditary dystonias named DYT

Symbol	Gene	Locus	Alternative name
DYT1	TOR1A	9q34	Early-onset torsion dystonia
DYT2	Unknown	Unknown	Autosomal recessive torsion dystonia
DYT3	TAF1	Xq13	X-linked dystonia-parkinsonism
DYT4	TUBB4	19p13.12-13	Autosomal dominant whispering dysphonia
DYT5a	GCH1	14q22.1-q22.2	Autosomal dominant dopamine-responsive dystonia
DYT5b	TH	11p15.5	Autosomal recessive dopamine-responsive dystonia
DYT6	THAP1	8p11.21	Autosomal dominant dystonia with cranio-cervical predilection
DYT7	Unknown	18p (questionable)	Autosomal dominant primary focal cervical dystonia
DYT8	MR1	2q35	Paroxysmal nonkinesigenic dyskinesia
DYT9	SLC2A1	1p35-p31.3	Episodic choreoathetosis/spasticity (now known to be synonymous with DYT18)
DYT10	PRRT2	16p11.2-q12.1	Paroxysmal kinesigenic dyskinesia
DYT11	SGCE	7q21	Myoclonic dystonia
DYT12	ATP1A3	19q12-q13.2	Rapid onset dystonia parkinsonism and alternating hemiplegia of childhood
DYT13	Unknown, near D1S2667	1p36.32-p36.13	Autosomal dominant cranio-cervical/upper limb dystonia in one Italian family
DYT14		14q	Dopa-responsive dystonia
DYT15	Unknown	18p11	Myoclonic dystonia not linked to SGCE mutations
DYT16	PRKRA	2q31.3	Autosomal recessive young onset dystonia parkinsonism
DYT17	Unknown, near D20S107	20p11.2-q13.12	Autosomal recessive dystonia in one family
DYT18	SLC2A1	1p35-p31.3	Paroxysmal exercise-induced dyskinesia
DYT19	Probably PRRT2	16q13-q22.1	Episodic kinesigenic dyskinesia, probably synonymous with DYT10
DYT20	Unknown	2q31	Paroxysmal nonkinesigenic dyskinesia
DYT21	Unknown	2q14.3-q21.3	Late-onset torsion dystonia
DYT23	ANO3	11p14.2	Autosomal dominant cranio-cervical dystonia with prominent tremor

Prior to considering DBS, brain MRI is always required to confirm diagnosis and assess structural abnormalities. Other imaging techniques, particularly functional imaging (Chernov et al. 2008), are used for research purposes (Thobois et al. 2011). There is no enough evidence to refuse or support consideration of DBS in patients with previous ablative procedures such as pallidotomy and thalamotomy (Bronte-Stewart et al. 2011).

10.4 Targets and Localization

The sensori-motor area of the globus pallidum interna (GPi) is the gold standard target of DBS for dystonia. However, we still do not know where the best point in the sensori-motor area of GPi is. The tentative target coordinate is 2 mm anterior to mid-commissural point, 4 mm below the commissural line, and 20 mm from the midline. The laterality is usually adjusted based on the relation of the optic tract on T2-weighted images of MRI. The target should lie just above the optic tract. This target is same as Laitinen's pallidotomy (Laitinen et al. 1992b), and it works in majority of cases, though if this point is best to control dystonia is debatable.

There are some reports that the subthalamic nucleus (STN) can be an alternative target of DBS for dystonias (Pahapill and O'Connell 2010; Kleiner-Fisman et al. 2007; Novak et al. 2008; Sun et al. 2007; Schrock et al. 2009). STN has both theoretical and clinical evidences as a target of DBS in PD. However, still the mechanisms of dystonia control are not well known. I consider that STN DBS for dystonia is not stimulating STN itself, but that fibers from internal pallidum to ventro-oral nucleus of the thalamus are stimulated at the rostral area to STN which is the lenticular fasciculus or Forel H field. This accounts for the facts that relatively low voltage stimulation is enough to control dystonic symptoms. In recent years in China, STN stimulation is more commonly performed than pallidal DBS for dystonias.

Data on thalamic DBS for dystonia are scarce. Although thalamic DBS may be effective for focal hand dystonia such as writer's cramp (Fukaya et al. 2007), I prefer Vo thalamotomy for such writer's and musician's focal hand dystonia, because the symptom is usually unilateral, patients are socially active, and there is no concern of hardware-related complications (Taira et al. 2003a, b; Horisawa et al. 2013).

10.5 Surgical Procedures

Surgical procedures of DBS differ from center to center (Abosch et al. 2013), and it is difficult to determine which the best is. Some neurosurgeons use frameless system or robotic device, while others are happy with the traditional stereotactic frames. Many neurosurgeons use intraoperative electrophysiological technique, and consider it very important, while some others rely on purely image-guided technique.

General anesthesia is often used for DBS for dystonias (Abosch et al. 2013) because dystonic movements may interfere accurate fixation of the stereotactic frame, MR scanning, and operative procedures. However, in my series of DBS for dystonias, we use general anesthesia only for small children, and did not use GA for adults. The only exception was a man who had a history of severe acute allergic reaction to lidocaine. This is because of availability of anesthetists and MR-compatible anesthetic devices. However, we seldom feel necessity of GA even in dystonia DBS. In our experience, we can easily fix the stereotactic frame and align the axes of the frame to the cerebral axes only with local anesthesia without sedation, even if dystonic symptom is severe. The frame is fixed in the sitting position on a wheel chair of which back-support can be reclined (Fig. 10.1). This is usually done in the ward. We used Leksell G frame (Elekta) and its ear-bars to align the frame. Fixing the frame takes about 10 min and then the patient is sent for MR scanning.

We use 1 mm thickness T1 axial and T2 coronal images without imaging gap or overwrap.

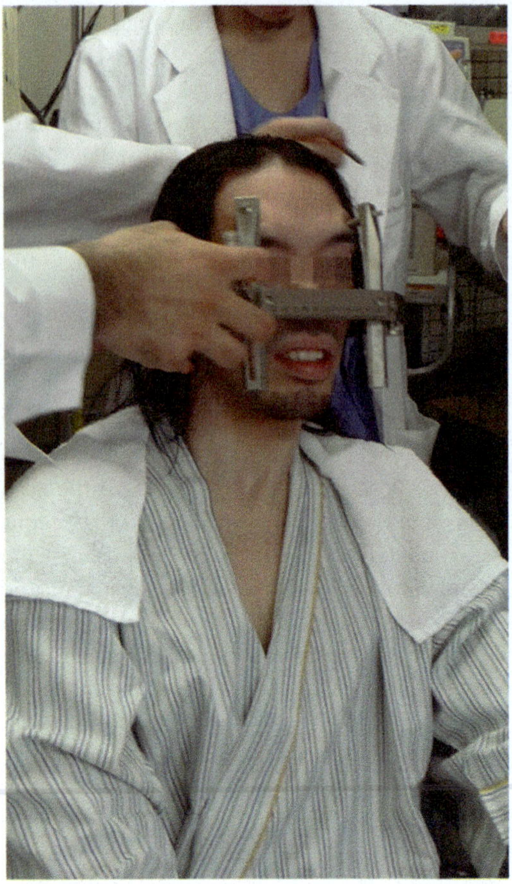

Fig. 10.1 Frame fixation in sitting position. Even if the patients head and neck move involuntary, fixation is not difficult without sedation

The image data are transferred online to the Surgiplan computer (Elekta). The GPi target is chosen at the point described already. The angle of trajectory is determined not to pass through the ventricles (Fig. 10.2). Usually, the location of bur holes come 3.5–4.0 cm from the midline and just anterior to the coronal suture.

In the operation room, the frame is fixed with Mayfield cramp to the operation table. Care should be taken not to flex the neck excessively to avoid airway obstruction. We may use mild sedation with intravenous diazepam or propofol, but this is exceptional. C-arm X-ray fluoroscope is set, and the patient head is sterilized with alcoholic and iodine solutions (Fig. 10.3). We do not shave the head totally but local hair clipping is enough, and this does not increase the risk of infection. After appropriate draping, two burr holes are opened symmetrically with 2.5 cm straight incisions, but the dura is not opened until the last minutes of electrode insertion. Once the electrode insertion is ready, the axes of X-ray fluoroscope are well aligned in right–left direction by using cross-hairline markers (Fig. 10.4).

We use a stainless-steel outer cannula (outer diameter: 2.1 mm, inner diameter: 1.5 mm, length: 20 cm) with a rigid inner stylet of 1.3 mm in diameter for DBS electrode placement. The stylet protrudes about 1.5 cm from the tip of the outer cannula. Once the tip of the stylet reaches

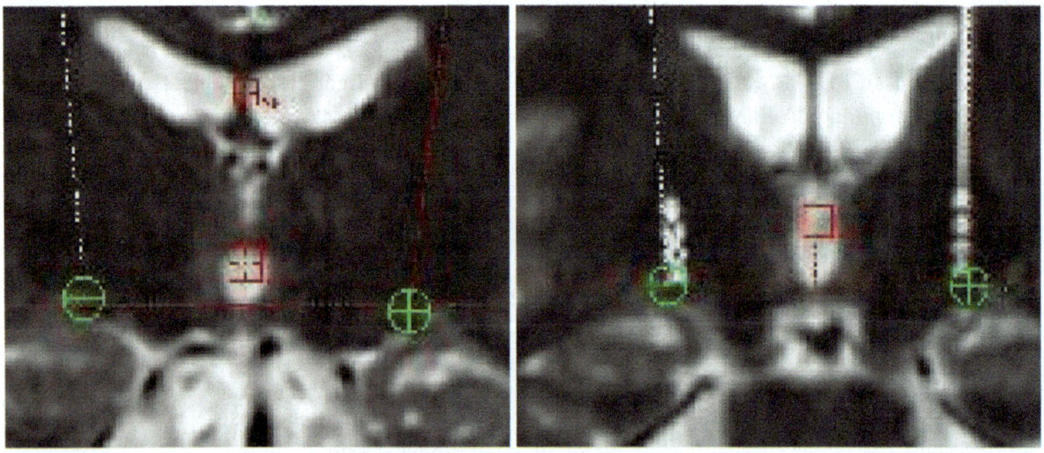

Fig. 10.2 *Left*: planning of GPi target. The target is just dorsal to the lateral edge of the optic tract. *Right*: Postoperative MR image showing accurate placement of the electrode

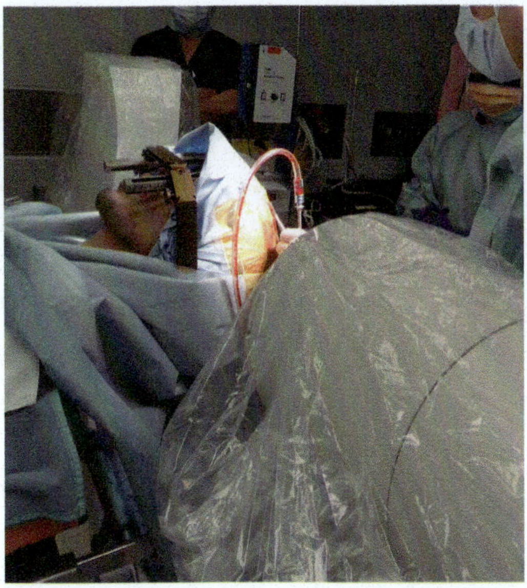

Fig. 10.3 Positioning of the patient and set-up of fluoroscope

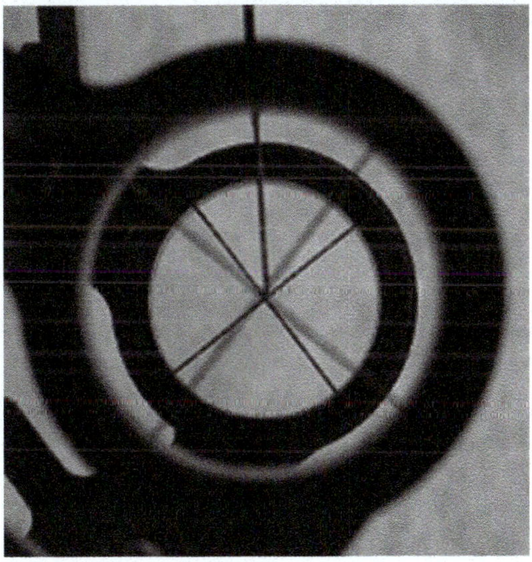

Fig. 10.4 X-ray beam should be aligned with cross-hairline markers before opening the dura

to the target, the stylet is replaced by DBS electrode (Model 3387, Medtronic) and then trial macro-stimulation is started. Initially, we usually use 0-1+ contacts with 130 Hz, 200 μs pulse width. The voltage is gradually increased until pyramidal symptoms appear. Usually this threshold is 4.0–4.5 V. For such intraoperative macrostimulation, we use a gas-sterilized DBS screening device (Fig. 10.5). This is very useful and handy, and we have been using it for more than 10 years and have not encountered dysfunction of the device despite gas sterilization. If pyramidal symptoms appear at voltage lower than 3.0, we check the contact 1-2+. If this combination of contacts shows lower threshold than 3.0 V, the trajectory is too close to the pyramidal tract, and we move the target 2 mm more laterally. Once the electrode is appropriately placed, we remove the outer cannula carefully so that the tip of the DBS electrode does not move. Then the DBS electrode is fixed to the skull with a titanium plate coved with a silastic tube (Fig. 10.6). A small piece of surgical is placed in the burr hole. We used to tunnel out the electrode for trial stimulation, but nowadays we just place the covered proximal end of the DBS electrode subcutaneously by making a separate small incision in the posterior parietal region. We can implant the pulse generator (IPG) immediately after placing DBS electrode, but again because of availability of anesthetists, we implant IPG about a week later. After surgery, the patient is always sent for MR and CT scanning to check the location of the electrode. Fusion images of both post operative MR and CT is useful to identify the actual location of every contact of the DBS electrode (Fig. 10.7). With the above technique, it take about less than 2 h for bilateral pallidal DBS from skin to skin, and 5 h from putting frame on and removing frame off.

For cosmetic reasons, we implant IPG with an incision under the axilla and place the IPG under the fascia of the pectoris muscle in the anterior chest (Fig. 10.8). For small children, abdominal subfascial placement may be preferred.

Many neurosurgeons use intraoperative micro-recording (MER) for verification of GPi, while others do not use MER and some even do not use intraoperative physiological confirmation in GPi DBS procedures (Vitek et al. 2011). The use of MER increases incidence of hemorrhagic complications (Zrinzo et al. 2012a). It is reported that image-verified DBS without MER may reduce risk without losing efficacy (Zrinzo et al. 2012b). Of

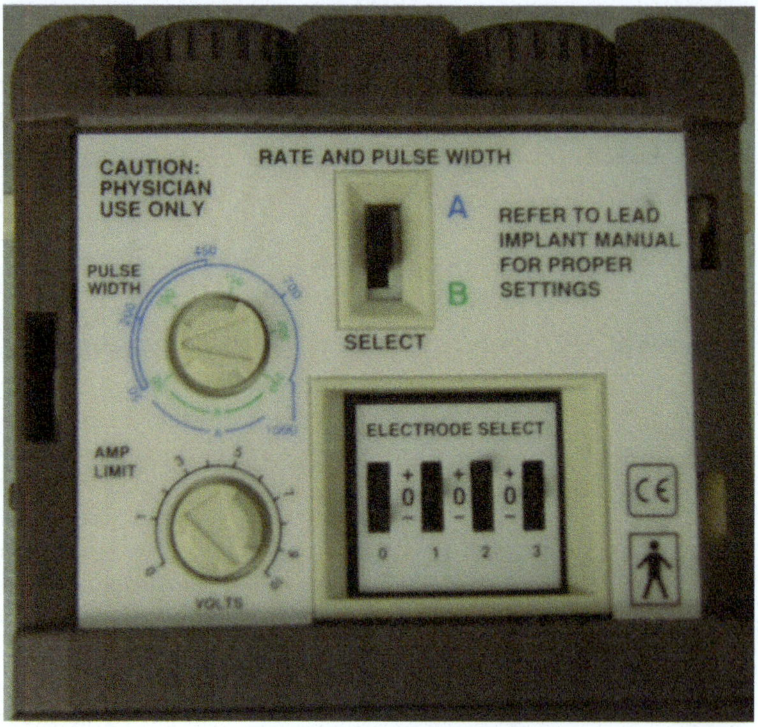

Fig. 10.5 Stimulation device for intraoperative test stimulation. This is gas-sterilized and controlled by the surgeon

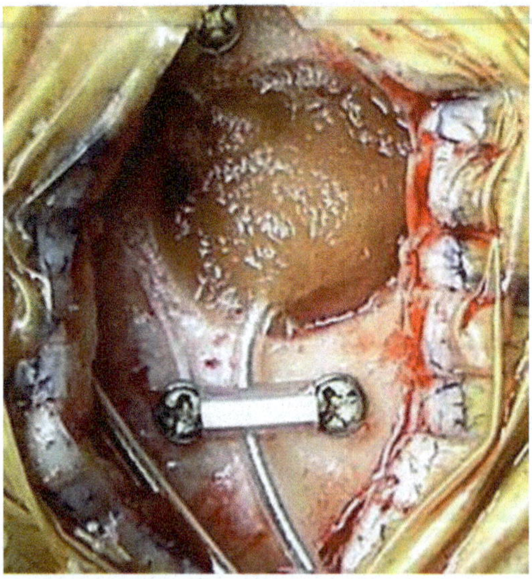

Fig. 10.6 Fixation of the DBS electrode to the skull. The mini-plate is covered with a silastic tube. If necessary, we may insert two or three DBS leads from a burr hole, and they can be fixed with this method

course, MER may be an interesting tool for research of basal ganglia pathophysiology in dystonia.

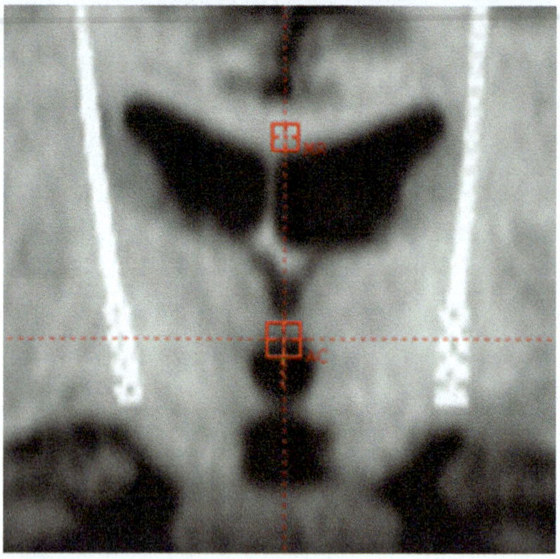

Fig. 10.7 Postoperative fusion image of MR and CT to identify the location of each contact. *AC* level of anterior commissure, *MR* midline reference

10.6 Stimulation Parameters

In general, stimulation parameters of pallidal DBS should be higher in dystonias than in PD. The most common parameters are 130–185 Hz,

210–450 μs pulse width, 1.5–5 V, but it varies from center to center. Some uses similar parameters as in PD, while others use very wide pulse width (450 μs) with relatively low voltage (1.5 V). There is no unanimous or standard parameters. If high frequency stimulation does not work well enough, one can try 60–80 Hz (Alterman et al. 2007a, b; Merola et al. 2013). We usually start stimulation with 0-1+ contacts, 185 Hz, 210 μs pulse width, and slightly lower voltage of pyramidal effect threshold (usually 3.0–3.5 V). If the clinical effect is inadequate, combination of 0-1-2+ is selected. I seldom use monopolar stimulation to avoid excessive current spread and to save battery energy.

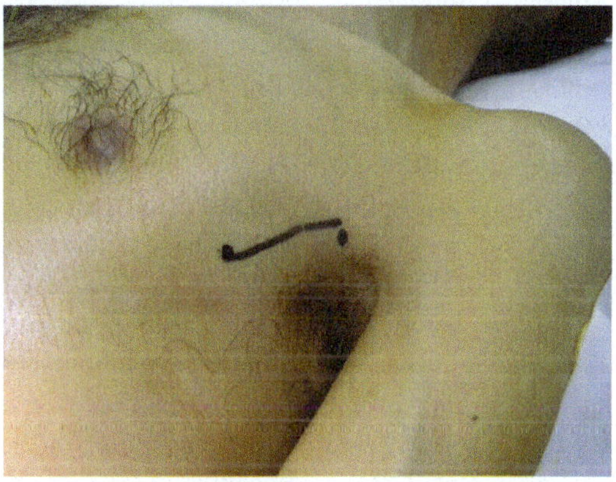

Fig. 10.8 Sub-axillar skin incision for placement of IPG

10.7 Side Effects and Complications

The most common side effect of bilateral GPi DBS is dysarthria. This is probably caused by current spread to the cortico-bulbar tract in the internal capsule located postero-medially to the GPi. To avoid such side effect, the electrode should be placed in the GPi where electrical macro-stimulation under 4.0 V does not elicit pyramidal tract symptoms such as dysarthria or increased tonus of the contralateral arm during surgery. Occasionally, some patients complain of dysarthria subjectively while speech sounds completely understandable and normal to others.

Hardware-related complications are the commonest issue in DBS, especially infection or rejection of the implanted leads and devices (Fig. 10.9). I have not experienced intracranial infection, but subcutaneous wires and device infection were seen in about 5 % of the patients. Conservative antibiotic treatment and local closure of the wound are generally ineffective. Once infection becomes apparent, all the subcutaneous hardware systems should be removed surgically. However, stopping stimulation may induce severe rebound dystonic storm. Therefore, we have to stop stimulation before removing the system to see what happened. If stopping stimulation induces uncontrollable dystonia, pallidotomy through DBS electrode should be considered. I have such experience in four cases,

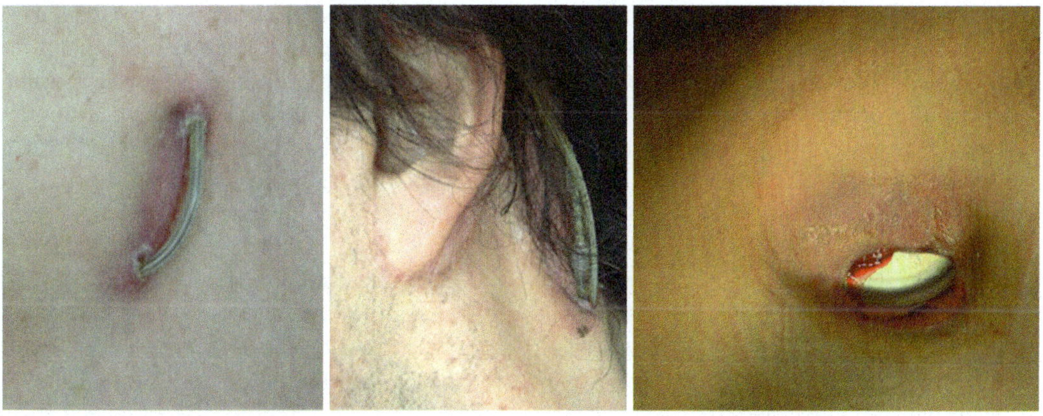

Fig. 10.9 Rejected DBS wires and IPG

and simultaneous bilateral pallidotomy excellently controlled dystonia without serious complications. Of course this is only possible with careful neurological examination during surgery under local anesthesia.

It was recently reported that GPi DBS may induce bradykinetic symptoms like parkinsonism in patients who receive effective stimulation for dystonia (Blahak et al. 2011; Berman et al. 2009). I have seen two similar patients and everyone should be aware of such rare complications.

10.8 Unexpected Improvement

The following is my unexpected experience in surgical management of dystonias. In clinical practice, unexpected things often happen and I hope such serendipity is important in any field of medicine. There are a few patients whose dystonic symptoms do not recur even after the battery of IPG is exhausted. I have experienced two such cases. Both were primary adult-onset axial dystonia and the duration of dystonia before surgery was 3 and 5 years respectively. When the patients came to the outpatient clinic for 3.5-year follow-up after successful control of dystonia by bilateral GPi DBS, we found the IPG battery had been completely flat. However, the patients had not noticed any changes and there were no dystonic symptoms. They were now followed up for 4 years without stimulation, and recurrence of dystonia has not been observed. Can we call such phenomena "complete cure of dystonia," or is it merely a transient "remission"? It has been considered that "dystonia" is incurable for many years. However, it may be appropriate to consider "the definition of cure" of dystonias.

I already reported disappearance of self-injury behavior in a patient with Lesch-Nyhan syndrome who underwent bilateral GPi DBS to control his dystonia (Taira and Hori 2003; Preston 2007). Several others have reconfirmed such effects of GPi DBS in this metabolic syndrome (Deon et al. 2012; Cif et al. 2007; Pralong et al. 2005).

Some patients with generalized dystonia have speech and swallowing problems as symptoms of dystonia. Even if axial or appendicular symptoms are controlled with DBS, their speech problem may persist. I performed bilateral GPi DBS for a patient with severe pharyngo-laryngeal dystonia who were unable to speak nor eat. He had been a school teacher and the symptom stared after his retirement. Immediately after the surgery, his speech and swallowing became completely normal. He has been followed up for 7 years now. Every time when his IPG battery is exhausted, the symptoms came back, and replacement of IPG resulted in good control of the symptoms.

10.9 Unsolved Issues

Although DBS is an established treatment for otherwise intractable dystonia, there are still many issues to be solved. For example, the current GPi target was originally chosen at the deepest part of GPi where ansa lenticularis fibers are focusing. However, in GPi DBS, many use not only contact 0 but often combinations of other contacts which are far from the ansa lenticularis (Fig. 10.10). This means that GPi DBS is stimulating the components of lenticular fasciculus that connect from GPi to the ventro-oral nucleus of the thalamus. Thus, we still do not know exactly where the best stimulation point in the sensori-motor GPi is. Recently, Moro et al. (2013) nicely pointed out and summarized such problems and raised the following questions: When is medical therapy not enough?, How do you select the best patients for the best outcome?, Is the internal segment of the globus pallidus the best target?, and Is there any role for pallidotomy? Then, they answered to these questions in detail by citing many papers. I would add to their comments the following: Is there any role of peripheral surgery for cervical dystonia? Are the patients actually happy with the improved rating score we measure for assessment of surgical treatments?, How should we manage more common type of dystonia such as writer's, musician's and occupational focal hand dystonia?, and Is DBS really the best? Moro et al. discussed about the role of DBS industries in the management of

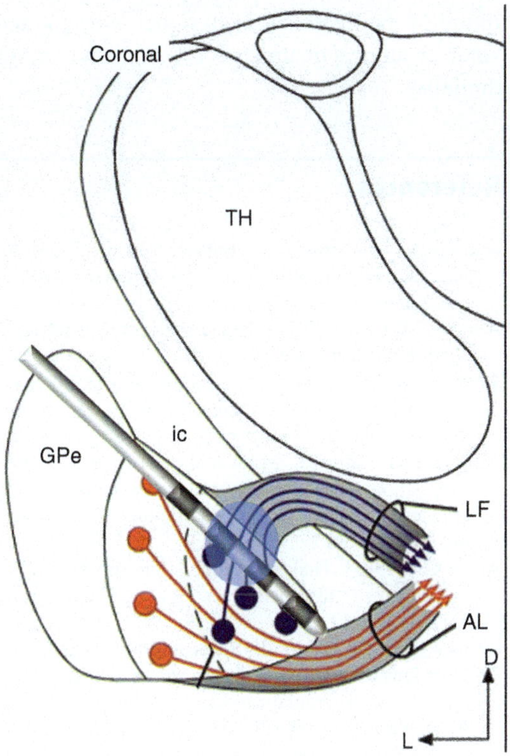

Fig. 10.10 Relation of the DBS electrode with the lenticular fasciculus (*LF*) and ansa lenticularis (*AL*). LF may be more important for the effect of GPi DBS. *TH* thalamus, *ic* internal capsule, *D* dorsal, *L* lateral, *GPe* globus pallidum externa

dystonias. Industries nowadays support financially DBS training courses, scientific meetings, large-scale clinical studies, and so on to push the use of DBS. Topics on the procedures that threaten disfavor of DBS, such as pallidotomy, thalamotomy, and peripheral denervation, are often left behind in sponsored meetings. Ablative procedures are technically more difficult for neurosurgeons and it takes more time for training. However, there remains a important role for pallidotomy for dystonia in more developed countries (Moro et al. 2013), and this is also true in case of thalamotomy and peripheral procedures. In my practice of treatment of dystonia, more than 520 patients underwent operations, and half of them are selective peripheral denervation for cervical dystonia, a quarter is pallidal DBS, and the remaining quarter is ventro-oral thalamotomy for task-specific focal hand dystonia. A few patients had intrathecal baclofen treatment. As "dystonia" is not a uniform disorder in terms of symptoms, distribution, severity, social burden, etiology, and so on, only a single procedure like DBS cannot solve the wide-range of problems in patients with dystonias. Those who treat dystonias at large should also pay attention to and armed with such other techniques, and it is very important to be able to select unbiased strategies.

10.10 Epilogue

When I was a registrar in Birmingham, UK in late 1980s, the head of the neurosurgical department, Professor Edward Hitchcock proposed me to study "neurosurgical management of dystonia." I thought it was nonsense, because I had not seen any patients with dystonia and I thought dystonia is too rare to study. I had to, however, obey the order of the professor. Then I reviewed clinical records of patients with dystonia treated by thalamotomy, examined such patients during followed-up visits, interviewed by phone, and finally reported in the Meeting of the World Society for Stereotactic and Functional Neurosurgery in 1989 (Taira and Hitchicock 1990). The report described "Immediate improvement occurred in patients with focal limb dystonia. … Improvement was sustained in patients with focal dystonia. …..Focal limb dystonia can be greatly improved by thalamotomy without any motor, sensory or intellectual disturbance." This fact is completely forgotten, and even I did not remember such a report when I started "modern" ventro-oral thalamotomy for task-specific focal hand dystonia in 2001 (Taira et al. 2003a; Horisawa et al. 2013). Today it is general belief that improvement of dystonia by GPi DBS is often delayed after surgery. However, immediate effect of thalamotomy on "focal hand" dystonia is described many years ago and it is a fact even today. The first patient I performed Vo-thalamotomy for writer's cramp was a young lady, who was a comic artist and had become unable to continue her job because of focal dystonia. After surgery she started working again and finally recorded in the Guinness Book as the most selling manga artist. Now I perform Vo-thalamotomy for focal hand dystonia almost every week.

In 1991, when I was a research fellow in University of Amsterdam in The Netherlands, Professor Andries Bosch kindly took me to Lueven in Belgium to see Professor Gybels' operation for spasmodic torticollis. The operation was selective peripheral denervation of the posterior neck muscles that was completely new for me. Even in the operation theater, watching the surgery, I was embarrassed that I could not understand the surgical anatomy at all. I started this operation, by chance, in 1995 and since then I have performed nearly 300 operations with my original modified technique (Taira et al. 2002). Now I see overwhelmingly many new patients with dystonia in my clinic, and realized that what I thought in Birmingham was completely wrong.

If we have effective and beneficial treatment modalities, many patients will come. If you have not seen patients with dystonia, this is not because dystonia is very rare but because you do not have methods, knowledge, or abilities to treat them. Although interest of industries may have played a role, introduction of botulinum toxin injections and deep brain stimulation has definitely played a very important role to make more doctors to be interested and involved in the treatment of dystonia, and patients with dystonia started coming to hospitals. Awareness of dystonia has been much improved over the past 10 years.

In Parkinson's disease, there will appear more effective new medical treatment in 10–20 years, and surgical treatment of PD including DBS has limitations because it does not stop progression of the disease itself. We know that most patients with PD finally deteriorate after so-called "honeymoon period" of DBS. In dystonia, animal models are inadequate and there is little hope of dramatically effective new drugs. Many types of dystonias are fortunately not degenerative disorder, and there is higher chance for us to bring "permanent cure." My longest follow-up of GPi DBS in dystonia is now 13 years, and even now DBS is working and the patients are enjoying normal life. Very long-term effect of DBS is much better in dystonias than PD. I hope the future of the treatment of dystonia is bright and value of surgical treatment for dystonia will never diminish.

References

Abosch A, Timmermann L, Bartley S et al (2013) An international survey of deep brain stimulation procedural steps. Stereotact Funct Neurosurg 91(1):1–11

Albanese A, Lalli S (2012) Update on dystonia. Curr Opin Neurol 25(4):483–490

Alterman RL, Miravite J, Weisz D et al (2007a) Sixty hertz pallidal deep brain stimulation for primary torsion dystonia. Neurology 69(7):681–688

Alterman RL, Shils JL, Miravite J et al (2007b) Lower stimulation frequency can enhance tolerability and efficacy of pallidal deep brain stimulation for dystonia. Mov Disord 22(3):366–368

Andy OJ (1983) Thalamic stimulation for control of movement disorders. Appl Neurophysiol 46(1–4):107–111

Berman BD, Starr PA, Marks WJ et al (2009) Induction of bradykinesia with pallidal deep brain stimulation in patients with cranial-cervical dystonia. Stereotact Funct Neurosurg 87(1):37–44

Bhatia KP, Marsden CD, Thomas DG (1998) Posteroventral pallidotomy can ameliorate attacks of paroxysmal dystonia induced by exercise. J Neurol Neurosurg Psychiatry 65(4):604–605

Blahak C, Capelle HH, Baezner H et al (2011) Micrographia induced by pallidal DBS for segmental dystonia: a subtle sign of hypokinesia? J Neural Transm 118(4):549–553

Bronte-Stewart H, Taira T, Valldeoriola F et al (2011) Inclusion and exclusion criteria for DBS in dystonia. Mov Disord 26(Suppl 1):S5–S16

Chang EF, Schrock LE, Starr PA et al (2010) Long-term benefit sustained after bilateral pallidal deep brain stimulation in patients with refractory tardive dystonia. Stereotact Funct Neurosurg 88(5):304–310

Chernov MF, Ochiai T, Taira T et al (2008) Serial (1) H-MRS of thalamus during deep brain stimulation of bilateral globus pallidus internus for primary generalized dystonia. Neuroradiology 50(12):1055–1059

Cif L, Biolsi B, Gavarini S et al (2007) Antero-ventral internal pallidum stimulation improves behavioral disorders in Lesch-Nyhan disease. Mov Disord 22(14):2126–2129

Cohen OS, Hassin-Baer S, Spiegelmann R (2007) Deep brain stimulation of the internal globus pallidus for refractory tardive dystonia. Parkinsonism Relat Disord 13(8):541–544

Comella C (2013) Classification and evaluation of dystonia. http://www.uptodate.com/contents/classification-and-evaluation-of-dystonia#H24

Cooper IS (1976) The victim is always the same. W. W. Norton & Company, New York

Cooper IS, Upton AR, Amin I (1980) Reversibility of chronic neurologic deficits. Some effects of electrical stimulation of the thalamus and internal capsule in man. Appl Neurophysiol 43(3–5):244–258

Delnooz CC, van de Warrenburg BP (2012) Current and future medical treatment in primary dystonia. Ther Adv Neurol Disord 5(4):221–240

Deon LL, Kalichman MA, Booth CL et al (2012) Pallidal deep-brain stimulation associated with complete remission of self-injurious behaviors in a patient with Lesch-Nyhan syndrome: a case report. J Child Neurol 27(1):117–120

Eltahawy HA, Feinstein A, Khan F et al (2004) Bilateral globus pallidus internus deep brain stimulation in tardive dyskinesia: a case report. Mov Disord 19(8):969–972

Fahn S, Bressman SB, Marsden CD (1998) Classification of dystonia. Adv Neurol 78:1–10

Filip P, Lungu OV, Bares M (2013) Dystonia and the cerebellum: a new field of interest in movement disorders? Clin Neurophysiol 124(7):1269–1276

Franzini A, Marras C, Ferroli P et al (2005) Long-term high-frequency bilateral pallidal stimulation for neuroleptic-induced tardive dystonia. Report of two cases. J Neurosurg 102(4):721–725

Fukaya C, Katayama Y, Kano T et al (2007) Thalamic deep brain stimulation for writer's cramp. J Neurosurg 107(5):977–982

Ge M, Zhang K, Ma Y et al (2011) Bilateral subthalamic nucleus stimulation in the treatment of neurodegeneration with brain iron accumulation type 1. Stereotact Funct Neurosurg 89(3):162–166

Gruber D, Trottenberg T, Kivi A et al (2009) Long-term effects of pallidal deep brain stimulation in tardive dystonia. Neurology 73(1):53–58

Haridas A, Tagliati M, Osborn I et al (2011) Pallidal deep brain stimulation for primary dystonia in children. Neurosurgery 68(3):738–743; discussion 743

Hariz MI, Blomstedt P, Zrinzo L (2010) Deep brain stimulation between 1947 and 1987: the untold story. Neurosurg Focus 29(2):E1

Hisatsune C, Miyamoto H, Hirono M et al (2013) P3R1 deficiency in the cerebellum/brainstem causes basal ganglia-independent dystonia by triggering tonic Purkinje cell firings in mice. Front Neural Circuits. doi:10.3389/fncir.2013.00156 2013

Horisawa S, Taira T, Goto S et al (2013) Long-term improvement of musician's dystonia after stereotactic ventro-oral thalamotomy. Ann Neurol 74(5):648–654

Iacono RP, Kuniyoshi SM, Lonser RR et al (1996) Simultaneous bilateral pallidoansotomy for idiopathic dystonia musculorum deformans. Pediatr Neurol 14(2):145–148

Isaias IU, Alterman RL, Tagliati M (2009) Deep brain stimulation for primary generalized dystonia: long-term outcomes. Arch Neurol 66(4):465–470

Islekel S, Zileli M, Zileli B (1999) Unilateral pallidal stimulation in cervical dystonia. Stereotact Funct Neurosurg 72(2–4):248–252

Jahanshahi M, Czernecki V, Zurowski AM (2011) Neuropsychological, neuropsychiatric, and quality of life issues in DBS for dystonia. Mov Disord 26(Suppl 1):S63–S78

Katsakiori PF, Kefalopoulou Z, Markaki E et al (2009) Deep brain stimulation for secondary dystonia: results in 8 patients. Acta Neurochir (Wien) 151(5):473–478; discussion 478

Kim JP, Chang WS, Park YS et al (2012) Effects of relative low-frequency bilateral globus pallidus internus stimulation for treatment of cervical dystonia. Stereotact Funct Neurosurg 90(1):30–36

Kleiner-Fisman G, Liang GS, Moberg PJ et al (2007) Subthalamic nucleus deep brain stimulation for severe idiopathic dystonia: impact on severity, neuropsychological status, and quality of life. J Neurosurg 107(1):29–36

Kline C (2009) The twists and turns of dystonia genes and loci: an update. http://www.movementdisorders.org/monthly_edition/2009/02/twists_and_turns.php

Koy A, Hellmich M, Pauls KA et al (2013) Effects of deep brain stimulation in dyskinetic cerebral palsy: a meta-analysis. Mov Disord 28(5):647–654

Krauss JK (2007) Deep brain stimulation for treatment of cervical dystonia. Acta Neurochir Suppl 97(Pt 2):201–205

Lai T, Lai JM, Grossman RG (1999) Functional recovery after bilateral pallidotomy for the treatment of early-onset primary generalized dystonia. Arch Phys Med Rehabil 80(10):1340–1342

Laitinen LV, Bergenheim AT, Hariz MI (1992a) Ventroposterolateral pallidotomy can abolish all parkinsonian symptoms. Stereotact Funct Neurosurg 58(1–4):14–21

Laitinen LV, Bergenheim AT, Hariz MI (1992b) Leksell's posteroventral pallidotomy in the treatment of Parkinson's disease. J Neurosurg 76(1):53–61

Lin JJ, Lin GY, Shih C et al (1999) Benefit of bilateral pallidotomy in the treatment of generalized dystonia. Case report. J Neurosurg 90(5):974–976

Lumsden DE, Kaminska M, Gimeno H et al (2013) Proportion of life lived with dystonia inversely correlates with response to pallidal deep brain stimulation in both primary and secondary childhood dystonia. Dev Med Child Neurol 55(6):567–574

Lyons MK, Birch BD, Hillman RA et al (2010) Long-term follow-up of deep brain stimulation for Meige syndrome. Neurosurg Focus 29(2):E5

Marks W, Bailey L, Reed M et al (2013) Pallidal stimulation in children: comparison between cerebral palsy and DYT1 dystonia. J Child Neurol 28(7):840–848

Mehrkens JH, Botzel K, Steude U et al (2009) Long-term efficacy and safety of chronic globus pallidus internus stimulation in different types of primary dystonia. Stereotact Funct Neurosurg 87(1):8–17

Mentzel CL, Tenback DE, Tijssen MA et al (2012) Efficacy and safety of deep brain stimulation in patients with medication-induced tardive dyskinesia and/or dystonia: a systematic review. J Clin Psychiatry 73(11):1434–1438

Merola A, Zibetti M, Artusi CA et al (2013) 80 Hz versus 130 Hz subthalamic nucleus deep brain stimulation:

effects on involuntary movements. Parkinsonism Relat Disord 19(4):453–456
Morgan JC, Sethi KD (2008) A single-blind trial of bilateral globus pallidus internus deep brain stimulation in medically refractory cervical dystonia. Curr Neurol Neurosci Rep 8(4):279–280
Moro E, Gross RE, Krauss JK (2013) What's new in surgical treatment for dystonia? Mov Disord 28(7):1013–1020
Mundinger F (1977) New stereotactic treatment of spasmodic torticollis with a brain stimulation system (author's transl). Med Klin 72(46):1982–1986
Novak KE, Nenonene EK, Bernstein LP et al (2008) Successful bilateral subthalamic nucleus stimulation for segmental dystonia after unilateral pallidotomy. Stereotact Funct Neurosurg 86(2):80–86
Ondo WG, Desaloms JM, Jankovic J et al (1998) Pallidotomy for generalized dystonia. Mov Disord 13(4):693–698
Ostrem JL, Racine CA, Glass GA et al (2011) Subthalamic nucleus deep brain stimulation in primary cervical dystonia. Neurology 76(10):870–878
Pahapill PA, O'Connell B (2010) Long-term follow-up study of chronic deep brain stimulation of the subthalamic nucleus for cervical dystonia. Neuromodulation 13(1):26–30
Panov F, Gologorsky Y, Connors G et al (2013) Deep brain stimulation in DYT1 dystonia:a 10-year experience. Neurosurgery 73(1):86–93
Pralong E, Pollo C, Coubes P et al (2005) Electrophysiological characteristics of limbic and motor globus pallidus internus (GPI) neurons in two cases of Lesch-Nyhan syndrome. Neurophysiol Clin 35(5–6):168–173
Preston R (2007) An error in the code: what can a rare disorder tell us about human behavior? New Yorker 13:30–36
Reese R, Gruber D, Schoenecker T et al (2011) Long-term clinical outcome in Meige syndrome treated with internal pallidum deep brain stimulation. Mov Disord 26(4):691–698
Sako W, Goto S, Shimazu H et al (2008) Bilateral deep brain stimulation of the globus pallidus internus in tardive dystonia. Mov Disord 23(13):1929–1931
Schrock LE, Ostrem JL, Turner RS et al (2009) The subthalamic nucleus in primary dystonia: single-unit discharge characteristics. J Neurophysiol 102(6):3740–3752
Sun B, Chen S, Zhan S et al (2007) Subthalamic nucleus stimulation for primary dystonia and tardive dystonia. Acta Neurochir Suppl 97(Pt 2):207–214
Tagliati M, Krack P, Volkmann J et al (2011) Long-Term management of DBS in dystonia: response to stimulation, adverse events, battery changes, and special considerations. Mov Disord 26(Suppl 1):S54–S62
Taira T, Hitchicock E (1990) Stereotactic thalamotomy for patients with dystonia. Stereotact Funct Neurosurg 54:212–223
Taira T, Hori T (2003) Stereotactic ventrooralis thalamotomy for task-specific focal hand dystonia (writer's cramp). Stereotact Funct Neurosurg 80(1–4):88–91
Taira T, Kobayashi T, Takahashi K et al (2002) A new denervation procedure for idiopathic cervical dystonia. J Neurosurg 97(2 Suppl):201–206
Taira T, Harashima S, Hori T (2003a) Neurosurgical treatment for writer's cramp. Acta Neurochir Suppl 87:129–131
Taira T, Kobayashi T, Hori T (2003b) Disappearance of self-mutilating behavior in a patient with lesch-nyhan syndrome after bilateral chronic stimulation of the globus pallidus internus. Case report. J Neurosurg 98(2):414–416
Thobois S, Taira T, Comella C et al (2011) Pre-operative evaluations for DBS in dystonia. Mov Disord 26(Suppl 1):S17–S22
Timmermann L, Pauls KA, Wieland K et al (2010) Dystonia in neurodegeneration with brain iron accumulation: outcome of bilateral pallidal stimulation. Brain 133(Pt 3):701–712
Trinh B, Ha AD, Mahant N et al (2014) Dramatic improvement of truncal tardive dystonia following globus pallidus pars interna deep brain stimulation. J Clin Neurosci 21(3):515–517. doi:10.1016/j.jocn.2013.03.035
Tronnier VM, Fogel W (2000) Pallidal stimulation for generalized dystonia. Report of three cases. J Neurosurg 92(3):453–456
Umemura A, Jaggi JL, Dolinskas CA et al (2004) Pallidal deep brain stimulation for longstanding severe generalized dystonia in Hallervorden-Spatz syndrome. Case report. J Neurosurg 100(4):706–709
Vitek JL, Bakay RA (1997) The role of pallidotomy in Parkinson's disease and dystonia. Curr Opin Neurol 10(4):332–339
Vitek JL, Zhang J, Evatt M et al (1998) GPi pallidotomy for dystonia: clinical outcome and neuronal activity. Adv Neurol 78:211–219
Vitek JL, Delong MR, Starr PA et al (2011) Intraoperative neurophysiology in DBS for dystonia. Mov Disord 26(Suppl 1):S31–S36
Walsh RA, Sidiropoulos C, Lozano AM et al (2013) Bilateral pallidal stimulation in cervical dystonia: blinded evidence of benefit beyond 5 years. Brain 136(Pt 3):761–769
Witt JL, Moro E, Ash RS et al (2013) Predictive factors of outcome in primary cervical dystonia following pallidal deep brain stimulation. Mov Disord 28(19):1384–1390. doi:10.10021/mds.25575
Yamada K, Hamasaki T, Hasegawa Y et al (2013) Long disease duration interferes with therapeutic effect of globus pallidus internus pallidal stimulation in primary cervical dystonia. Neuromodulation 16(3):219–225; discussion 225
Yoshor D, Hamilton WJ, Ondo W et al (2001) Comparison of thalamotomy and pallidotomy for the treatment of dystonia. Neurosurgery 48(4):818–824; discussion 824–816
Zrinzo L, Foltynie T, Limousin P et al (2012a) Reducing hemorrhagic complications in functional neurosurgery: a large case series and systematic literature review. J Neurosurg 116(1):84–94
Zrinzo L, Foltynie T, Limousin P et al (2012b) Image-verified deep brain stimulation reduces risk and cost with no apparent impact on efficacy. Mov Disord 27(12):1585–1586; author reply 1586–1587

11 Deep Brain Stimulation for Essential Tremor

Ryoma Morigaki and Satoshi Goto

11.1 Introduction

Essential tremor (ET) is the most common movement disorder in adults (Deuschl et al. 2011). The postural and action–intention components affecting distal and proximal musculature are the typical manifestations of advanced ET. ET affects the upper extremities, head, voice, legs, and trunk. The primary treatment for ET is pharmacotherapy. Two drugs, primidone and propranolol, have been established as effective (level-A evidence by the criteria of the American Academy of Neurology) (Zesiewicz et al. 2011). However, 30–50 % of patients will not respond to both drugs (Koller and Vetere-Overfield 1989). Five drugs, topiramate, alprazolam, atenolol, gabapentin, and sotalol, have been shown to be compatible to level-B evidence (probably effective). Irrespective of these medications, 25–55 % of patients manifest medication-refractory ET (Louis 2001). Around 10 % of patients experience significant physical impairment and markedly decreased quality of life. Although the evidence for surgical therapies remains at level C (possibly effective) due to a lack of class-I and class-II studies, thalamotomies and deep brain stimulations have been applied to drug-resistant ET patients, and they have been reported to be highly efficacious for upper limb tremor in patients with ET (Deuschl et al. 2011).

Although the therapeutic efficacy of ablation surgery may be comparable to that of DBS (Schuurman et al. 2000, 2008), DBS is currently preferred over thalamotomy due to its reversibility and adjustability and to the undesirable and irreversible tissue damage that is caused by the ablation surgery (Tasker 1998). The ventral intermediate (VIM) nucleus of the thalamus has been used as a classic target for ET since 1987 (Miocinovic et al. 2013). However, axial tremor, the action component of distal tremor, and proximal tremor respond poorly to VIM DBS (Benabid et al. 1991, 1996). In addition, VIM DBS manifests a high incidence of dysarthria and disequilibrium (Benabid et al. 1991, 1996; Pahwa et al. 1999; Taha et al. 1999) and tolerance to the stimulation (i.e., habituation) (Benabid et al. 1991, 1996; Hariz et al. 1999). The posterior subthalamic area (PSA), which is composed of the prelemniscal radiation (Raprl) and the caudal zona incerta (cZI), has been a target of early ablation surgery in patients with tremor (Ito 1975; Krauss et al. 1994; Mundinger 1969; Velasco et al. 1972). Recently, this structure has been revived as another option for DBS for ET (Lehman and Augustine 2013). Subthalamic nucleus (STN) DBS has also been considered for ET (Lind et al. 2008).

R. Morigaki, MD • S. Goto, MD, PhD (✉)
Department of Motor Neuroscience and Neurotherapeutics, Institute of Health Bioscience, Graduate School of Medical Science, University of Tokushima, Tokushima City, Tokushima Prefecture, Japan
e-mail: sgoto@clin.med.tokushima-u.ac.jp

T. Itakura (ed.), *Deep Brain Stimulation for Neurological Disorders: Theoretical Background and Clinical Application*, DOI 10.1007/978-3-319-08476-3_11,

11.2 Pathophysiology of Essential Tremor

The precise pathogenesis of ET is poorly understood. In the harmaline animal model, abnormally synchronized (4–10 Hz) oscillations have been identified in the inferior olivary nucleus (ION), and these are transmitted to the dentate and interpositus nuclei in the cerebellum (Park et al. 2010; Wilms et al. 1999). The calcium-dependent neuronal synchrony in the ION is sufficient to drive the cerebellothalamocortical circuit to produce tremor (Park et al. 2010), and a functional imaging study has shown the abnormal activation of the ION in ET (Boecker et al. 1996). These results suggest the dysfunction of the olivocerebellar circuit is the primary cause of ET (Deuschl and Bergman 2002). There are no morphological changes in the ION, supporting the idea that ET is due to a functional abnormality within the central nervous system (Deuschl et al. 2001; Louis et al. 2013). The ION adjusts or modulates planned movements during their execution in response to unconditioned afferent information; in other words, it is a movement error detector (Plaha et al. 2004).

The cerebellar nuclei connect to the ventrolateral thalamus through the cerebellothalamic tract and consecutively to the motor cortex. Plaha et al. (2008) have presumed that excessive movement correction in response to limb displacement detection and overcorrection might create abnormal oscillation in the ION in ET. Louis and Vonsattel (2008) have proposed that the cerebellum is integrally involved in the pathophysiology of ET, and some neurodegenerative features in the cerebellum have been shown (Louis et al. 2009). This hypothesis is supported by the findings of a recent neuroimaging study that ET is associated with γ-aminobutyric acid (GABA)ergic neurotransmission dysfunction in the cerebellum (Boecker et al. 2010; Gironell et al. 2012).

Although the olivocerebellar system and the thalamus are key structures, corticomuscular coherence studies have suggested the existence of several central pacemakers in the cerebellum, thalamus, and motor cortex (Govindan et al. 2006; Hua and Lenz 2005; Raethjen and Deuschl 2012; Schelter et al. 2009; Schnitzler et al. 2009). Recent studies using magnetoencephalography (MEG) have revealed that all of the centers simultaneously work and are not fixed and that its constituents may vary over time (Raethjen et al. 2007; Schnitzler et al. 2009; Raethjen and Deuschl 2012). The intermittent cortical involvement may shift the mode of cooperation between all of the constituents of the tremor network (Raethjen et al. 2007; Raethjen and Deuschl 2012). The so-called burst and tonic modes of activity have been observed in thalamic neurons. In the burst mode, the transfer of information has a high signal-to-noise ratio that is conveyed in a nonlinear manner such that new signals are readily identifiable but not readily analyzed. In the tonic mode, there is a linear transfer of the activity of specific afferents, but the signal-to-noise ratio is low (Godwin et al. 1996). These patterns of activity have been seen in the lateral thalamus (Tsoukatos et al. 1997; Zirh et al. 1998). The interaction within the network seems to determine the emerging type of movement (Raethjen and Deuschl 2012), including ET.

The contribution of the basal ganglia loop in generating ET has been controversial (Gerasimou et al. 2012; Lou and Jankovic 1991). The fact that the stimulation of VIM, PSA, and STN could also affect neurons and fibers that are included in the basal ganglia loop has suggested that stimulation of both the cerebellothalamic and pallidothalamic fibers might be responsible for the therapeutic effects on tremor (Deuschl and Bergman 2002).

11.3 Anatomy and Electrophysiology of DBS Surgery

The VIM nucleus, which receives strong cerebellothalamic afferents, is a major target of tremor in functional neurosurgery (Asanuma et al. 1983a, b; Ilinsky and Kultas-Ilinsky 2002; Kultas-Ilinsky and Ilinsky 1991). VIM DBS has demonstrated promising results for the treatment of ET (Rehncrona et al. 2003; Sydow et al. 2003). Recently, many studies have demonstrated that the PSA (Fytagoridis et al. 2012; Kitagawa et al. 2000; Murata et al. 2003; Plaha et al. 2004, 2008, 2011; Velasco et al. 2001) and STN (Blomstedt et al. 2011a, b; Lind et al. 2008; Stover et al. 2005) could be alternative targets. Recent evidence has revealed that the effects of DBS for ET in these subthalamic structures yielded good results.

11.3.1 The VIM Nucleus

11.3.1.1 Functional Anatomy of VIM

The ventrolateral (VL) thalamus is comprised of ventral oral posterior (Vop) nucleus, ventralis oralis internus (Voi), and the VIM nucleus (Hassler 1959). Anterior and lateral to these nuclei lie the reticular nucleus of the thalamus and the internal capsule (El-Tahawy et al. 2004). The VL thalamus mediates motor control. It receives afferent fibers from the cerebellum, basal ganglia, cerebral cortices, and spinal cord, and it projects efferent fibers to the cerebral cortices and basal ganglia. The VL has two subcortical afferent territories: the pallidothalamic and cerebellothalamic territories (Ilinsky and Kultas-Ilinsky 1987; Kuo and Carpenter 1973; Nakano 2000; Sidibé et al. 1997). The density of the pallidothalamic territory decreases in an anterior to posterior gradient and that of the cerebellothalamic territory decreases in a posterior to anterior gradient in the VL thalamus (Sakai et al. 1996). These two territories are widely interdigitated (Asanuma et al. 1983a, b; Sakai et al. 1996). The Vop preferentially receives inhibitory pallidothalamic inputs from the globus pallidus internus (GPi), and the VIM predominantly receives excitatory inputs from the cerebellum. The efferents from the VIM nucleus preferentially project to the primary motor, premotor, and proper supplementary motor area, which, in turn, provide reciprocal excitatory corticothalamic inputs (Bromberg et al. 1981; Hoover and Strick 1999). The VIM nucleus projects predominantly to the deep cortical areas of the motor cortex (Area 4 and possibly, Area 3a), which respond to the passive motor movements of joints (Anderson and Turner 1991; Butler et al. 1992; Jones 2007; Miyagishima et al. 2007; Vitek et al. 1994). The VIM neurons are somatotopographically organized; the face, forelimb, and hindlimb receptive fields are arranged medially to laterally (Strick 1976; Vitek et al. 1994; Kurata 2005). The Vc nucleus, which is the major termination structure of the medial lemniscus, projects to the primary somatosensory cortex (El-Tahawy et al. 2004). The subthalamic area (STA) is located ventrally to the VL thalamus.

11.3.1.2 Electrophysiological Findings During VIM DBS

As the microelectrode descends toward the thalamic target, the caudate has a very slow rate of spontaneous discharge (0–10 Hz) (Vitek et al. 1998), and the thalamus is relatively quiet in the awake patient but shows occasional slow bursting activity (Starr et al. 1998). Microelectrode entry into the motor thalamus can be indicated by the identification of movement-responsive cells and/or cells discharging at tremor frequency (Lenz et al. 1994). Microelectrode recording can identify the Vc nucleus, which is a tactile relay nucleus, and its anterior border with VIM as well as the ventral border with STA (El-Tahawy et al. 2004). Neurons that respond to voluntary movements (voluntary cells) are predominantly present in the Voa and Vop (El-Tahawy et al. 2004). Voluntary cells do not respond to verbal commands but rather to the voluntary act itself, and they are sometimes difficult to distinguish from kinesthetic cells (El-Tahawy et al. 2004; Raeva et al. 1999). Kinesthetic cells receive afferents from muscle spindles that are located in the tendons and muscle bellies or from stretch receptors that are located in the tendons, joint capsules or deep tissues, and they respond to passive joint movements and proprioceptive afferents. These cells are located just anterior to the tactile receptive field (Ohye and Narabayashi 1979; Ohye et al. 1989). Tactile cells in the Vc nucleus respond to superficial light touch. Stimulation of the Vc nucleus induces paresthesia due to activation of the medial lemniscal axons (El-Tahawy et al. 2004).

11.3.1.3 Surgical Anatomy of VIM for Essential Tremor

VIM DBS reduces abnormal tremor-electromyography coherence in ET postural tremor (Vaillancourt et al. 2003). The ideal target for abolishing the tremor is supposed to be located in the area where kinesthetic and tremor cells coexist (Lenz et al. 1994; Atkinson et al. 2002). The kinesthetic zone is located in the lower and lateral part of the VIM nucleus, which is a region of confluence of cerebellothalamic and spinothalamic tracts and which sends the majority of its axons to the motor cortex (Percheron et al. 1996). Ohye and colleagues have postulated that this area is optimal for radiofrequency lesioning to abolish tremor (Ohye and Narabayashi 1979; Ohye et al. 1989). Kiss et al. (2003) have reported that there is an expansion of the representation of movement-related (kinesthetic and deep-responding) neurons anteriorly in patients with tremor. Although DBS of the lateral portion of the VIM nucleus, where tremor cells might play a predominant role, provides the best control of parkinsonian tremor, as suggested previously (Atkinson et al. 2002; Hariz and Hirabayashi 1997), this is not the case for ET and post-stroke tremor, in which, presumably, the tremor cells are spread out in wide areas (Katayama et al. 2005) and they involve more proximal muscle components, which are represented more anteriorly and dorsally in the VIM nucleus (Ohye et al. 1989). A clinical study that examined the relationship between lead location and clinical outcome of 57 leads in 37 ET patients revealed that the lead locations in the anterior margin of the VIM nucleus corresponded to significant improvements in tremor scores (Papavassiliou et al. 2004). In such cases, thalamic DBS with bipolar stimulation or a low angle of the DBS electrode to the anterior commissure–posterior commissure (AC–PC) line (~45°) is advocated, as this could cover the more anterior (Katayama et al. 2005; Kobayashi et al. 2010; Yamamoto et al. 2004; Kiss et al. 2003) and dorsal areas (Kiss et al. 2003; Nguyen and Degos 1993).

11.3.2 Posterior Subthalamic Area (PSA)

11.3.2.1 Functional Anatomy of the PSA

The PSA and its vicinity comprises the nuclei area, which includes the Zi, the STN, and substance Q of Sano, and the fiber area, which includes the ansa lenticularis, Forel's fields H, H1, and H2, Raprl, perirubral fibers, and rubrothalamic fibers (Carrillo-Ruiz et al. 2012). There also exist extended nuclei from mesencephalon that correspond to the substantia nigra (SN) and red nucleus (RN). The PSA is situated anterolateral of the red nucleus, posteromedial of the STN, inferior of the ventral thalamic nuclei, superior of the SN, and anteromedial of the posterior limb of the internal capsule (Xie et al. 2012; Fytagoridis et al. 2013a).

The Zi consists of four territories: rostral, dorsal, ventral, and caudal. Rostral Zi, which is attributed to visceral control, is located dorsomedial to the pallidofugal fibers and STN. Dorsal Zi is attributed to the wake and ventral Zi is under the guidance of the eye and head movements (Carrillo-Ruiz et al. 2012). The cZi, which is called the motor part of the Zi, extends posterior to the STN (Carrillo-Ruiz et al. 2012). The cZi is situated ventral to the Va thalamic nucleus, just ventral to the fascicularis thalamicus (Forel's fields H), and dorsal to the fascicularis lenticularis (Forel's fields H2) (Morel 2007; Plaha et al. 2008). Medial to the cZi is situated the cerebellothalamic tract and the red nucleus, and, lateral to the cZi, exists the internal capsule. The Zi receives inputs from motor, associative, and limbic cortices, the interpositus nucleus of the cerebellum, the substantia nigra reticulata (SNr), the globus pallidus internus (GPi), and the ascending reticular activating system, and it then connects to the centromedian and parafascicular (CM/Pf) and VL nuclei of the thalamus, SNr, GPi, the parvocellular RN, ION, the medial reticular formation, the pedunculopontine tegmental nucleus, the interpositus nucleus of the cerebellum, hypothalamus, the brainstem, including the pedunculopontine nucleus, the spinal cord, and the cerebral cortices (Carrillo-Ruiz et al. 2012; Heise and Mitrofanis 2004; Mitrofanis et al. 2004; Mitrofanis 2005; Plaha et al. 2008). cZI is an extension of the reticular thalamic nucleus, and it predominantly consists of GABAergic neurons. It affects both the basal ganglia and cerebellar outputs, medial reticular formation, and midbrain reticular formation, which are involved in controlling axial and proximal limb muscles (Blomstedt et al. 2009; Plaha et al. 2008). Current theories suggest that the cZi might play a key role in transmitting GABAergic input from the basal ganglia to the cerebellothalamocortical circuits and that DBS might alter or inhibit abnormal oscillations (Blomstedt et al. 2009; Fytagoridis et al. 2012; Plaha et al. 2008). Plaha et al. (2008) have suggested that Zi is an effective target for various types of tremors.

The Raprl is situated inferior to the Vo and VIM thalamic nuclei, in front of the lemniscus pathway, externally is the thalamic reticular nucleus, Zi, and STN, and the medial side is bordered by the RN (Carrillo-Ruiz et al. 2008, 2012; Lehman and Augustine 2013; Morel 2007). The Raprl contains cerebellothalamic, pallidothalamic, renticulothalamic, and rubrothalamic fibers (Carrillo-Ruiz et al. 2008, 2012).

11.3.2.2 Electrophysiological Findings During PSA DBS

When PSA DBS is performed, the transfrontal trajectory to the target is ~45° to the AC–PC plane, and an abrupt increase in impedance (from 400–500 to 600–700 Ω) is experienced when the electrode is passed beyond the ventral boundary of the thalamus into the subthalamic white matter (Murata et al. 2003; Plaha et al. 2008). Alternatively, single-unit-activity recordings have demonstrated frequencies of at least 15 Hz and/or responses to somatosensory stimulation or joint movements in the thalamus, while single-unit activity is absent or below 5 Hz with low background activity and does not respond to outer stimuli in the subthalamic area (Raprl) (Herzog et al. 2007; Kiss et al. 2003). In awake humans, late components of the somatosensory evoked potential from median nerve stimulation can be recorded from Raprl (Blomstedt et al. 2009). The extracellular action potential characteristics of the anterior thalamus and Zi are similar: low frequency and irregular discharge. The major difference is the neuronal density or the distance traversed before extracellular action potentials are encountered (Baker et al. 2004). In the Zi, the neuronal density is lower than that of the anterior thalamus. When the microelectrode enters into the STN, high frequency irregular discharges and increases in background activity are notably observed (Theodosopoulos et al. 2004). Just outside the bottom of the STN is an electrically quiet zone. When the microelectrode enters into the SNr, high frequency regular discharges with decreased background activity are detected.

11.3.3 Surgical Anatomy of the Subthalamic Area (STA) and STN

Herzog et al. (2007) have reported that most contacts that disrupt tremor-electromyography synchronization are located within the PSA, although they are still present in the VL thalamus. Stimulation of the PSA significantly increases the tremor frequency, which reflects a reduced contribution of the pathological central tremor oscillator (Deuschl and Bergman 2002; Herzog et al. 2007). The cerebellothalamic fibers pass through the lateral portion of the red nucleus and the bulk of fibers that continue in the rostrolateral direction pass through the field H of Forel and Raprl and enter the thalamus (Ilinsky and Kultas-Ilinsky 1984; Herzog et al. 2007). The fasciculus thalamicus (pallidothalamic tract) includes the fasciculus and ansa lenticularis (Forel H1 and H2, respectively). These two fibers merge and form the fasciculus thalamicus (Forel H) (Morel 2007). Therefore, the PSA is largely comprised of these two fibers: the cerebellothalamic fibers and Forel H. These fibers, especially the cerebellothalamic fibers, pass through the Zi and the Raprl (Morel 2007). Therefore, the effects of cZi stimulation on tremor might, in part, be due to the stimulation of cerebellothalamic and/or pallidothalamic fibers. In patients suffering from ET over the long term, the tremor and kinesthetic cells spread into Vo segments (Katayama et al. 2005; Kiss et al. 2003). The intention component of ET is supposed to be intensively affected by cerebellothalamic afferents to the VIM nucleus (Pedrosa et al. 2013). These facts suggest that it might be better to stimulate cerebellothalamic fibers themselves in order to alleviate ET. The most effective electrode might be situated in the border zone of the PSA and VIM for ET. This situation has been shown to be true for Parkinson's disease (PD); the border zone of the cZi and the STN was most effective for DBS (Deuschl and Bergman 2002).

According to the stereotactic target of the STN proposed by Blomstedt et al. (2011a), the stimulation site is located at the border of the STN and fasciculus lenticularis from Morel's atlas, and this location is close to the Zi and the fasciculus thalamicus. The effect of STN DBS might affect the tonic activation of adjacent tracts, as well as the cZi, which might lead to a tonic activation of VIM neurons and disrupt the tremor synchronous activity (Stover et al. 2005; Miocinovic et al. 2013). Stover et al. (2005) have postulated that this hypothesis is compatible with the results that the short-latency excitation of thalamic neurons begins just after STN stimulation in MPTP PD model monkeys. Lind et al. (2008) have reported that the most effective contacts are situated in the mid (56.3 %) and ventral (31.3 %) side of the STN.

11.4 Tentative Stereotactic Coordinates for DBS in Patients with ET

The current surgical targets for ET are the VIM (Fig. 11.1), STA (Fig. 11.2), and STN (Fig. 11.3). The tentative stereotactic coordinate for VIM DBS is 15 mm lateral to the midline at the level of the intercommissural line (ICL) and 6 mm anterior to the PC (Benabid et al. 1996). The Guiot approach that is widely used in France is the following: (11.0 or 11.5 + 1/2 or 1/3 of the third ventricular width) mm lateral to the midline at the level of the AC–PC plane and one-fourth of the AC–PC length anterior to the PC (Bardinet et al. 2011).

In most studies, the PSA has been targeted directly (Murata et al. 2003; Plaha et al. 2008; Blomstedt et al. 2010). Murata et al. (2003) have

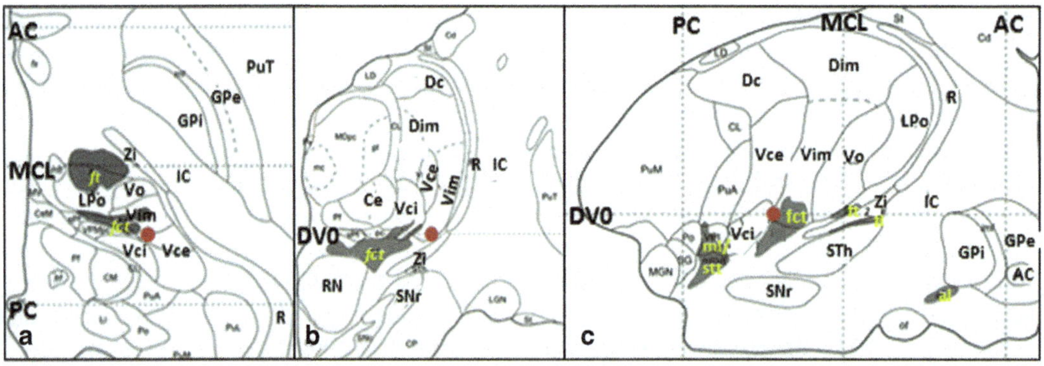

Fig. 11.1 Stereotactic coordinate modified from Morel's atlas (2007) illustrating the location of the Vim nucleus (●). (**a**) Axial plane, on the AC–PC plane. (**b**) Coronal plane, 6 mm anterior to the PC. (**c**) Sagittal plane, 14.5 mm lateral to the median plane (From Morel (2007) with permission.) Abbreviations: *AC* anterior commissure, *al* ansa lenticularis, *Ce* nucleus centralis externus, *Dc* nucleus dorsocaudalis, *Dim* nucleus dorsointermedius, *DVO* AC-PC plane, *fct* fasciculus cerebello-thalamicus, *fl* fasciculus lenticularis, *ft* fasciculus thalamicus, *GPi* globus pallidus, internal segment, *GPe* globus pallidus, external segment, *LPo* nucleus lateropolaris thalami, *stt* spinothalamic tract, *IC* internal capsule, *MCL* midcommissural line, *ml* medial lemniscus, *PC* posterior commissure, *PuT* putamen, *R* reticular thalamic nucleus, *RN* red nucleus, *SNr* substantia nigra, pars reticulata, *STh* Subthalamic nucleus, *Vce* & *Vci* nucleus ventrocaudalis externus & internus, *Vim* nucleus ventrointermedius, *Vo* nucleus ventrooralis, *Zi* zona incerta

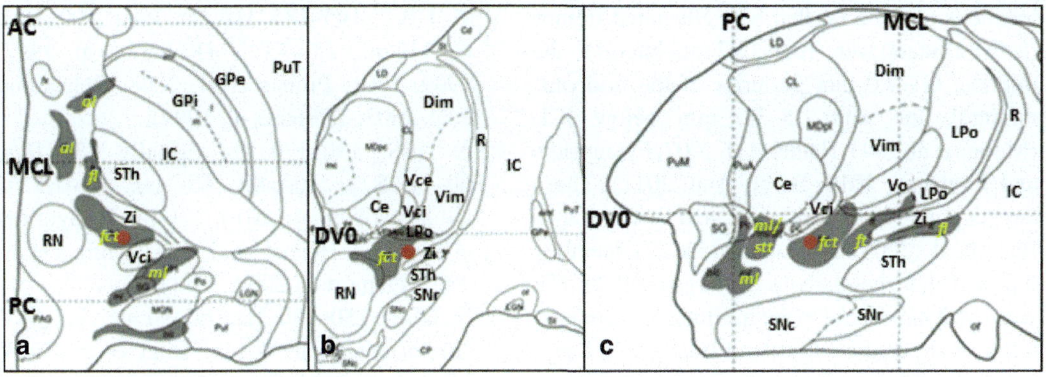

Fig. 11.2 Stereotactic coordinate modified from Morel's atlas (2007) illustrating the location of the STA (•). (**a**) Axial plane, 2.7 mm ventral to the AC-PC plane. (**b**) Coronal plane, 7 mm anterior to the PC. (**c**) Sagittal plane, 11.8 mm lateral to the median plane (From Morel (2007) with permission.) Abbreviations: *AC* anterior commissure, *al* ansa lenticularis, *Ce* nucleus centralis externus, *Dim* nucleus dorsointermedius, *DVO* AC-PC plane, *fct* fasciculus cerebello-thalamicus, *fl* fasciculus lenticularis, *ft* fasciculus thalamicus, *GPi* globus pallidus, internal segment, *GPe* globus pallidus, external segment, *LPo* nucleus lateropolaris thalami, *stt* spinothalamic tract, *IC* internal capsule, *MCL* midcommissural line, *ml* medial lemniscus, *PC* posterior commissure, *PuT* putamen, *R* reticular thalamic nucleus, *RN* red nucleus, *SNc* substantia nigra, pars compacta, *SNr* substantia nigra, pars reticulata, *STh* Subthalamic nucleus, *Vce & Vci* nucleus ventrocaudalis externus & internus, *Vim* nucleus ventrointermedius, *Vo* nucleus ventrooralis, *Zi* zona incerta

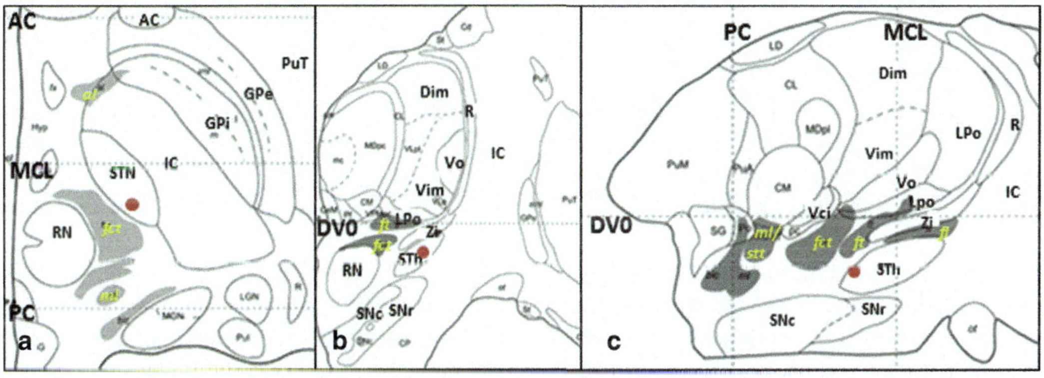

Fig. 11.3 Stereotactic coordinate modified from Morel's atlas (2007) illustrating the location of the STh (•). (**a**) Axial plane, 3.6 mm ventral to the AC-PC plane. (**b**) Coronal plane, 9 mm anterior to the PC. (**c**) Sagittal plane, 11.8 mm lateral to the median plane (From Morel (2007) with permission.) Abbreviations: *AC* anterior commissure, *al* ansa lenticularis, *Dim* nucleus dorsointermedius, *DVO* AC-PC plane, *fct* fasciculus cerebello-thalamicus, *fl* fasciculus lenticularis, *ft* fasciculus thalamicus, *GPi* globus pallidus, internal segment, *GPe* globus pallidus, external segment, *LPo* nucleus lateropolaris thalami, *stt* spinothalamic tract, *IC* internal capsule, *MCL* midcommissural line, *ml* medial lemniscus, *PC* posterior commissure, *PuT* putamen, *R* reticular thalamic nucleus, *RN* red nucleus, *SNc* substantia nigra, pars compacta, *SNr* substantia nigra, pars reticulata, *STh* Subthalamic nucleus, *Vci* nucleus ventrocaudalis internus, *Vim* nucleus ventrointermedius, *Vo* nucleus ventrooralis, *Zi* zona incerta

reported the PSA coordinates as approximately 10 mm lateral and 3–4 mm behind the posterior border of the STN on the axial slice with the greatest STN diameter. Plaha et al. (2004) have targeted the point medial to the posterior dorsal third of the STN. Blomstedt et al. (2010) have targeted the cZi with thin-slice T2-weighted magnetic resonance images: slightly posteromedial to the tail of the STN at the level of the maximal diameter of the red nucleus. The stereotactic locations of the STA that best alleviated tremor (active contact) were 10.9–12.7 mm lateral to the midline, 6.1–7.0 mm posterior of the midcommissural line, and 1.5–3.0 mm below ICL (Murata et al. 2003; Hamel et al. 2007; Fytagoridis and Blomstedt 2010; Barbe et al. 2011). These targets are supposed to be located in the Raprl. Plaha et al. (2008) have targeted the cZi, and they reported that the stereotactic targets of the cZi were 14.2 mm lateral to the midline, 5.7 mm posterior to the mid-commissural line, and 2.1 mm below the ICL.

Blomstedt et al. (2011a, b) have targeted the STN with thin-slice T2-weighted images at the level of the maximal diameter of the red nucleus, at a line joining the anterior borders of these nuclei, and around 1.5 mm lateral from the visualized medial border of the STN. Lind et al. (2008) have reported that the position of active contact is 12 mm lateral to the midline, 16 mm posterior to the AC, and 4 mm below the ICL.

11.5 Definition of the Active Target During DBS Surgery

Intraoperative macrostimulation under local anesthesia is a reliable method to evaluate the effects of the optimal locations for each patient. The tremor stops immediately after the stimulation. Adverse events, such as dysesthesia and limb ataxia, which diminish within 10 s during the stimulation (200–300 Hz, 1 s trains of 0.1- or 0.2-ms pulse widths, the stimulation current is usually limited to a maximum of ~100 μA with high-impedance microelectrodes), are acceptable (El-Tahawy et al. 2004; Krack et al. 2002; Morigaki et al. 2010). Electrode model 3389 (Medtronic, Inc., Minneapolis, MN, USA) is usually used for VIM and STN, and model 3387 or 3389 is used for STA as it enabled stimulation of the VL thalamus alternatively (Plaha et al. 2004).

11.6 Stimulation Parameters

The mean parameters used in VIM, PSA, and STN DBS for ET are the following:

VIM DBS: 145–185 Hz (at least 100 Hz), 60–117 μs, 2.0–3.7 V (Koller et al. 1997, 1999, 2001; Pilitsis et al. 2008; Rehncrona et al. 2003; Tröster et al. 1999).

PSA DBS: 130–170 Hz (usually 130 Hz), 60–112.5 μs (usually 60 μs), 1.9–2.5 V (Blomstedt et al. 2010, 2011a; Fytagoridis et al. 2013a; Herzog et al. 2007; Murata et al. 2003; Plaha et al. 2004, 2011).

STN DBS: 130–180 Hz, 60–90 μs, 1.5–3 V (Blomstedt et al. 2011a; Lind et al. 2008; Meng et al. 2013; Stover et al. 2005).

11.7 The Possible Mechanisms by Which DBS Alleviates Tremor

Several hypotheses have been proposed with regard to the mechanisms of high-frequency DBS. Conduction or depolarization block is the simplest hypothesis, and it is supported by the findings that ablation surgery has similar effects as DBS (Benabid et al. 1996). Activation of inhibitory presynaptic afferents and inhibition of projection neurons (Wu et al. 2001; Anderson et al. 2006), inhibition of neuronal activity near the stimulation site and activation of axonal elements that leave the target structure (Vitek 2002), activation of adjacent fiber tracts surrounding or running through the stimulated site (Johnson et al. 2009), and the superposition of continuous stimuli onto rhythmically oscillating subcortical–cortical loops (Montgomery and Baker 2000) are other hypotheses. Some authors have hypothesized that high-frequency stimulation in the VIM increases glutamate release from glial cells and excites local interneurons, thereby increasing the production of inhibitory neurotransmitters (e.g., GABA and glycine) and resulting in a decrease in the firing rates of projection neurons (Kang et al. 1998; Tawfik et al. 2010; Tian et al. 2005). When we consider the effect of VIM, as well as PSA (especially Rarpl) stimulation, the conduction or depolarization block might be a plausible mechanism. However, positron emission tomography analyses have demonstrated that VIM DBS increases regional blood flow in the supplemental motor area (Ceballos-Baumann et al. 2001; Perlmutter et al. 2002). Taking into consideration that the cerebellothalamic and thalamocortical fibers are both glutamatergic (excitatory), a different mechanism might be at work. DBS might modulate abnormal oscillation coupling by superposing continuous stimuli onto rhythmically oscillating loops (Montgomery & Baker's theory) or activate adjacent or surrounding fiber components (Vitek's or Johnson's theory).

11.8 Patient Selection

Factors to consider in DBS include tremor severity, refractoriness to medication, tremor type, patient characteristics, including age, comorbid conditions, surgical risk, patient preference, social and employment factors, and social support (Cooper and Bowes 2012). One of the most important aspects is cognitive function. This is especially important for bilateral procedures, particularly bilateral STN DBS (Hariz 2002). Patients with borderline mental conditions have experienced irreversible and unadjustable dementia after bilateral STN DBS. Although most cases involve unilateral surgery (left side), VIM, Raprl, and cZi DBS have not been shown to affect higher cognitive processes as long as in 6-year follow-up periods (Heber et al. 2013).

Unilateral thalamotomy could be an option when a patient does not want to implant devices, a patient has difficulty in consulting medical care frequently, extensive lesioning is predicted due to a proximal inclusion, a patient has an increased risk of infection (immune-compromised patients), and habituation or tolerance occurs after DBS (Bahgat et al. 2013).

With regard to VIM DBS, tremor-suppressing medications could be discontinued after bilateral VIM DBS, but they should be continued after unilateral DBS. Unilateral VIM DBS is insufficient to eliminate the necessity for tremor-suppressing medications, and discontinuation has been shown to worsen the tremor (Favilla et al. 2013).

11.9 Therapeutic Impact of DBS for ET

In general, resting tremors are better controlled than action tremors, distal limb tremors are better than proximal limb tremors, and upper limb tremors are better than lower limb tremors (Benabid et al. 1996, 1998; Lozano 2000). The short- and long-term efficacy of VIM DBS is promising. However, tolerance to the stimulation and insufficient effects on axial and proximal tremor are the biggest problems. The PSA is an effective target for tremor suppression in early ablation surgery (Spiegel et al. 1963). Although there are not enough results concerning long-term efficacy, PSA DBS seems promising in a number of recent publications. Moreover, PSA stimulation showed a powerful effect, even for axial and proximal tremor, and several short-term and a few long-term results have described that ET patients with PSA DBS did not manifest tolerance to the stimulation. Here, we review the short- and long-term outcomes that are related to VIM, PSA (Raprl & cZi), and STN DBS for patients with ET.

11.9.1 Therapeutic Impact of VIM DBS

Only one randomized controlled trial with a direct comparison of thalamotomy with DBS is available (Schuurman et al. 2000, 2008). The results demonstrated that VIM DBS was equally effective as VIM thalamotomy. However, half of the ET patients experienced diminished effects of the stimulation over the 5-year follow-up (Schuurman et al. 2008).

11.9.1.1 Short-Term Efficacy

Tremor Reduction (Assessors Blind)

Numerous case series are available, and the short- and long-term effects of VIM DBS are usually favorable (Morigaki et al. 2010). Among them, blinded assessments have shown a marked reduction in tremor scores and significant improvements in disability scores (Koller et al. 1997, 1999, 2001; Lyons et al. 1998; Pahwa et al. 1999;

Tröster et al. 1999; Schuurman et al. 2000; Hariz 2002; Rehncrona et al. 2003; Fields et al. 2003).

Schuurman et al. (2000) have reported that the contralateral tremors of 13 ET patients were completely suppressed at 6 months postoperatively. In Koller's series (Koller et al. 1997), VIM stimulation resulted in 31 % of the ET patients obtaining contralateral tremor remission, and 79 % of the ET patients experienced marked tremor improvement (50–100 %) at the 3-month follow-up. Hariz et al. (2002) have reported that unilateral VIM DBS improved the total Fahn-Tolosa-Marin (FTM)-tremor rating scale (TRS) tremor score by 47 % from baseline at the 12-month follow-up. Unilateral VIM DBS improved the FTM-TRS tremor scores by 50.8–78.0, 53–78.7, and 20.6 % from baseline at the 3-, 12-, and 24-month follow-ups, respectively (Fields et al. 2003; Hariz 2002; Rehncrona et al. 2003; Tröster et al. 1999). The improvement in upper limb tremors contralateral to the DBS improved 79 % at the 12-month follow-up (Hariz 2002). Both the contralateral upper postural and activity/intention components improved 66.7 % at the 24-month follow-up (Rehncrona et al. 2003). Bilateral VIM DBS improved the FTM-TRS motor scores (items 1–10) and the postural + intention tremor by 64.9 and 66.7 %, respectively, at the 3-month follow-up (Pahwa et al. 1999). Head tremor was improved in 71 % of patients (Koller et al. 1999).

Although the assessors were not blind, several publications have indicated the efficacy of bilateral VIM DBS for axial tremors (Koller et al. 1999; Limousin et al. 1999; Obwegeser et al. 2000; Ondo et al. 1998; Putzke et al. 2005; Sydow et al. 2003; Taha et al. 1999). However, its therapeutic efficacy has been reported to vary. With respect to voice tremor, some studies have reported a significant and marked (more than 80 %) improvement (Obwegeser et al. 2000; Taha et al. 1999), whereas others have reported minimal changes in either short- or long-term follow-up studies (Limousin et al. 1999; Putzke et al. 2005; Sydow et al. 2003).

Motor Function of the Upper Limb

VIM stimulation improved FTM-TRS writing, spiral-drawing, straight line-drawing, and liquid-pouring scores by 56.7, 48.4, 56.3, and 63.3 %, respectively, at the 3-month follow-up (Koller et al. 1997). Unilateral VIM DBS improved FTM-TRS hand function scores by 39 % at the 12-month follow-up (Hariz 2002).

Improvement in Activity of Daily Living/Disability Scores

The therapeutic effects have been reported with several different scales. The Frenchay activity index score improved by 18 % at the 6-month follow-up after VIM DBS (Schuurman et al. 2000). VIM stimulation improved the global disability score by 57.6 % at the 3-month follow-up (Koller et al. 1997). Unilateral VIM DBS improved the Parkinson's Disease Questionnaire (PDQ-39) Activities of Daily Living (ADL) score by 55.5 and 43.6 % at the 3- and 12-month follow-ups, respectively (Fields et al. 2003). Unilateral VIM DBS improved the FTM-TRS ADL score (items 15–21) by 54 % at the 12-month follow-up (Hariz 2002). Several factors of the ADL taxonomy scale significantly improved (Hariz 2002).

Improvements in Other Symptoms

VIM DBS has been shown to improve cognitive screening measures, visual attention, fine visuomotor and visuoperceptual functions, verbal memory, delayed prose recall, social life, interest/hobbies, and mood state/emotional reactions 3 and 12 months after unilateral VIM DBS (Fields et al. 2003; Hariz 2002; Tröster et al. 1999). However, Heber et al. (2013) have reported that neither stereotactic surgery nor electric stimulation affected higher cognitive functions, including memory and verbal fluency, at 1- and 6-year follow-up evaluations.

11.9.1.2 Long-Term Efficacy

There has been two publication with a blind assessment. Rehncrona et al. (2003) have found that FTM-TRS tremor (item 1–9) and hand function (items 11–14) scores improved by 47 and 71 %, respectively, compared to those presurgery at a mean follow-up period of 6.5 years after unilateral VIM DBS. The contralateral upper postural and activity/intention components improved 66.7 and 50 %, respectively.

Several publications with unblinded assessors have shown similar results. Sydow et al. (2003) have reported a 41 % reduction in FTM-TRS tremor scores and a 39 % improvement in the ADL scores with a follow-up period of 6.5 years. Pahwa et al. (2006) have reported that VIM DBS at a 5-year follow-up period resulted in a 75 % improvement in targeted hand tremors by unilateral stimulation, a 65 % improvement in the left limb, and an 86 % improvement in the right limb by bilateral stimulation, with a 36 and 51 % improvement in ADL scores by unilateral and bilateral stimulation, respectively. Total FTM-TRS, tremor score, contralateral hand function, and ADL scores improved significantly, except for voice tremor, at the 86-month follow-up (Blomstedt et al. 2007; Hariz et al. 2008). However, the DBS efficacy on tremor decreased, and almost all of the improvements in ADL at 1 year were no longer sustained (Hariz et al. 2008). Zhang et al. (2010) have reported a 80.4 and 69.7 % improvement of FTM-TRS tremor and handwriting scores, respectively, in a series of 34 patients (bilateral/unilateral DBS; 11/23 patients) with a follow-up period of about 5 years. Hariz et al. (2008) have reported an 18 % reduction in FTM-TRS total scores in a follow-up period of 7 years by unilateral stimulation. Nazzaro et al. (2012) have reported a 55, 44, and 31 % significant reduction in FTM-TRS total tremor scores for the follow-up periods of 1, 4, and 9 years by unilateral stimulation, respectively. FTM-TRS ADL improved 73, 52, and 37 %, and the PDQ-39 quality of life domains of the ADLs improved 27, 23, and 19 %, respectively. The PDQ-39 evaluation revealed ADL, emotional well-being, stigma, and cognition were significantly improved up to 7 years, but only stigma remained significant at 9 years and the mobility score significantly worsened.

11.9.2 Therapeutic Impact of PSA DBS

In a few early studies, the subthalamic area has been identified as a better location than the thalamus for alleviating ET (Mohadjer et al. 1990; Mundinger 1969; Velasco et al. 1972). The short-term results of DBS in this area seem promising, and the results include tremors that are difficult to be controlled by VIM DBS, such as proximal postural tremors and distal intention tremors (Xie et al. 2012). Publications concerning long-term results are limited (Fytagoridis et al. 2012).

11.9.2.1 Short-Term Efficacy of PSA DBS for ET

Tremor Reduction

Murata et al. (2003) have reported that unilateral PSA (Raprl and cZi) DBS immediately alleviated intractable proximal and distal tremors in patients with eight ET by 81 % as assessed with the modified tremor rating scale (FTM-TRS), and no worsening was observed during the mean 22-month follow-up periods. Voice, neck, and/or orthostatic axial tremors were also improved.

Using the FTM-TRS evaluation method and comparing the results with tremor severity at baseline, unilateral PSA DBS improved total tremor scores by 60–80.1 % at 12 months (Blomstedt et al. 2010; Plaha et al. 2004). The tremor score (items 1–9) improved by 61.2–84.2 % (Blomstedt et al. 2010; Plaha et al. 2004); upper limb postural and action components improved by 84.4 % (Plaha et al. 2004). Unilateral PSA DBS improved intention tremor by 63.4 and 68.4 % for a left- and right-side tremor, respectively, in patients with eight ET, two multiple sclerosis (MS), and one spinocerebellar ataxia (SCA) (Hamel et al. 2007).

Bilateral PSA DBS reduced the FTM-TRS total tremor scores by 63.5 % at a mean of 17 months postoperatively in patients with 10 ET (Herzog et al. 2007). The ipsilateral upper tremor improved by 8.7 % and the contralateral upper tremor improved by 95 %; the rest, postural, and activity/intention components improved by 100, 83.3, and 94.1 %, respectively (Herzog et al. 2007).

Unilateral cZi DBS improved total tremor scores by 60.9–76.9 %, tremor scores by 59.4–65.1 %, upper extremity tremors by 95.0–100 % (rest, postural, and action/intention components improved by 100, 95.8–100, and 93.8–94.1 %, respectively) 1 year postoperatively (Blomstedt et al. 2011a, b; Fytagoridis et al. 2012; Sandvik et al. 2012).

Bilateral cZi DBS improved total tremor scores by 75.9 % and upper extremity tremors by 85.6 % in six ET patients 1 year postoperatively (Plaha et al. 2008). Both distal (75.9 %) and proximal (71.2 %) intention tremors have been reported to be improved. Another study has shown that bilateral cZi DBS improved total tremor scores by 73.8 %, upper extremity tremors by 86.6 % (postural and action components by 88.2 and 82.2 %, respectively) at a 31.7-month follow-up (Plaha et al. 2011).

Some studies have adopted a more objective index. PSA DBS reduced the total power of accelerometry by 99 %, whereas DBS at the ventral thalamic border reduced it by 68 % and DBS at thalamus proper reduced it by 2.5 % at least 6 months after the operation (Herzog et al. 2007). Using a 3D ultrasound kinematic analysis tool in 21 ET patients, bilateral PSA DBS improved hand tremors by 86 % at least 3 months after the operation (Barbe et al. 2011).

Head tremor has been reported to be greatly improved: 75.0–100 % in short-term studies and 75 % in one long-term (48.5 months) follow-up study as well (Blomstedt et al. 2010, 2011b; Fytagoridis et al. 2012; Plaha et al. 2004, 2008, 2011). Face and trunk tremors were improved by 90.4 and 100 %, respectively, in Plaha's series (cZi DBS, 31.7-month follow-up) (Plaha et al. 2011). The effects of PSA DBS on voice tremor seem to be worsening over the years: 66.7–98.7 % improvements in short-term follow-up periods (Blomstedt et al. 2010, 2011b; Fytagoridis et al. 2012), while a 33.3 % improvement was observed in a long-term follow-up duration (Fytagoridis et al. 2012; Plaha et al. 2011). However, we should be aware of the small sample size in the study of the long-term results.

Motor Function of the Upper Limb

Two early case series demonstrated that unilateral PSA DBS improves hand writing in all patients (Kitagawa et al. 2000; Murata et al. 2003). Using FTM-TRS, unilateral PSA DBS improved motor function scores of the upper limb (items 10–14); writing, spiral drawing, pouring water, and drawing lines improved by 68, 66.7, 76.9, and 58.3 %, respectively (Plaha et al. 2004), while bilateral cZi DBS improved them by 60.1–64.2, 81.9, 52.9 and 71.7 %, respectively (Blomstedt et al. 2011b; Plaha et al. 2008, 2011). Unilateral cZi DBS improved contralateral hand function (items 11–14) by 78.8–100 % at a 1-year follow-up (Blomstedt et al. 2011a, b; Fytagoridis et al. 2012; Sandvik et al. 2012).

Improvement in Activity of Daily Living Scores

Unilateral PSA DBS improved FTM-TRS ADL scores (items 15–21) by 66.4–88.8 % 12 months postoperatively (Blomstedt et al. 2010; Plaha et al. 2004). Bilateral PSA DBS improved ADL scores by 85.7 % in patients with eight ET, two MS, and one SCA (Hamel et al. 2007). Unilateral cZi DBS improved ADL scores by 64.1–76.5 % at a 1-year follow-up (Fytagoridis et al. 2012; Blomstedt et al. 2011a; Sandvik et al. 2012). Bilateral cZi DBS improved ADL scores by 80–84.5 % (Plaha et al. 2008, 2011).

A SF-36-survey physiological component score was improved by 23.7 %, and the mental component score improved by 22.4 % (Plaha et al. 2011). In another report, cZi DBS did not improve SF-36 subscores, and the authors postulated that SF-36 might be unsuitable for evaluating changes in ET patients in this condition (Sandvik et al. 2012).

The Quality of Life in Essential Tremor Questionnaire (QUEST) score 1 year after cZi DBS was improved in the summary index (SI), ADL, and psychosocial scores by 35.5, 40.2, and 40.9 %, respectively (Sandvik et al. 2012).

11.9.2.2 Long-Term Efficacy of PSA DBS for ET

With regard to the long-term efficacy, three ET patients (mean 5-year follow-up duration) with unilateral cZi DBS exhibited improved total tremor scores by 57.4 %, improved tremor scores (items 1–9) by 46.9 %, improved contralateral hand tremor by 100 %, improved hand function (items 11–14) by 87.5 %, and improved ADL scores (items 15–21) by 76.5 % (Blomstedt et al. 2011a). Eighteen ET patients (mean 48.5-month follow-up duration) with unilateral cZi DBS exhibited improved total tremor scores by 52.4 %, improved tremor scores (items 1–9) by 48.0 %, improved hand tremors by 91.8 % (improved rest, postural, and action/intention components by 100, 95.8, 85.3 %, respectively), improved hand function (items 11–14) by 39 % (contralateral side, 78.5 %; ipsilateral side, −13 %), and improved ADL scores by 65.8 % (Fytagoridis et al. 2012). Four ET patients with bilateral cZi DBS exhibited improved total tremor scores by 72.6 %, improved tremor scores (items 1–9) by 81.5 %, improved total hand function (items 11–14) by 60 %, and improved ADL scores (items 15–21) by 82.4 % with a mean 6.25-year follow-up duration (Plaha et al. 2011).

11.9.2.3 PSA DBS in Patients with Failed VIM DBS

Kitagawa et al. (2000) have reported the efficacy of unilateral PSA DBS in an ET patient with failed unilateral VIM thalamotomy. High-frequency (120–130 Hz) stimulation totally abolished the patient's tremor. Blomstedt et al. (2012) have described two patients with early failure of VIM DBS and three failures after several years of good effects. It was confirmed that the failure in these patients was not due to the misplacement of electrodes. Before cZi DBS, VIM DBS improved total tremor scores and hand tremor/functions (items 5, 11–14) by 17 and 28.7 %, respectively. Unilateral cZi DBS moderately improved them: 31.7 and 54.3 % from baseline, respectively. Combined cZi and VIM stimulation that was tried in a single patient further improved these scores.

11.9.3 Therapeutic Impact of STN DBS for ET

Almost all publications about STN DBS are related to Parkinson's tremor, and those that are associated with ET tremor are limited. However, some authors have postulated that STN DBS is also effective for ET (Stover et al. 2005; Lind et al. 2008; Blomstedt et al. 2011a; Meng et al. 2013).

Unilateral STA DBS improved FTM-TRS total tremor scores by 72.5 %, improved tremor scores (items 1–9) by 33.3 %, improved contralateral hand tremors by 66.7 %, improved hand function (items 11–14) by 77.8 %, and improved ADL by 100 % 1 year after the operation in a single patient (Blomstedt et al. 2011a). Meng et al. (2013) have described one patient with unilateral STN and another with bilateral STN DBS. The former exhibited an improved total tremor score by 75.5 % after a 6-month follow-up, and the latter exhibited a 66.7 % improved after a 24-month follow-up. Lind has described ten ET patients with unilateral STN DBS with a 1- to 3-year follow-up. They reported that all of the patients experienced favorable effects (slight tremor to complete disappearance of the tremor), but one patient changed to VIM DBS due to the development of a dystonic twist, two experienced minor speech disturbances, and two experienced balance disturbances (Lind et al. 2008). Lind et al. (2008) have reported complete tremor disappearance in all three patients with long-term follow-up (mean, 8.7 years).

11.10 Microlesioning and Stimulation-Related Problems

Stimulation-induced side effects are important because they determine the intensity of the stimulation and whether it can be used or not. Generally, sensory side effects have a high degree of habituation over time and are not a major threat to the therapeutic results (Fytagoridis et al. 2013a). Motor side effects are less susceptible to habituation and more prone to impede the results of the treatment. Theoretically, stimulation of the internal capsule (corticospinal or corticobulbar tracts) causes muscle contraction and dysarthria (Baker et al. 2004; Tamma et al. 2002). Dysarthria can also be induced by stimulation of cerebellothalamic fibers (Fytagoridis et al. 2013a). Stimulation of the medial lemniscus or Vc thalamic nucleus could result in paresthesia (Murata et al. 2003). Stimulation of the third nerve complex results in conjugate and disconjugate eye movements or eyelid closure (Baker et al. 2004). Stimulation of the oculomotor region of the STN just medial to the somatic sensorimotor region or rostral interstitial nucleus causes the same adverse effects (Tamma et al. 2002). Horizontal gaze deviation is considered to be a motor side effect of the corticofugal tract, which transverses the anterior limb of the internal capsule (Tamma et al. 2002). Cerebellar signs, such as limb ataxia, hypotonia, gait disturbance, and disequilibrium, are attributed to the stimulation of cerebellothalamic fibers. Hyperhydrosis might be due to the disruption of sympathetic efferent fibers in the Zi or activation of basal and posteromedial structures of the STN (Fytagoridis and Blomstedt 2010; Lind et al. 2008; Lipp et al. 2005; Tamma et al. 2002).

11.10.1 Adverse Effects Related to VIM DBS

According to a recent systematic review, the stimulation-related complications of 430 patients who received Vim DBS were paresthesia (18.84 %), dysarthria (8.84 %), headache (7.21 %), disequilibrium (3.95 %), and paresis (3.02 %) (Flora et al. 2010). The stimulation-related adverse events concerning long-term (more than 5 years) follow-ups have been described as follows: paresthesias (0–38 %), dysarthria (0–36 %), gait disturbance (0–19 %), dystonia/hypertonia (0–16 %), balance disturbance (0–8 %), and cognitive dysfunction (0–3 %) (Rehncrona et al. 2003; Sydow et al. 2003; Pahwa et al. 2006; Tarsy et al. 2005; Hariz et al. 2008; Schuurman et al. 2008). Most adverse events were mild and could be adjusted (Flora et al. 2010). Among these adverse effects, the nonadjustable and long-lasting complications included paresthesia (0–19 %), dysarthria (0–19 %), dystonia (0–6 %), gait disturbance (0–4 %), and upper limb ataxia (0–4 %). Bilateral stimulation can cause persistent complications that include dysarthria, disequilibrium, and gait disturbance, even if the stimulus parameters are optimized (Pahwa et al. 2006). Therefore, unilateral or staged bilateral procedures are safe and recommended.

11.10.2 Adverse Events Related to PSA DBS

Transient dysphasia (22.5 %), clumsiness (5 %), hemiparesis (2.5 %), and persistent dizziness (2.5 %) have been reported as nonstimulation-induced (due to microlesioning) complications after PSA surgery (Fytagoridis and Blomstedt 2010). The high rate of transient dysphasia might be due to a microlesional effect/edema caused by the passage of the electrode into the thalamus of the dominant hemisphere (Fytagoridis and Blomstedt 2010). When the active electrode is placed too close to the red nucleus, nonadjustable visual disturbances and dizziness occur (Fytagoridis and Blomstedt 2010). Fytagoridis et al. (2013b) have reported reduced verbal fluency that was statistically significant at 3 days and not significant at 1 year after cZi DBS in 17 patients. They hypothesized that this might have been due to microlesion/edema of the ventral thalamus.

Paresthesia (hand ≒ face>leg ≒ arm), dizziness, blurred vision, muscle contractures, dysarthria, ataxia/dysmetria, diplopia, ptosis, and hyperhidrosis are stimulation-induced side effects (Fytagoridis et al. 2013a). There exists a large anatomical variation in their emergence, or, in other words, it is hard to predict the adverse events that will occur from the anatomical location of the contacts (Fytagoridis et al. 2013a). This might be due to the stimulation of axonal components that spread electrical impulses farther than expected (Johnson et al. 2009). These side effects are totally reversible, adjustable, and usually do not affect the final results.

Bilateral lead implantation in Raprl induced somnolence in all five patients with PD and the deterioration of depression in two out of five patients with PD (Carrillo-Ruiz et al. 2008), and it has been reported to induce a 40 % incidence of hypophonic speech and disequilibrium (Plaha et al. 2011). Similarly, bilateral cZi stimulation induced dysarthria and hypophonic speech in three out of the 15 ET patients (20 %) in a relatively long-term (mean, 31 months) follow-up study (Plaha et al. 2011). These side effects were completely reversible but persistent and present at all times in one patient (6.7 %). In this study, the anatomical location of this side effect was supposed to be induced by stimulation that was dorsomedial to the STN (Plaha et al. 2006). PSA DBS bears a risk of speech, balance, and sensory disturbances, which is more pronounced with bilateral procedures. Staged surgery for bilateral PSA DBS might be safe and recommended.

11.10.3 Adverse Events Related to STN DBS

The adjustable complications induced by STN-DBS include arm dystonia, dysarthria, dizziness, and balance disturbances (Lind et al. 2008; Blomstedt et al. 2011a, b). Motor contraction and dysarthria are frequent (81 %), paresthesia occurs (32.5 %), and oculomotor side effects (24 %) are caused by stimulation of the third nerve or the rostral interstitial nucleus (Tamma et al. 2002). Vegetative side effects (nausea, heat sensation, sweating, or bradycardia) are also common (40.5 %). One patient experienced an unadjustable dystonic twist of the contralateral foot (Lind et al. 2008). Bilateral stimulation did not cause further side effects (Plaha et al. 2008, 2011).

11.11 Tolerance (Habituation)

The recurrence of ET seems to be higher than that of PD tremors (Benabid et al. 1996; Tasker 1998; Pilitsis et al. 2008). Poor outcomes have been documented in up to 40 % of ET patients with VIM DBS (Hariz and Hirabayashi 1997; Benabid et al. 1998; Hariz et al. 1999; Koller et al. 2001; Kumar et al. 2003). A gradual loss of tremor control is due to suboptimal lead placement, misdiagnosis, disease progression, and habituation (Deuschl et al. 2011). The tolerance could be explained by disease progression or the adaptation of the biological response by the stimulated neuronal network (Benabid et al. 1996; Deuschl et al. 2011; Barbe et al. 2011; Shih et al. 2013). Therefore, the intermittent use of implantable pulse generators is recommended in order to avoid the development of habituation and to save battery life (Morigaki et al. 2010, Lozano and Levy 2012). Acute changes of the stimulation parameters could suppress the habituated tremor. However, it adapts to the changed parameters over a time of 10 weeks, which causes tremor recurrence (Barbe et al. 2011). Barbe et al. (2011) have hypothesized that frequently switching between two equivalent but slightly different stimulation settings might be useful for reducing habituation. The prevalence of tolerance for VIM DBS has been estimated to be 10–40 % (Pahwa et al. 2006; Benabid et al. 1998; Papavassiliou et al. 2004; Pilitsis et al. 2008; Benabid et al. 1996). A recent long-term follow-up study (mean, 55.9 months) with strict criteria demonstrated that 73.3 % of the patients with 45 ET experienced waning benefits of VIM DBS over time (Shih et al. 2013). In contrast, many authors referred to the fact that there was no or less tolerance to the maintenance of the constant chronic stimulation of the PSA (Kitagawa et al. 2000; Murata et al. 2003; Plaha et al. 2004, 2008, 2011). Although we need further evidence, the loss of habituation might be a potential benefit of PSA DBS.

11.12 Which Is the Optimal Target in the Treatment for ET?

PSA (Raprl and cZi) DBS showed better tremor control and hand function with the use of lower voltages, which resulted in a reduction of side effects, such as dysarthria and disequilibrium (Lozano and Levy 2012). Using the same electrode different contacts, PSA stimulation preceded thalamic stimulation in patients with ET (Murata et al. 2003; Hamel et al. 2007; Herzog et al. 2007; Barbe et al. 2011). One study with 34 VIM DBS and 34 PSA DBS for ET patients implied that PSA DBS preceded to VIM DBS. However, there is no statistical evidence so far (Blomstedt et al. 2011b). Blomstedt et al. have compared the effects of cZi with STN DBS in ET by implanting two ipsilateral electrodes simultaneously, one in the STN and one in the cZi (Blomstedt et al. 2011a). Although they reported that both STN and cZi DBS were effective, cZi was the preferable target because the best effect was achieved at lower energy consumption with less adverse events.

VIM DBS developed tolerance (habituation) to stimulation despite the amplitude increase, and tremor recurrence may occur within weeks or years (Plaha et al. 2004). Plaha et al. (2011) have postulated that tolerance was a major property of VIM itself. Although further evidence with more patients is required for PSA DBS with both short- and long-term follow-up periods, PSA DBS might be preceded by VIM DBS in efficacy and safety. There might be a possibility that VIM and PSA DBS manifest synergic effects on ET (Blomstedt et al. 2012).

Conclusions

VIM DBS is a standard target for medically intractable tremor. Its short- and long-term efficacies are promising. PSA is a new target for DBS. Short-term efficacy of PSA DBS seems the same or better than VIM DBS, and two publications have reported satisfactory long-term outcomes. The complications and side effects related to PSA are limited, and notably, PSA DBS has been reported to be effective for proximal tremor and free from tolerance. In these points, PSA might be a preferred target for ET. However, further short- and long-term studies with large numbers of patients are required, and it is necessary to compare the effects and complications of PSA DBS with the established target of VIM DBS to elucidate its real therapeutic impact.

Acknowledgements This work was supported in part by the Grants from the Ministry of Education, Culture, Sports, Science and Technology of Japan (grant-in-aid for Scientific Research, 23500428; 21390269; 23659458; 24390223; 26461272).

References

Anderson ME, Turner RS (1991) Activity of neurons in cerebellar-receiving and pallidal-receiving areas of the thalamus of the behaving monkey. J Neurophysiol 66:879–893

Anderson TR, Hu B, Iremonger K et al (2006) Selective attenuation of afferent synaptic transmission as a mechanism of thalamic deep brain stimulation-induced tremor arrest. J Neurosci 26:841–850

Asanuma C, Thach WR, Jones EG (1983a) Distribution of cerebellar terminations and their relation to other afferent terminations in the ventral lateral thalamic region of the monkey. Brain Res 286:237–265

Asanuma C, Thach WT, Jones EG (1983b) Anatomical evidence for segregated focal groupings of efferent cells and their terminal ramifications in the cerebellothalamic pathway of the monkey. Brain Res 286: 267–297

Atkinson JD, Collins DL, Bertrand G et al (2002) Optimal location of thalamotomy lesions for tremor associated with Parkinson disease: a probabilistic analysis based on postoperative magnetic resonance imaging and an integrated digital atlas. J Neurosurg 96:854–866

Bahgat D, Magill ST, Berk C et al (2013) Thalamotomy as a treatment option for tremor after ineffective deep brain stimulation. Stereotact Funct Neurosurg 91: 18–23

Baker KB, Boulis NM, Rezai AR et al (2004) Target selection using microelectrode recording. In: Israel Z, Burchiel KJ (eds) Microelectrode recording in movement disorder surgery. Thieme, New York, pp 138–151

Barbe MT, Liebhart L, Runge M et al (2011) Deep brain stimulation of the ventral intermediate nucleus in patients with essential tremor: stimulation below intercommissural line is more efficient but equally effective as stimulation above. Exp Neurol 230:131–137

Bardinet E, Belaid H, Grabli D et al (2011) Thalamic stimulation for tremor: can target determination be improved? Mov Disord 26:307–312

Benabid AL, Pollak P, Gervason C et al (1991) Long-term suppression of tremor by chronic stimulation of the ventral intermediate thalamic nucleus. Lancet 337: 403–406

Benabid AL, Pollak P, Gao D et al (1996) Chronic electrical stimulation of the ventralis intermedius nucleus of the thalamus as a treatment of movement disorders. J Neurosurg 84:203–214

Benabid AL, Benazzouz A, Hoffmann D et al (1998) Long-term electrical inhibition of deep brain targets in movement disorders. Mov Disord 13(Suppl 3):s119–s125

Blomstedt P, Hariz GM, Hariz MI et al (2007) Thalamic deep brain stimulation in the treatment of essential tremor: a long-term follow-up. Br J Neurosurg 21: 504–509

Blomstedt P, Sandvik U, Fytagoridis A et al (2009) The posterior subthalamic area in the treatment of movement disorders: Past, present, and future. Neurosurgery 64:1029–1042

Blomstedt P, Sandvik U, Tisch S (2010) Deep brain stimulation in the posterior subthalamic area in the treatment of essential tremor. Mov Disord 25:1350–1356

Blomstedt P, Sandvik U, Linder J et al (2011a) Deep brain stimulation of the subthalamic nucleus versus the zona incerta in the treatment of essential tremor. Acta Neurochir 153:2329–2335

Blomstedt P, Sandvik U, Hariz MI et al (2011b) Influence of age, gender and severity of tremor on outcome after thalamic and subthalamic DBS for essential tremor. Parkinsonism Relat Disord 17:617–620

Blomstedt P, Lindvall P, Linder J et al (2012) Reoperation after failed deep brain stimulation for essential tremor. World Neurosurg 78:554E1–554E5

Boecker H, Wills AJ, Ceballos-Baumann A et al (1996) The effect of ethanol on alcohol-responsive essential tremor: a positron emission tomography study. Ann Neurol 39:650–658

Boecker H, Weindl A, Brooks DJ et al (2010) GABAergic dysfunction in essential tremor: an ^{11}C-flumazenil PET study. J Nucl Med 51:1030–1035

Bromberg MB, Penny JB Jr, Stephenson BS et al (1981) Evidence for glutamate as the neurotransmitter of corticothalamic and corticorubral pathways. Brain Res 215:369–374

Butler EG, Horne MK, Hawkins NJ (1992) The activity of monkey thalamic and motor cortical neurones in a skilled, ballistic movement. J Physiol 445:25–48

Carrillo-Ruiz JD, Velasco F, Jimènez F et al (2008) Bilateral electrical stimulation of prelemniscal radiations in the treatment of advanced Parkinson's disease. Neurosurgery 62:347–359

Carrillo-Ruiz JD, Velasco F, Jiménez F et al (2012) Prelemniscal radiations neuromodulation in Parkinson disease's treatment. In: Carrillo-Ruiz J (ed) Topics in neuromodulation treatment. InTech, Rijeka, Croatia, pp 63–86. ISBN 978-953-51-0395-0

Ceballos-Baumann AO, Boecker H, Fogel W et al (2001) Thalamic stimulation for essential tremor activates motor and deactivates vestibular cortex. Neurology 56:1347–1354

Cooper S, Bowes M (2012) Surgical considerations for tremor and dystonia. Cleve Clin J Med 79(Suppl 2): S40–S43

Deuschl G, Bergman H (2002) Pathophysiology of nonparkinsonian tremors. Mov Disord 17:S41–S48

Deuschl G, Raethjen J, Lindemann M et al (2001) The pathophysiology of tremor. Muscle Nerve 24:716–735

Deuschl G, Raethjen J, Hellriegel H et al (2011) Treatment of patients with essential tremor. Lancet Neurol 10: 148–161

El-Tahawy H, Lozano AM, Dostrovsky JO (2004) Electrophysiological findings in Vim and Vc. In: Israel Z, Burchiel KJ (eds) Microelectrode recording in movement disorder surgery. Thieme, New York, 4:pp 63–71

Favilla CG, Topiol DD, Zesiewicz TA et al (2013) Impact of discontinuing tremor suppressing medications following thalamic deep brain stimulation. Parkinsonism Relat Disord 19:171–175

Fields JA, Tröster AI, Woods SP et al (2003) Neuropsychological and quality of life outcomes 12 months after unilateral thalamic stimulation for essential tremor. J Neurol Neurosurg Psychiatry 74: 305–311

Flora ED, Perera CL, Cameron AL et al (2010) Deep brain stimulation for essential tremor: a systematic review. Mov Disord 25:1550–1559

Fytagoridis A, Blomstedt P (2010) Complications and side effects of deep brain stimulation in the posterior subthalamic area. Stereotact Funct Neurosurg 88: 88–93

Fytagoridis A, Sandvik U, Åström M et al (2012) Long term follow-up of deep brain stimulation of the caudal zona incerta for essential tremor. J Neurol Neurosurg Psychiatry 83:258–262

Fytagoridis A, Åström M, Wårdell K et al (2013a) Stimulation-induced side effects in the posterior subthalamic area: distribution, characteristics and visualizaion. Clin Neurol Neurosurg 115:65–71

Fytagoridis A, Sjöberg RL, Åström M et al (2013b) Effects of deep brain stimulation in the caudal zona incerta on verbal fluency. Stereotact Funct Neurosurg 91:24–29

Gerasimou G, Costa DC, Papanastasiou E et al (2012) SPECT study with I-123-ioflupane (Da TSCAN) in patients with essential tremor. Is there any correlation with Parkinson's disease. Ann Nucl Med 26:337–344

Gironell A, Figueiras FP, Pagonabarraga J et al (2012) Gaba and serotonin molecular neuroimaging in essential tremor: a clinical correlation study. Parkinsonism Relat Disord 18:876–880

Godwin DW, Vaughan JW, Sherman SM (1996) Metabotropic glutamate receptors switch visual response mode of lateral geniculate nucleus cells from burst to tonic. J Neurophysiol 76:1800–1816

Govindan RB, Raethjen J, Arning K et al (2006) Time delay and partial coherence analyses to identify cortical connectivities. Biol Cybern 94:262–275

Hamel W, Herzog J, Kopper F et al (2007) Deep brain stimulation in the subthalamic area is more effective than nucleus ventralis intermedius stimulation for bilateral intention tremor. Acta Neurochir (Wien) 149:749–758

Hariz MI (2002) Complications of deep brain stimulation surgery. Mov Disord 17(Suppl 3):s162–s166

Hariz MI, Hirabayashi H (1997) Is there a relationship between size and site of the stereotactic lesion and symptomatic results of pallidotomy and thalamotomy? Stereotact Funct Neurosurg 69:28–45

Hariz MI, Shamsgovara P, Johansson F et al (1999) Tolerance and tremor rebound following long-term chronic thalamic stimulation for Parkinsonian and essential tremor. Stereotact Funct Neurosurg 72:208–218

Hariz GM, Blomstedt P, Koskinen LO (2008) Long-term effect of deep brain stimulation for essential tremor on activities of daily living and health-related quality of life. Acta Neurol Scand 118:387–394

Hassler R (1959) Introduction to stereotaxic operation with an atlas of the human brain. In: Schaltenbrand G,

Bailey P (eds) Anatomy of the thalamus. Thieme, Stuttgart, pp 230–290
Heber IA, Coenen VA, Reetz K et al (2013) Cognitive effects of deep brain stimulation for essential tremor: evaluation at 1 and 6 years. J Neural Transm 120: 1569–1577
Heise CE, Mitrofanis J (2004) Evidence for a glutamatergic projection from the zona incerta to the basal ganglia of rats. J Comp Neurol 468:482–495
Herzog J, Hamel W, Wenzelburger R et al (2007) Kinematic analysis of thalamic versus subthalamic neurostimulation in postural and intention tremor. Brain 130:1608–1625
Hoover JE, Strick PL (1999) The organization of cerebellar and basal ganglia outputs to primary motor cortex as revealed by retrograde transneuronal transport of herpes simplex virus type 1. J Neurosci 19:1446–1463
Hua SE, Lenz FA (2005) Posture-related oscillations in human cerebellar thalamus in essential tremor are enabled by voluntary motor circuits. J Neurophysiol 93:117–127
Ilinsky IA, Kultas-Ilinsky K (1984) An autoradiographic study of topographical relationships between pallidal and cerebellar projections to the cat thalamus. Exp Brain Res 54:95–106
Ilinsky IA, Kultas-Ilinsky K (1987) Sagittal cytoarchitectonic maps of the Macaca mulatta thalamus with a revised nomenclature of the motor-related nuclei validated by observasions on their connectivity. J Comp Neurol 262:331–364
Ilinsky IA, Kultas-Ilinsky K (2002) Motor thalamic circuits in primates with emphasis on the area targeted in treatment of movement disorders. Mov Disord 17(Suppl 3):s9–s14
Ito Z (1975) Stimulation and destruction of the prelemniscal radiation or its adjacent area in various extrapyramidal disorders. Cofin Neurol 37:41–48
Johnson MD, Vitek JL, McIntyre CC (2009) Pallidal stimulation that improves parkinsonian motor symptoms also modulates neuronal firing patterns in primary motor cortex in the MPTP-treated monkey. Exp Neurol 219:359–362
Jones EG (2007) The thalamus, vol II, 2nd edn. Cambridge University Press, New York, pp 1297–1447
Kang J, Jiang L, Goldman SA et al (1998) Astrocyte-mediated potentiation of inhibitory synaptic transmission. Nat Neurosci 1:683–692
Katayama Y, Kano T, Kobayashi K et al (2005) Difference in surgical strategies between thalamotomy and thalamic deep brain stimulation for tremor control. J Neurol 252(Suppl 4):17–22
Kiss ZH, Davis KD, Tasker RR et al (2003) Kinaesthetic neurons in thalamus of humans with and without tremor. Exp Brain Res 150:85–94
Kitagawa M, Murata J, Kikuchi S et al (2000) Deep brain stimulation of subthalamic area for severe proximal tremor. Neurology 55:114–116
Kobayashi K, Katayama Y, Sumi K et al (2010) Effects of electrode implantation angle on thalamic stimulation for treatment of tremor. Neuromodulation 13:31–36
Koller WC, Vetere-Overfield B (1989) Acute and chronic effects of propranolol and primidone in essential tremor. Neurology 39:1587–1588
Koller W, Pahwa R, Busenbark K et al (1997) High-frequency unilateral thalamic stimulation in the treatment of essential and parkinsonian tremor. Ann Neurol 42:292–299
Koller WC, Lyons KE, Wilkinson SB et al (1999) Efficacy of unilateral deep brain stimulation of the VIM nucleus of the thalamus for essential head tremor. Mov Disord 14:847–850
Koller WC, Lyons KE, Wilkinson SB et al (2001) Long-term safety and efficacy of unilateral deep brain stimulation of the thalamus in essential tremor. Mov Disord 16:464–468
Krack P, Dostrovsky J, Ilinsky I et al (2002) Surgery of the motor thalamus: problems with the present nomenclatures. Mov Disord 17(Suppl 3):2–8
Krauss JK, Mohadjer M, Nobbe F et al (1994) The treatment of posttraumatic tremor by stereotactic surgery. Symptomatic and functional outcome in a series of 35 patients. J Neurosurg 80:810–819
Kultas-Ilinsky K, Ilinsky IA (1991) Fine structure of the ventral lateral nucleus (VL) of the Macaca mulatta thalamus: cell types and synaptology. J Comp Neurol 314:319–349
Kumar R, Lozano AM, Sime E et al (2003) Long-term follow-up of thalamic deep brain stimulation for essential and parkinsonian tremor. Neurology 61: 1601–1604
Kuo JS, Carpenter MB (1973) Organization of pallidothalamic projections in the rhesus monkey. J Comp Neurol 151:201–236
Kurata K (2005) Activity properties and location of neurons in the motor thalamus that project to the cortical motor areas in monkeys. J Neurophysiol 94:550–566
Lehman RM, Augustine JR (2013) Evolution and rebirth of functional stereotaxy in the subthalamus. World Neurosurg 80:521–533
Lenz FA, Kwan HC, Martin RL et al (1994) Single unit analysis of the human ventral thalamus nuclear group. Tremor related activity in functionally identified cells. Brain 117:531–543
Limousin P, Speelman JD, Gielen F et al (1999) Multicentre European study of thalamic stimulation in parkinsonian and essential tremor. J Neurol Neurosurg Psychiatry 66:289–296
Lind G, Schechtmann G, Lind C et al (2008) Subthalamic stimulation for essential tremor. Short- and long-term results and critical target area. Stereotact Funct Neurosurg 86:253–258
Lipp A, Tank J, Trottenberg T et al (2005) Sympathetic activation due to deep brain stimulation in the region of the STN. Neurology 65:774–775
Lou RS, Jankovic J (1991) Essential tremor: clinical correlates in 350 patients. Neurology 41:234–238
Louis ED (2001) Clinical practice. Essential tremor. N Engl J Med 345:887–891
Louis ED, Vonsattel JP (2008) The emerging neuropathology of essential tremor. Mov Disord 23:174–182

Louis ED, Yi H, Erickson-Davis C et al (2009) Structural study of Purkinje cell axonal torpedoes in essential tremor. Neurosci Lett 450:287–291

Louis ED, Babij R, Cortés E et al (2013) The inferior olivary nucleus: a postmortem study of essential tremor. Case versus controls. Mov Disord 28:779–786

Lozano AM (2000) Vim thalamic stimulation for tremor. Arch Med Res 31:266–269

Lozano AM, Levy R (2012) Reoperation of deep brain stimulation in patients with essential tremor. World Neurosurg 78:442–444

Lyons KE, Pahwa R, Busenbark KL et al (1998) Improvements in daily functioning after deep brain stimulation of the thalamus for intractable tremor. Mov Disord 13:690–692

Meng FG, Kao CC, Chen N et al (2013) Deep brain stimulation of the subthalamic nucleus for essential tremor. Chin Med J (Engl) 126:395–396

Miocinovic S, Somayajula S, Chitnis S et al (2013) History, applications, and mechanisms of deep brain stimulation. JAMA Neurol 70:163–171

Mitrofanis J (2005) Some certainty for the "zone of uncertainty"? Exploring the function of the zona incerta. Neuroscience 130:1–15

Mitrofanis J, Ashkan K, Wallace BA et al (2004) Chemoarchitectonic heterogeneities in the primate zona incerta: clinical and functional implications. J Neurocytol 33:429–440

Miyagishima T, Takahashi A, Kikuchi S et al (2007) Effect of ventralis intermedius thalamotomy on the area in the sensorimotor cortex activated by passive hand movements: fMR imaging study. Stereotact Funct Neurosurg 85:225–234

Mohadjer M, Goerke H, Milios E et al (1990) Long-term results of stereotaxy in the treatment of essential tremor. Stereotact Funct Neurosurg 54–55:125–129

Montgomery EB Jr, Baker KB (2000) Mechanisms of deep brain stimulation and future technical developments. Neurol Res 22:259–266

Morel A (2007) Subthalamic fiber tracts. In: Morel A (ed) Stereotactic atlas of the human thalamus and basal ganglia. Informa Healthcare USA, Inc., New York, pp 111–118

Morigaki R, Nagahiro S, Kaji R et al (2010) Current use of thalamic surgeries for treating movement disorders. In: Song JL (ed) Thlamus: anatomy, functions and disorders. Nova Science Publisher, New York, pp 1–31

Mundinger F (1969) Results f 500 subthalamotomies in the region of the zona incerta. In: Third Symposium on Parkinson's disease. E & S Livingstone, Edinburgh/London, pp 261–265

Murata J, Kitagawa M, Uesugi H et al (2003) Electrical stimulation of the posterior subthalamic area for the treatment of intractable proximal tremor. J Neurosurg 99:708–715

Nakano K (2000) Neural circuits and topographic organization of the basal ganglia and related regions. Brain Dev 22(Suppl 1):S5–S16

Nazzaro JM, Pahwa R, Lyons KE (2012) Long-term benefits in quality of life after unilateral thalamic deep brain stimulation for essential tremor. J Neurosurg 117:156–161

Nguyen JP, Degos JD (1993) Thalamic stimulation and proximal tremor. A specific target in the nucleus ventrointermedius thalami. Arch Neurol 50:498–500

Obwegeser AA, Uitti RJ, Turk MF (2000) Thalamic stimulation for the treatment of midline tremors in essential tremor patients. Neurology 54:2342–2344

Ohye C, Narabayashi H (1979) Physiological study of presumed ventralis intermedius neurons in the human thalamus. J Neurosurg 50:290–297

Ohye C, Shibazaki T, Hirai T (1989) Further physiological observations on the ventralis intermedius neurons in the human thalamus. J Neurophysiol 61:488–500

Ondo W, Jankovic J, Schwartz K et al (1998) Unilateral thalamic deep brain stimulation for refractory essential tremor and Parkinson's disease tremor. Neurology 51:1063–1069

Pahwa R, Lyons KL, Wilkinson SB et al (1999) Bilateral thalamic stimulation for the treatment of essential tremor. Neurology 53:1447–1450

Pahwa R, Lyons KE, Wilkinson SB et al (2006) Long-term evaluation of deep brain stimulation of the thalamus. J Neurosurg 104:506–512

Papavassiliou E, Rau G, Heath S et al (2004) Thalamic deep brain stimulation for essential tremor: relation of lead location to outcome. Neurosurgery 54: 1120–1129

Park YG, Park HY, Lee CJ et al (2010) Ca(V)3.1 is a tremor rhythm pacemaker in the inferior olive. Proc Natl Acad Sci U S A 107:10731–10736

Pedrosa DJ, Auth M, Eggers C et al (2013) Effects of low-frequency thalamic deep brain stimulation in essential tremor patients. Exp Neurol 248:205–212

Percheron G, François C, Talbi B et al (1996) The primate motor thalamus. Brain Res Rev 22:93–181

Perlmutter JS, Mink JW, Bastian AJ et al (2002) Blood flow responses to deep brain stimulation of thalamus. Neurology 58:1388–1394

Pilitsis JG, Metman LV, Toleikis JR et al (2008) Factors involved in long-term efficacy of deep brain stimulation of the thalamus for essential tremor. J Neurosurg 109:640–646

Plaha P, Patel NK, Gill SS (2004) Stimulation of the subthalamic region for essential tremor. J Neurosurg 101:48–54

Plaha P, Ben-Shlomo Y, Patel NK et al (2006) Stimulation of the caudal zona incerta is superior to stimulation of the subthalamic nucleus in improving contralateral parkinsonism. Brain 129:1732–1747

Plaha P, Khan S, Gill SS (2008) Bilateral stimulation of the caudal zona incerta nucleus for tremor control. J Neurol Neurosurg Psychiatry 79:504–513

Plaha P, Javed S, Agombar D et al (2011) Bilateral caudal zona incerta nucleus stimulation for essential tremor: outcome and quality of life. J Neurol Neurosurg Psychiatry 82:899–904

Putzke JD, Uitti RJ, Obwegeser AA et al (2005) Bilateral thalamic deep brain stimulation: midline tremor control. J Neurol Neurosurg Psychiatry 76:684–690

Raethjen J, Deuschl G (2012) The oscillating central network of essential tremor. Clin Neurophysiol 123:61–64
Raethjen J, Govindan RB, Kopper F et al (2007) Cortical involvement in the generation of essential tremor. J Neurophysiol 97:3219–3228
Raeva SN, Vainberg NA, Dubynin VA et al (1999) Changes in the spike activity of neurons in the ventrolateral nucleus of the thalamus in humans during performance of a voluntary movement. Neurosci Behav Physiol 29:505–513
Rehncrona S, Johnels B, Widner H et al (2003) Long-term efficacy of thalamic deep brain stimulation for tremor: double-blind assessments. Mov Disord 18:163–170
Sakai ST, Inase M, Tanji J (1996) Comparison of cerebellothalamic and pallidothalamic projections in the monkey (Macaca fuscata): a double anterograde labeling study. J Comp Neurol 368:215–228
Sandvik U, Hariz GM, Blomstedt P (2012) Quality of life following DBS in the caudal zona incerta in patients with essential tremor. Acta Neurochir 154:495–499
Schelter B, Timmer J, Eichler M (2009) Assessing the strength of directed influences among neural signals using renormalized partial directed coherence. J Neurosci Methods 179:121–130
Schnitzler A, Münks C, Butz M et al (2009) Synchronized brain network associated with essential tremor as revealed by magnetoencephalography. Mov Disord 24:1629–1635
Schuurman PR, Bosch DA, Bossuyt PM et al (2000) A comparison of continuous thalamic stimulation and thalamotomy for suppression of severe tremor. N Engl J Med 342:461–468
Schuurman PR, Bosch DA, Merkus MP et al (2008) Long-term follow-up of thalamic stimulation versus thalamotomy for tremor suppression. Mov Disord 23:1146–1153
Shih LC, LaFaver K, Lim C et al (2013) Loss of benefit in VIM thalamic deep brain stimulation (DBS) for essential tremor (ET): how prevalent is it? Parkinsonism Relat Disord 19:676–679
Sidibé M, Bevan MD, Bolam JP et al (1997) Efferent connections of the internal globus pallidus in the squirrel monkey: I. Topography and synaptic organization of the pallidothalamic projection. J Comp Neurol 382:323–347
Spiegel EA, Wycis HT, Szekely EG et al (1963) Campotomy in various extrapyramidal disorders. J Neurosurg 20:871–884
Starr PA, Vitek JL, Bakay RA (1998) Ablative surgery and deep brain stimulation for Parkinson's disease. Neurosurgery 43:989–1013
Stover NP, Okun MS, Evatt ML et al (2005) Stimulation of the subthalamic nucleus in a patient with Parkinson disease and essential tremor. Arch Neurol 62:141–143
Strick PL (1976) Activity of ventrolateral thalamic neurons during arm movement. J Neurophysiol 39: 1032–1044
Sydow O, Thobois S, Alesch F et al (2003) Multicentre European study of thalamic stimulation in essential tremor: a six year follow up. J Neurol Neurosurg Pscychiatry 74:1387–1391
Taha JM, Janszen MA, Favre J (1999) Thalamic deep brain stimulation for the treatment of head, voice, and bilateral limb tremor. J Neurosurg 91:68–72
Tamma F, Caputo E, Chiesa V et al (2002) Anatomo-clinical correlation of intraoperative stimulation-induced side-effects during HF-DBS of the subthalamic nucleus. Neurol Sci 23(Suppl 2):s109–s110
Tarsy D, Scollins L, Corapi K et al (2005) Progression of Parkinson's disease following thalamic deep brain stimulation for tremor. Stereotact Funct Neurosurg 83:222–227
Tasker RR (1998) Deep brain stimulation is preferable to thalamotomy for tremor suppression. Surg Neurol 49:145–153
Tawfik VL, Chang SY, Hitti FL et al (2010) Deep brain stimulation results in local glutamate and adenosine release: investigation into the role of astrocytes. Neurosurgery 67:367–375
Theodosopoulos PV, Turner RS, Starr PA (2004) Electrophysiological findings in STN and SNr. In: Israel Z, Burchiel KJ (eds) Microelectrode recording in movement disorder surgery. Thieme, New York, pp 82–89
Tian GF, Azmi H, Takano T et al (2005) An astrocytic basis of epilepsy. Nat Med 11:973–981
Tröster AI, Fields JA, Pahwa R et al (1999) Neuropsychological and quality of life outcome after thalamic stimulation for essential tremor. Neurology 53:1774–1780
Tsoukatos J, Kiss ZH, Davis KD et al (1997) Patterns of neuronal firing in the human lateral thalamus during sleep and wakefulnee. Exp Brain Res 113:273–282
Vaillancourt DE, Sturman MM, Verhagen Metman L et al (2003) Deep brain stimulation of the VIM thalamic nucleus modifies several features of essential tremor. Neurology 61:919–925
Velasco FC, Molina-Negro P, Bertrand C et al (1972) Further definition of the subthalamic target for arrest of tremor. J Neurosurg 36:184–191
Velasco F, Jiménez F, Pérez ML et al (2001) Electrical stimulation of the prelemniscal radiation in the treatment of Parkinson's disease: an old target revised with new techniques. Neurosurgery 49:293–308
Vitek JL (2002) Mechanisms of deep brain stimulation: excitation or inhibition. Mov Disord 17(Suppl 3):s69–s72
Vitek JL, Ashe J, DeLong MR et al (1994) Physiologic properties and somatotopic organization of the primate motor thalamus. J Neurophysiol 71:1498–1513
Vitek JL, Bakay RA, Hashimoto T et al (1998) Microelectrode-guided pallidotomy: technical approach and its application in medically intractable Parkinson's disease. J Neurosurg 881027–1043
Wilms H, Sievers J, Deuschl G (1999) Animal models of tremor. Mov Disord 14:557–571
Wu YR, Levy R, Ashby P et al (2001) Does stimulation of the GPi control dyskinesia by activating inhibitory axons? Mov Disord 16:208–216

Xie T, Bernard J, Warnke P (2012) Post subthalamic area deep brain stimulation for tremors: a mini-review. Transl Neurodegener 1:20
Yamamoto T, Katayama Y, Kano T et al (2004) Deep brain stimulation for the treatment of parkinsonian, essential, and poststroke tremor: a suitable stimulation method and changes in effective stimulation intensity. J Neurosurg 101:201–209
Zesiewicz TA, Elble RJ, Louis ED et al (2011) Evidence-based guideline update: treatment of essential tremor: report of the Quality Standards subcommittee of the American Academy of Neurology. Neurology 77:1752–1755
Zhang K, Bhatia S, Oh MY et al (2010) Long-term results of thalamic deep brain stimulation for essential tremor. J Neurosurg 112:1271–1276
Zirh TA, Lenz FA, Reich SG et al (1998) Patterns of bursting occurring in thalamic cells during parkinsonian tremor. Neuroscience 83:107–121

Spinal Cord Stimulation for Intractable Pain

12

Gustavo Polo, Patrick Mertens, and Marc Sindou

12.1 Introduction and Historical Background

Chronic pain is a very difficult problem that the neurosurgeon has frequently to deal with. Treatment is very arduous; a majority of affected patients harbor disabling neurological disorders together with severe neuropsychological handicaps. Chronic pain may be present in different clinical situations such as long survival cancer, complex regional pain syndrome (CRPS), visceral pain (peripheral vascular disease and angina pectoris), and neuropathic pain.

Medications, physical therapy, and psychotherapies often become insufficient to reduce the pain to a bearable level; in some well-defined circumstances functional neurosurgery may provide solution. Neuromodulative techniques aim at enhancing the physiological control of pain; they include electrostimulation and drug delivery systems. Also, there are lesioning techniques that consist of making selective lesions in well-defined targets involved in sustaining-pain mechanisms. Before surgery be indicated and the most appropriate procedure chosen, the anatomical and physiological mechanisms at the origin of the pain in every particular patient must be analyzed. This needs solid basic and clinical knowledge.

Spinal cord stimulation (SCS) is a modulative reversible neurosurgical method, which enhances the inhibitory control of the dorsal horn, through activation of the large primary afferent fibers. Historically, the rationale was based on the gate control theory (Melzack and Wall 1965; Wall and Sweet 1967). In 1967 Shealy et al. first introduced stimulation of the dorsal columns of the spinal cord to control lower extremity chronic neuropathic pain. The electrodes were applied directly at the contact of the dorsal columns in the subdural space. Because of complications due to subdural approach, Burton (1975) then introduced epidural positioning of the electrodes.

12.2 Physiological Effects

The fact that SCS produces paresthesias had raised the question whether a superimposed placebo effect contributes, at least partly, to the analgesic effect. Evidence of objective modifications of spinal responses to noxious stimuli under SCS had been documented by Garcia-Larrea et al. (1989). The authors carried out recordings of the RIII flexion reflexes in the hamstring muscles in response to painful stimuli applied to the sensory sural nerve. They found depression of the RIII reflex during SCS, especially when the method was clinically effective (Fig. 12.1). Also

G. Polo, MD, MSc (✉) • P. Mertens, MD, PhD
M. Sindou, MD, PhD
Department of Neurosurgery, Neurological Hospital Lyon, Lyon, France
e-mail: gustavo.polo@chu-lyon.fr

T. Itakura (ed.), *Deep Brain Stimulation for Neurological Disorders: Theoretical Background and Clinical Application*, DOI 10.1007/978-3-319-08476-3_12,

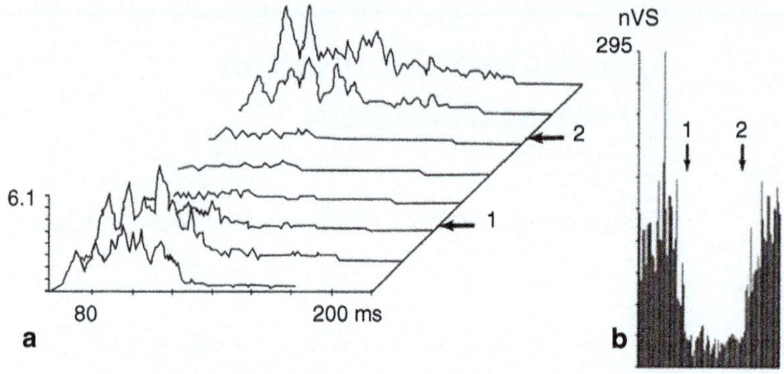

Fig. 12.1 (**a**) (surface histogram) The depression of RIII ("nociceptive") flexion reflexes induced by SCS in a 35-year-old woman with electrodes at T10 level. Each trace is the rectified average of five single responses recorded at 15-s intervals. (**b**) Note that RIII was strongly depressed during stimulation (*1*) and regained basal values almost immediately after end of stimulation (*2*)

experimental data in rats showed an inhibition of long-term potentiation of the wide dynamic range neurons of the dorsal horn following SCS (Wallin et al. 2003; Kim et al. 2001; Yakhnitsa et al. 1999). Besides, experimental studies in rats on modifications in the neurotransmission of the dorsal horn through SCS demonstrated inhibition of excitatory amino acid through GABAergic secretion (Cui et al. 1997; Meyerson et al. 1997; Stiller et al. 1996).

12.3 Material and Technique

There are two methods to implant electrode leads: percutaneous and open surgery. Different models of electrodes can be chosen according to clinical situations (Fig. 12.2). After multi-step assessment, the selected patients are operated on either through an open interlaminar approach or percutaneously.

12.3.1 Percutaneous Stimulation Test and Implantation

The patient is placed in prone position on radio-transparent table. The epidural space is entered with a Tuohy needle. Under fluoroscopic control, the electrode is pushed through the needle to cranial direction in the posterior epidural

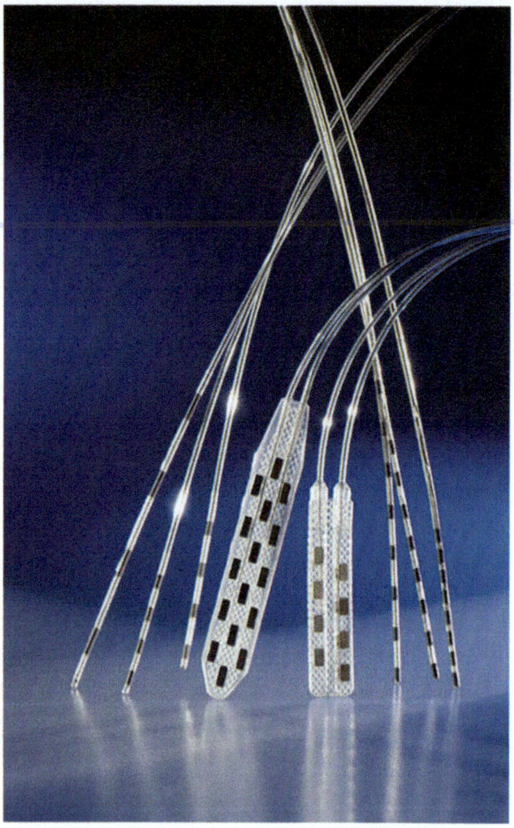

Fig. 12.2 Electrodes for percutaneous and surgical approaches. *Left*: three different models of percutaneous electrodes with four contacts. *Center*: Specify 5-6-5 with 16 contacts for lumbar pain and hinged 2×4 electrode for radicular pain. *Right*: percutaneous electrodes with eight contacts. Different sizes and distances between contacts (©Medtronic France, 2013)

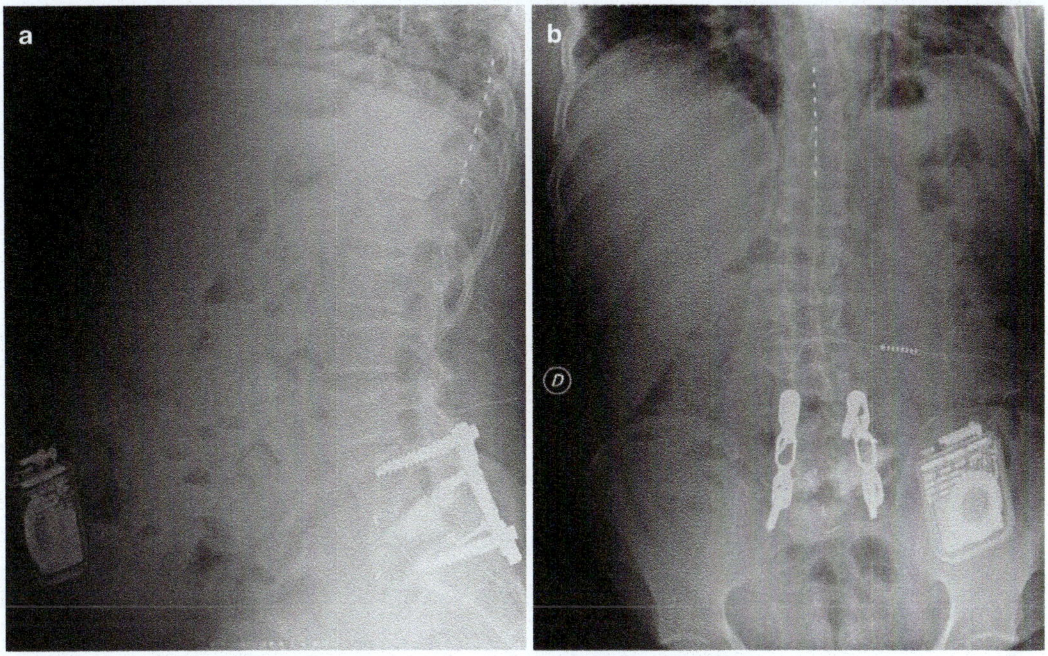

Fig. 12.3 SCS at T8–T9 level in a 39-year-old man with left sciatic and lumbar pain following twice lumbar disk surgery with no evidence of lumbar disk recurrence on CT. Pain was resistant to all medical treatments and transcutaneous electrical nerve stimulation. Patient had 75 % sciatic and 75 % lumbar pain relief after SCS. Implantation was using percutaneous technique (**a**) profile X-ray, (**b**) front X-ray

space. The electrode is connected to an external stimulator. The best location for the electrode is at the upper level of the spinal cord segments corresponding to the painful territory. For lower thoracic positioning of the electrode (Fig. 12.3), percutaneous technique is preferred, with an entry point to the epidural space distal to the conus medullaris to lessen neurological risk. The percutaneous technique has the advantage to insert and place the electrode under local anesthesia. The most effective location is the one which induces evoked paresthesias to stimulation in the whole painful territory. The Tuohy needle is then withdrawn and the electrode is fixed to the subcutaneous tissue at the site of puncture. The electrode is switched to an external stimulator by a temporary cable tunneled distally. This temporary system is used for testing, for 3 days on average, before decision. If pain relief is obtained, the temporary cable is removed and the pulse generator is implanted under general anesthesia. If there is no evidence of pain relief the electrode is removed.

12.3.2 Surgical Implantation of the Spinal Cord System

Open implantation requires general anesthesia. The patient is placed in the prone position. For high thoracic and cervical positioning of the electrode for pain in upper limb (Fig. 12.4), an open surgical unilateral interlaminar approach is preferable. As a matter of fact the percutaneous technique at these levels would be less safe; it must only be reserved to very experienced hands. For pain in lower limbs, especially when lumbar pain is associated, midline interlaminar approach between T10–T11 and electrode placement in front of T8 vertebral body are favored, whatever percutaneous or open implantation (Fig. 12.5). In case of open surgery, under general anesthesia, absence of postoperative induced paresthesias or partial covering of the pain territory necessitate electrode repositioning. In all circumstances the best location of the electrode is at the upper level of the spinal cord segments corresponding to the painful territory.

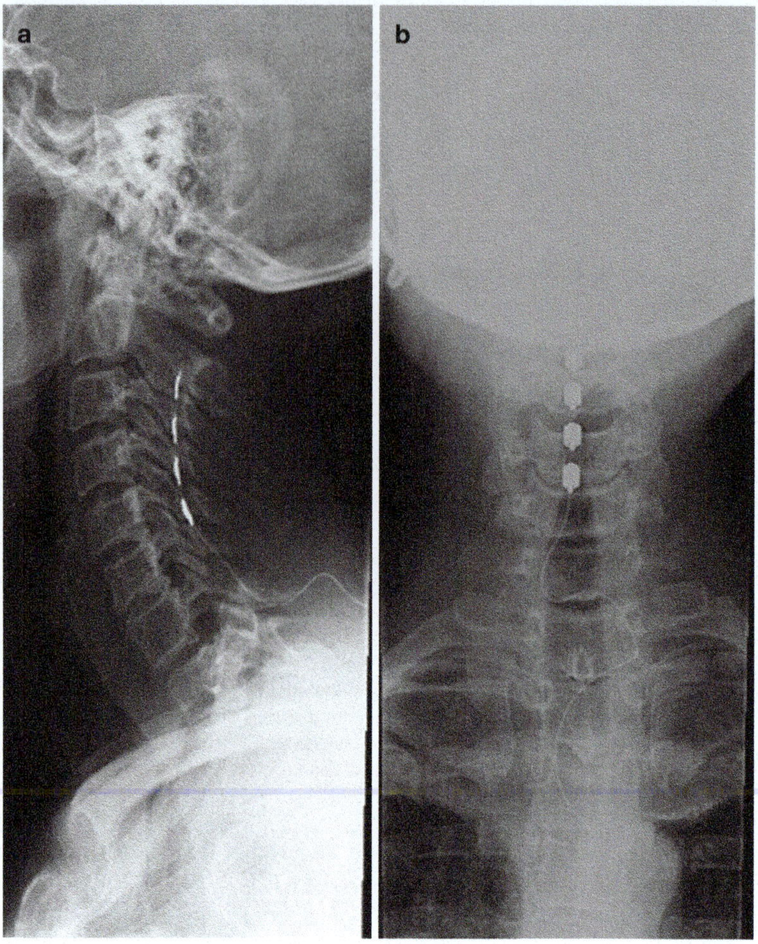

Fig. 12.4 Open interlaminar approach for a C5–C6 right insertion of a Resume TL (Medtronic) quadripolar electrode (**a**) profile X-ray, (**b**) front X-ray

12.4 Indications, Selection of Patients, and Result

12.4.1 Neuropathic Pain

Neuropathic pain is defined as "the pain associated with primary injury of neural tissues – peripheral (peripheral nerves or roots) or central (spinal cord or brain)" (Gybels and Sweet 1989).

Mechanism of Action of Stimulation

The neurophysiological effect of electrostimulation is most likely due to activation of the large primary afferents through stimulation of the dorsal columns (Burton 1975; Brown et al. 1973; Handwerker et al. 1975; Lindblom et al. 1977). Before considering indication for stimulation one must be sure that enough dorsal column fibers up to the brainstem are present and functionally valid. In a retrospective study of our series correlating the long-term effect of SCS on pain and the anatomical location of the pathological lesion, we found that interruption of primary afferent neurons at the radicular level, centrally to the dorsal root ganglion or at the spinal cord level, was associated with a high rate of failure of SCS (Keravel and Sindou 1985) (Fig. 12.6).

Indications

According to literature, neuropathic pain syndromes for which SCS can be helpful include: persistent pain due to radiculopathies in the frame of the so-called failed back surgery syndrome

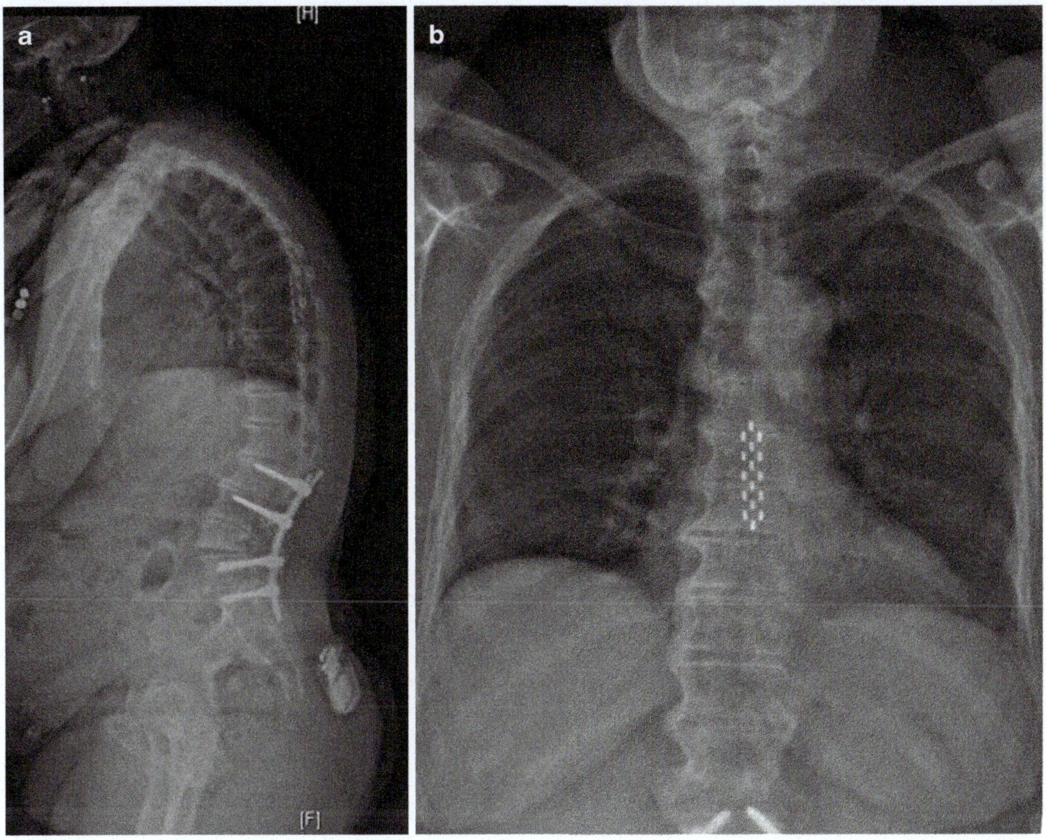

Fig. 12.5 Specify 5-6-5 lead (Medtronic) at T8 level for failed back surgery syndrome including lumbar pain and radicular pain. (**a**) profile X-ray, (**b**) front X-ray

(FBSS), pain after peripheral nerve lesions, and post-amputation pain. SCS may be also indicated in diabetic neuropathy refractory to medical treatment except when autonomic neuropathy is present (Tesfaye et al. 1996; Kumar et al. 1996; Siegfried and Lazorthes 1982; Turner et al. 1995; Krainick et al. 1980).

Selection of Patients

Clinical and imaging examinations should determine whether the dorsal column fibers between the dorsal root ganglion (DRG) and the cuneate gracilis relay nuclei of brainstem are intact. The Somatosensory evoked potentials (SSEPs) examination is a valuable tool to assess their functional status (Mertens et al. 1992). Dorsal column function was assessed by measuring the central conduction time (CCT), namely the N13–N20 interval for the upper limb and the N22–P39 interval for the lower limb (Fig. 12.7). Sindou et al. (2003) established the value of SSEPs for predicting the long-lasting effects on pain after SCS. When preoperative CCT was significantly abnormal, the success rate of SCS, defined as at least 50 % long-term pain relief, was nil, whereas it was 75.4 % in patients with normal preoperative CCT (Table 12.1). Authors concluded that SSEPs are a useful tool for preoperative patient selection, and that if CCT is abolished or significantly altered, as seen in the presented illustrative case, the patient should not undergo SCS (Fig. 12.8).

Results

In FBSS, results are better when pain is radicular and anatomically limited rather than diffuse,

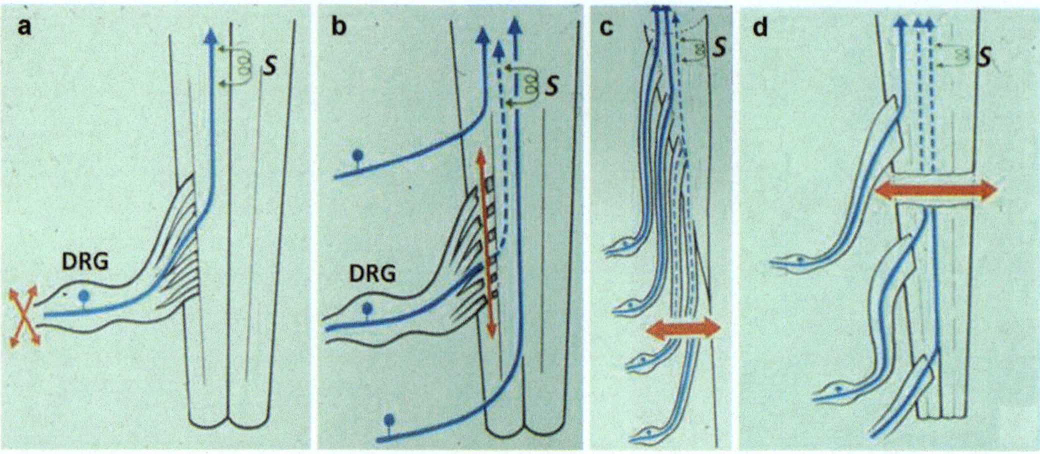

Fig. 12.6 Anatomical bases for SCS: functionality of the dorsal column fibers. When the lesion (*orange arrows*) is at the peripheral nerve level or at the radicular level distally to the dorsal root ganglion (*DRG*), axons going up to the brainstem sensory relay nuclei, through the dorsal columns, are intact (**a**). When the lesion interrupts the fibers centrally to the DRG, as for instance in brachial plexus avulsion (**b**), the dorsal column fibers had degenerated (*dotted blue lines*) up to the brainstem. When a lesion damaged the root centrally to the DRG at the lumbosacral level, as does a lumbar disc herniation not removed early enough, for instance, fibers had centrally degenerated (**c**). Same applies for spinal cord lesions (**d**). If dorsal column fibers are totally interrupted, SCS cannot be effective. Consideration of the location of the causal lesion, together with the degree of completeness of interruption of the dorsal column fibers, is of prime importance to predict effectiveness of SCS (*S*)

and when unilateral rather than bilateral. For FBSS, pain relief greater than 50 % is obtained in 60–75 % of the patients. North et al. (1993) found 52 % of patients with more than 50 % pain reduction at 7 years of follow-up. Low back pain in FBSS was considered in early series as a poor prognostic factor for SCS. However a high positioning of the electrode, between the seventh and tenth thoracic vertebrae, seems to give good results in at least 50 % of the patients so implanted. SCS can also be indicated in diabetic neuropathies refractory to medical treatment. In contrast, post-herpetic pain and intercostal neuralgias seem to respond less favorably.

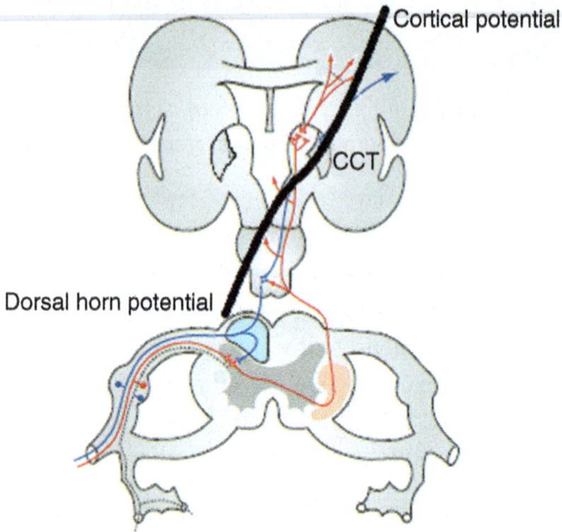

Fig. 12.7 Assessment of neural conduction in the dorsal columns with the use of somatosensory evoked potentials (SSEPs). The central conduction time (*CCT*) measures the time from dorsal horn potential and cortical potential

12.4.2 CRPS

CRPS is a regional pain that affects the foot and the hand, which appears after surgery, trauma or even after immobilization. Excruciating pain results in functional impairment and trophic changes. When there is no evidence of nerve injury, the condition is defined as CRPS type I. When pain is associated with nerve injury, the condition is referred to as CRPS type II (Causalgia) (Stanton-Hicks 2006). Diagnostic criteria were established by International

Table 12.1 Pain relief, according to preoperative CCT

Pre-operative CCT↓	Post-op pain relief ≥50 %	Post-op pain relief <50 %
Normal CCT (n=111)	93 (84 %)	18 (16 %)
Abnormal CCT (n=32)	0 (0 %)	32 (100 %)
Total (n=143)	93 (65 %)	50 (35 %)

Overall results after 18.8 months follow-up
Chi=40.3, $p<0.005$
CCT central conduction time

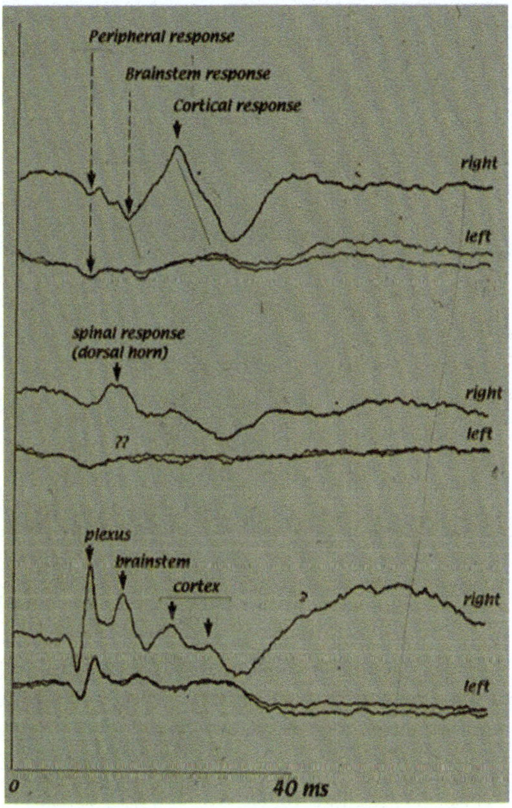

Fig 12.8 Somato-sensory evoked potentials to median nerve stimulation in a patient with left brachial plexus avulsion; main locus of impaired transmission was central to the dorsal ganglion. In such case SCS would not be effective, according to authors' experience

Association for the Study of Pain (Merskey and Bogduk 1994) (Table 12.2).

Mechanism of Action of Stimulation

Is not really known. Pathophysiology of CRPS remains unclear. Implication of the autonomic nervous system explains the frequent at least transitory response of sympathetic blockage. Temporary relief from pain following a sympathetic nerve block is a reliable prediction for beneficial effect of SCS in CRPS I (Kumar et al. 1997; Harke and Gretenkort 2005). In chronic cases SCS can be effective to reduce pain.

Treatment of CRPS Type I

Sympathetic blocks and transcutaneous electrical stimulation are first proposed to improve function, concurrently with conventional pain medications and physical therapy. Psychological disability and inability to work of these patients must be considered through a multidisciplinary approach. When pain is resistant, SCS can be considered. The treatment of chronic CRPS-I with SCS and physical therapy is more effective than physical therapy alone (Kemler et al. 2008).

Treatment of CRPS Type II

Primary factors causing pain must be identified to be treated first. Functional restoration is facilitated by psychological and medical interventions (Stanton-Hicks et al. 2002). SCS may alleviate pain. The percutaneous technique is preferred, with a test stimulation period, considering that SCS does not guarantee improvement of allodynia. When resistant to SCS, and if paroxysmal and/or allodynic pain components are predominant, lesioning techniques, especially DREZ surgery, may be considered.

Results

Kemler et al. (2000) reported that spinal cord stimulation was successful in 56 % of patients with CRPS and concluded after test stimulation that in carefully selected patients, SCS can reduce pain and improve health-related quality of life.

12.4.3 Peripheral Vascular Disease (PVD) and Angina Pectoris

12.4.3.1 PVD

In PVD the pain can be at rest or during walking. In critical leg ischemia (CLI), manifested by ischemic rest pain and/or ischemic tissue loss,

Table 12.2 Diagnostic criteria for CRPS-I and CRPS-II, according to International Association for the Study of Pain

CRPS-I (reflex sympathetic dystrophy)	CRPS-II (Causalgia)
1. The presence of an initiating noxious event, or a cause of immobilization	1. The presence of continuing pain, allodynia, or hyperalgesia after a nerve injury, not necessarily limited to the distribution of the injured nerve
2. Continuing pain, allodynia, or hyperalgesia with which the pain is disproportionate to any inciting event	2. Evidence at some time of edema, changes in skin blood flow, or abnormal sudomotor activity in the region of the pain
3. Evidence at some time of edema, changes in skin blood flow, or abnormal sudomotor activity in the region of the pain	3. This diagnosis is excluded by the existence of conditions that would otherwise account for the degree of pain and dysfunction
4. This diagnosis is excluded by the existence of conditions that would otherwise account for the degree of pain and dysfunction	
Note: Criteria 2–4 must be satisfied	Note: All three criteria must be satisfied

SCS is an alternative for patients who cannot have blood vessel surgery (Ubbink and Vermeulen 2006).

Mechanism of Action of Stimulation

The first to notice autonomic changes in patients with stimulation of the spinal cord was Cook; he interpreted that regional increase in blood flow might be the underlying mechanism of SCS (Cook et al. 1976). Also, Dooley and Kasprak (1976) observed increased blood flow using transcutaneous electrical stimulation; transcutaneous electro-stimulation resulted in a fall of impedance that was assumed as increase in blood flow. Tallis et al. (1992) suggested three possible mechanisms for SCS to influence blood flow:

1. Pain relief reverses the sympathetic vasoconstriction,
2. SCS induces electrical sympathetic paralysis,
3. Antidromic stimulation of dorsal root afferents causes sustained vasodilatation.

Indications

Chronic pain conditions which are refractory to medication and revascularization can benefit from SCS. Also, non-eligible patients for vascular reconstruction can be treated by SCS. To assess blood flow two parameters can be used: systolic pressure and transcutaneous pO2 measures. *CLI* patients with ankle systolic pressure ≤50 mmHg or less, or a toe pressure of 30 mmHg or less, or an ankle/brachial index (≤30 %) can benefit from SCS. Patients with transcutaneous pO2 (TcpO2) values between 10 and 30 mmHg can also benefit from SCS.

Technique

The tip of the electrode is positioned at T10–T11. The stimulation must generate paresthesias in the ischemic area of the leg.

Results

Spincemaille et al. (2001) published that in randomized studies standard treatment resulted in limb salvage of 40–50 % after 2 years follow-up whilst with SCS limb salvage was of 55–65 %. TcpO2 was the parameter most frequently used to evaluate microcirculation. Limb survival of patients with intermediate TcpO2 value was 76 % for SCS, compared to 52 % with the conservatively treated patients ($p = 0.08$). A rise in TcpO2 after trial stimulation of at least 15 % resulted in limb salvage of 77 % at 18 months ($p = 0.01$). The alleviation of pain appears to be due to improved local microcirculation of the skin and healing of ulcers. Relief of pain results in improvement in mobilization of the patient. Therefore, the need for amputation would decrease. SCS also reduces the need for oral analgesics and improves quality of life (De Vries et al. 2007).

12.4.3.2 Chronic Angina Pectoris

Angina pectoris is a chronic condition characterized by the presence of angina, caused by coronary insufficiency in the presence of coronary artery disease, which cannot be adequately controlled by a combination of medical therapy, angioplasty and coronary artery surgery. The presence of reversible myocardial ischemia should be clinically established to be the cause of symptoms (Mannheimer et al. 2002).

Mechanism of Action of Stimulation

The modulation of the autonomic nervous system is supposed to produce anti-ischemic effect of SCS. SCS decreases the frequency of angina attacks and nitrate consumption (Murphy and Giles 1987).

Indications

Disabling chest pain during effort or even at rest despite pharmacological treatment and revascularization interventions. Pain should be considered therapeutically refractory to treatment intended to decrease metabolic demand or following revascularization procedures. Different studies have demonstrated an anti-ischemic effect, SCS is an alternative to coronary artery bypass grafting if patient has high risk for surgical procedures. Electrical neuromodulation is accepted as an additional therapy for refractory angina pectoris by the American College of Cardiology/American Heart Association guidelines (Gibbons et al. 2003).

Technique

The procedure is similar to the method used for other SCS indications. Under local anesthesia, a percutaneous puncture is performed between T4 and T8 to reach T1 or T2 with the tip of the electrode, slightly left to the spinal midline. Evoked paresthesias must cover the area of angina. The proper position of the electrode is essential to the success of SCS.

Results

Murray et al. (1999) analyzed the need for acute admissions for chest pain in patients with refractory angina pectoris. Annual admission rate after revascularization was 0.97/patient/year versus 0.27/patient/year in the SCS group ($p=0.02$). The average time the patients was in the hospital after revascularization was 8.3 days/year versus 2.5 days/year after SCS ($p=0.04$). Authors concluded that SCS patients with refractory angina have less hospital admissions, without masking warning signal of myocardial infarction. SCS improves quality of life without influencing mortality and morbidity. Reducing angina pectoris in its frequency and intensity increases exercise capacity, and does not seem to mask the warning signs of a myocardial infarction (De Vries et al. 2007).

12.5 How to Avoid Complications

Careful patient selection is crucial. The most important prerequisites for choosing the appropriate neurosurgical procedure in neuropathic pain are the underlying mechanism(s) of the pain and the topographic level of the lesion. Clinical examination together with imaging investigations has to determine whether the dorsal column fibers are intact between the DRG and the cuneate-gracilis relay nuclei of the brainstem. SSEP recordings are a valuable tool to assess the functional status of the dorsal columns and the lemniscal system (North et al. 1993). When CCT – i.e., the time course between the dorsal horn potential and the cortical potential – is significantly altered, the patient should not undergo SCS. When CCT is normal, electrode implantation can be performed without a preliminary percutaneous surgical trial. When clinical, imaging and electrophysiological assessment cannot be certain of the integrity of the fibers to be stimulated, a percutaneous stimulation test has to be performed for a few hours or for a longer period, despite a potentially subsequent higher rate of infection.

The neurosurgeon dealing with the treatment of chronic pain must be able to use all techniques: percutaneous as well as open surgery procedures, according to the particular features of the referred patient. Bipolar electrostimulation has greater clinical reliability and fewer side-effects than unipolar systems in terms of uncomfortable, sometimes unbearable, paresthesias and motor twitches by diffusion of current to the neighboring sensory and motor rootlets, respectively. Complications of SCS include: infection, in the order of 5 %, despite prophylactic administration of antibiotics, and the need for revision of the system in 13 % on average. Complications and technical problems in early systems are nowadays less common thanks to evolved technologies. Migration of electrode is observed in 7 % of the cases with recent multi-channel electrodes and is mainly observed in association with the percutaneous technique.

Conclusions

Whatever pain syndromes the neurosurgeon is confronted with, indications for surgery must be considered within the framework of the entire armamentarium of pain surgery (Burchiel 2002; Gybels and Sweet 1989; Tasker 1984; White 1969) and discussed through a multidisciplinary team (Fig. 12.9).

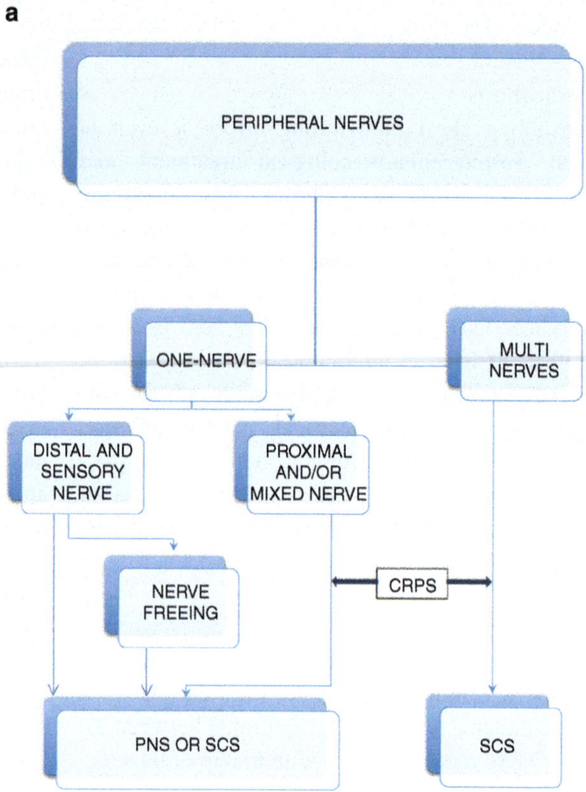

Fig. 12.9 Algorithms. Decision-making for spinal cord stimulation (*SCS*) according to the topography of the causal lesion. Lesioning techniques, especially DREZ surgery, can be useful for deafferentation pain, especially root avulsion pain, and segmental pain after spinal cord/cauda equina lesions, and occasionally for pain after peripheral nerve lesions when paroxysmal and/or allodynic pain components are predominant and SCS failed (**a**) peripheral nerves, (**b**) radiculopathies

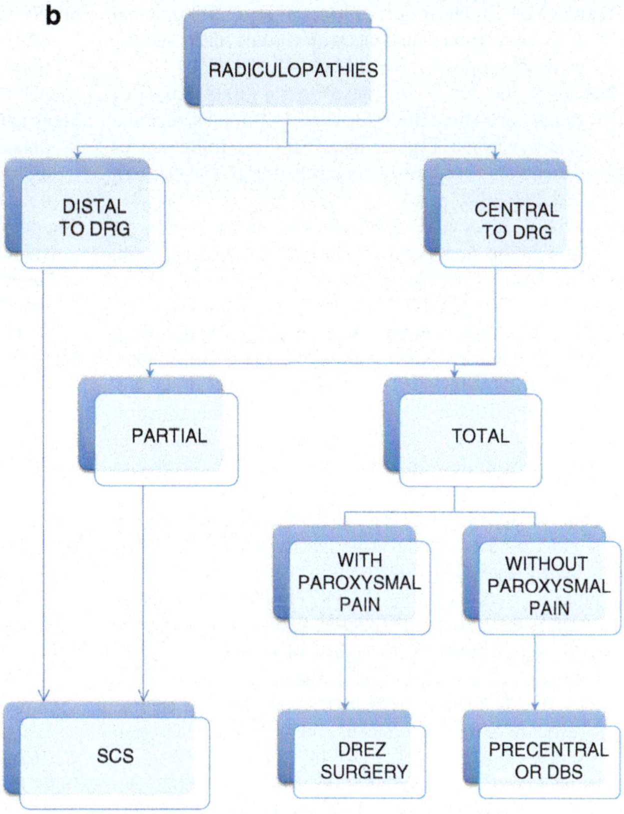

Fig. 12.9 (continued)

References

Brown AG, Hamann WC, Martin HF (1973) Interactions of cutaneous myelinated (A) and non-myelinated (C) fibres on transmission through the spinocervical tract. Brain Res 53(1):222–226

Burchiel KJ (2002) Surgical management of pain. Thieme, New York

Burton C (1975) Dorsal column stimulation: optimization of application. Surg Neurol 4:171–176

Cook AW, Oygar A, Baggenstos P et al (1976) Vascular disease of extremities: electrical stimulation of spinal cord and posterior roots. N Y State J Med 76: 366–378

Cui JG, O'Connor WT, Ungerstedt U et al (1997) Spinal cord stimulation attenuates augmented dorsal horn release of excitatory amino acids in mononeuropathy via a GABAergic mechanism. Pain 73(1):87–95

De Vries J, De Jongste MJL, Spincemaille G et al (2007) Spinal cord stimulation for ischemic heart disease and peripheral vascular disease. In: Pickard JD (ed) Advances and technical standards in neurosurgery, vol 32. Springer, Wien/New York, pp 63–89

Dooley D, Kasprak M (1976) Modifications of blood flow to the extremities by electrical stimulation of the nervous system. South Med J 69:1309–1311

Garcia-Larrea L, Sindou M, Maugière F (1989) Nociceptive flexion reflexes during analgesic stimulation in man. Pain 39:145–156

Gibbons RJ, Abrams J, Chatterjee K (2003) ACC/AHA 2002 guideline update for the management of patients with chronic stable angina-summary article: a report of the American College of Cardiology/American Heart Association Task Force on Practice Guidelines (Committee on the Management of Patients with Chronic Stable Angina). Circulation 107(1):149–158

Gybels JM, Sweet WH (1989) Neurosurgical treatment of persistant pain. In: Gildenberg PL (ed) Pain and headache, vol 2. Karger, Basel, pp 293–302

Handwerker HO, Iggo A, Zimmermann M (1975) Segmental and supraspinal actions on dorsal horn neurons responding to noxious and non-noxious skin stimuli. Pain 1(2):147–165

Harke H, Gretenkort P (2005) Spinal cord stimulation in sympathetically maintained complex region pain type I with disability. A prospextive clinical study. Eur J Pain 9(4):363–373

Kemler MA, Barendse G, Van Kleef M et al (2000) Spinal cord stimulation in patients with chronic reflex sympathetic dystrophy. N Engl J Med 343:618–624

Kemler M, De Vet H, Barendse G et al (2008) Effect of spinal cord stimulation for chronic complex regional pain syndrome Type I: five year final follow-up of patients in a randomized controlled trial. J Neurosurg 108:292–298

Keravel Y, Sindou M (1985) Indications and limits of stimulation treatments in chronic neurological pain. Rev Prat 35(21):1247–1254

Kim SH, Tasker RR, Oh MY (2001) Spinal cord stimulation for nonspecific limb pain versus neuropathic pain and spontaneous versus evoked pain. Neurosurgery 48(5):1056–1064

Krainick JU, Thoden U, Riechert T (1980) Pain reduction in amputees by long-term spinal cord stimulation: long-term follow-up study over 5 years. J Neurosurg 52:346–350

Kumar K, Toth C, Nath RK (1996) Spinal cord stimulation for chronic pain in peripheral neuropathy. Surg Neurol 46(4):363–369

Kumar K, Nath RK, Toth C (1997) Spinal cord stimulation is effective in the management of reflex sympathetic dystrophy. Neurosurgery 40(3):503–509

Lindblom U, Tapper DN, Wiesenfeld Z (1977) The effect of dorsal column stimulation on the nociceptive response of dorsal horn cells and its relevance for pain suppression. Pain 4(2):133–144

Mannheimer C, Camici P, Chester MR et al (2002) The problem of chronic refractory angina. Report from the ESC Joint Study Group on the treatment of refractory angina. Eur Heart J 23:355–370

Melzack R, Wall PD (1965) Pain mechanisms: a new theory. Science 150(699):971–979

Merskey H, Bogduk N (eds) (1994) Classification of chronic pain: descriptions of chronic pain syndromes and definitions of pain terms, 2nd edn. IASP Press, Seattle

Mertens P, Sindou M, Gharios B et al (1992) Spinal cord stimulation for pain treatment: prognostic value of somesthesic potentials. Acta Neurochir 117:90–91

Meyerson BA, Cui JG, Yakhnitsa V et al (1997) Modulation of spinal pain mechanisms by spinal cord stimulation and the potential role of adjuvant pharmacotherapy. Stereotact Funct Neurosurg 68(1–4 Pt 1): 129–140

Murphy DF, Giles KE (1987) Dorsal column stimulation for pain relief from intractable angina pectoris. Pain 28:365–368

Murray S, Carson KG, Ewings PD et al (1999) Spinal cord stimulation significantly decreases the need for acute hospital admission for chest pain in patients with refractory angina pectoris. Heart 82:89–92

North RB, Kidd DH, Zahurak M et al (1993) Spinal cord stimulation for chronic, intractable pain: two decades' experience. Neurosurgery 32:384–395

Shealy CN, Mortimer JT, Reswick JB (1967) Electrical inhibition of pain by stimulation of the dorsal columns: preliminary clinical report. Anesth Analg 46: 489–491

Siegfried J, Lazorthes Y (1982) Long-term follow-up of dorsal cord stimulation for chronic pain syndrome after multiple lumbar operations. Appl Neurophysiol 45:201–204

Sindou MP, Mertens P, Bendavid U et al (2003) Predictive value of somatosensory evoked potentials for long-lasting pain relief after spinal cord stimulation: practical use for patient selection. Neurosurgery 52(6):1374–1383

Spincemaille G, de Vert H, Ubbink T et al (2001) The results of spinal cord stimulation in critical limb ischaemia. Eur J Vasc Endovasc Surg 20:99–105

Stanton-Hicks M (2006) Complex regional pain syndrome: manifestations and role of neurostimulation in its management. J Pain Symptom Manage 31(4 Suppl): 20–24

Stanton-Hicks MD, Burton AW, Bruehl SP et al (2002) An updated interdisciplinary clinical pathway for CRPS: report of an expert panel. Pain Pract 2(1): 1–16

Stiller CO, Cui JG, O'Connor WT et al (1996) Release of gamma-aminobutyric acid in the dorsal horn and suppression of tactile allodynia by spinal cord stimulation in mononeuropathic rats. Neurosurgery 39(2): 367–375

Tallis R, Jacobs M, Miles J (1992) Spinal cord stimulation in peripheral vascular disease (Editorial). Br J Neurosurg 6:101–105

Tasker RR (1984) Deafferentation. In: Wall PD, Melzack R (eds) Textbook of pain. Churchill – Livingstone, Edinburgh, pp 119–132

Tesfaye S, Watt J, Benbow SJ et al (1996) Electrical spinal-cord stimulation for painful diabetic peripheral neuropathy. Lancet 21–28; 348(9043): 1698–1701

Turner JA, Loeser JD, Bell KG (1995) Spinal cord stimulation for chronic low back pain: a systematic literature synthesis. Neurosurgery 37:1088–1096

Ubbink D, Vermeulen H (2006) Spinal cord stimulation for critical leg ischemia: a review of effectiveness and optimal patient selection. J Pain Symptom Manage 31:S30–S35

Wall PD, Sweet WH (1967) Temporary abolition of pain in man. Science 155(3758):108–109

Wallin J, Fiska A, Tjolsen A et al (2003) Spinal cord stimulation inhibits long-term potentiation of spinal wide dynamic range neurons. Brain Res 973(1):39–43

White JC, Sweet WH (1969) Pain and the neurosurgeon. A forty year experience. CC Thomas, Springfield

Yakhnitsa V, Linderoth B, Meyerson BA (1999) Spinal cord stimulation attenuates dorsal horn neuronal hyperexcitability in a rat model of mononeuropathy. Pain 79(2–3):223–233

Deep Brain Stimulation for Psychiatric Disorders

13

Nir Lipsman and Andres M. Lozano

13.1 Introduction

The global burden of neuropsychiatric disease is substantial, and expected to rise significantly in the next few decades. The World Health Organization (WHO) estimates that one in four patients who seek medical help do so for a mental or behavioural illness, with major depressive disorder (MDD) ranking as the third most important cause of global disease burden (Kessler et al. 2003, 2005). As the population ages, and the prevalence of these conditions increases, there will be an urgent need to develop novel therapeutic interventions.

For patients with the most common forms of mental illness, including MDD and obsessive–compulsive disorder (OCD), some effective treatments are available, including pharmacological and psychotherapeutic options whether alone or in combination. For example, current guidelines for the management of MDD emphasize a stepwise, graded approach to medical management, which achieves a satisfactory clinical response in up to two-thirds of patients (Kennedy et al. 2009; Lam et al. 2009). Despite these and other available therapies, however, a substantial proportion of patients remain resistant to treatment (Giancobbe et al. 2009; Kennedy et al. 2009). For these patients neuromodulation may be an option.

Brain circuit-based neuromodulation for psychiatric illness is not new, and its history extends to the 1930s with the early development of electroconvulsive therapy (ECT). The idea that electrical currents can be used to 'reset' activity in pathological brain structures took hold early, and with significant advances in anaesthesia, patient monitoring, and psychopharmacology, ECT today is an important part of the treatment algorithm for several psychiatric conditions (Lipsman et al. 2013a). Other non-invasive approaches currently under active investigation include repetitive transcranial magnetic stimulation (rTMS), deep TMS and magnetic seizure therapy (MST).

Alternatives to non-invasive neuromodulation are invasive surgical procedures which can more directly target pathological circuits and structures. Early operations, such as limbic leucotomy, have now been supplanted by far more refined, safer and image-guided procedures. Deep brain stimulation (DBS) is one such procedure. The last 15 years have seen a surge of interest in DBS for psychiatric disorders, an interest that has been driven primarily by three factors:

1. Safety and efficacy: DBS is part of the standard treatment of patients with Parkinson's disease (PD), dystonia and essential tremor, with over 100,000 patients treated globally to date (Lozano et al. 2013). In properly selected patients, and guided by expert

N. Lipsman, MD, PhD (✉) • A.M. Lozano, MD, PhD
Department of Neurosurgery,
Toronto Western Hospital, Toronto, ON, Canada
e-mail: nir.lipsman@utoronto.ca

T. Itakura (ed.), *Deep Brain Stimulation for Neurological Disorders: Theoretical Background and Clinical Application*, DOI 10.1007/978-3-319-08476-3_13,

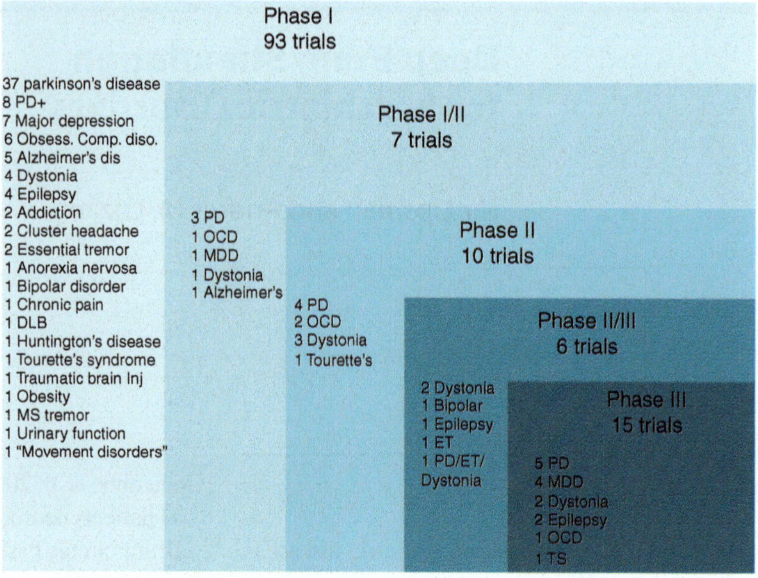

Fig. 13.1 Clinical trials in deep brain stimulation, according to the National Institute of Health (NIH) clinical trials registry (From Lozano and Lipsman (2013) with permission)

multi-disciplinary teams, DBS is effective in controlling symptoms and improving quality of life in these disorders. The ability of DBS to reversibly modulate activity in motor circuits has led to its investigation in other circuit-based conditions, including psychiatric disorders.

2. Neuroimaging: Advances in structural and functional neuroimaging are providing insights into the mechanisms of psychiatric conditions. Imaging studies have helped generate hypothesis-driven investigations of neural circuitry and suggested critical nodes within disrupted circuits that can be targeted with DBS.
3. Definition of treatment-resistance: Although pharmacological treatments are available for most psychiatric illnesses, a large minority of patients remains treatment-resistant. Specific approaches for these patients, who are susceptible to the effects of both polypharmacy and chronic mental illness, are required.

DBS is currently under investigations for a number of neurological and psychiatric conditions. A survey of the National Institutes of Health (NIH) clinical trial registry reveals that at least 21 distinct indications are now under Phase I, 'first-in-man', investigation (Fig. 13.1). Several of these, such as Parkinson's disease, epilepsy and depression, have progressed to Phase III, randomized controlled, multi-centre trials. It appears therefore that the fastest growing indications for investigative DBS are psychiatric, which as of today are among the strongest drivers of progress in DBS research. There are currently trials investigating DBS for major depression, bipolar disorder, OCD, Tourette's syndrome, anorexia nervosa, schizophrenia, obesity, Alzheimer's disease and addiction. This chapter will focus on two of the most common indications, MDD and OCD, and provide an overview of the circuitry of these conditions, the targets currently employed, and a summary of results to date. We also discuss some of the emerging indications in the last 5 years, and hypothesize about the future psychiatric DBS, and neuromodulation for these disorders.

13.2 MDD

13.2.1 Epidemiology and Phenomenology

MDD is among the most common psychiatric conditions, with a lifetime prevalence of up to 16 % in the general adult population (Kessler et al. 2003). The condition is highly heterogeneous, and encompasses much more than just depressed mood. Patients often endorse varying degrees of amotivation, apathy, and anhedonia, as well as lack of energy, and sleep and appetite disturbances. The involvement of multiple 'systems' including mood, cognitive, perceptual and vegetative functions suggests broad circuit dysfunction involving several, primarily limbic, networks. It is not possible, therefore, to ascribe MDD to dysfunction of a specific structure, but instead MDD should be viewed as a network disorder, much like Parkinson's disease. Similarly, it is not possible to link MDD to dysfunction in one neurotransmitter system, such as serotonin. Indeed, neurobiological models suggest that dopaminergic and noradrenergic dysfunction contribute in important ways to MDD, as evidenced, in part, by the successful use of anti-depressants that target these systems (Lam et al. 2009). An improved understanding of MDD aetiology, and the development of novel therapies, would therefore need to account for its heterogeneous clinical and neurobiological picture.

13.2.2 Neurocircuitry

Much of the progress in elucidating MDD circuitry has been driven by advances in neuroimaging, and particularly functional imaging which permits a real-time view of the active brain. These studies have identified critical 'nodes' in primarily limbic circuits that are dysfunctional in the pathologically depressed state. For example, metabolic imaging with fluorodeoxyglucose (FDG)-PET has shown that the subcallosal cingulate (SCC) region is hyperactive in unmedicated depressed patients as well as in healthy subjects experiencing sadness (Kennedy et al. 2007; Mayberg 1997; Mayberg et al. 1999). This hyperactivity normalizes with remission of the depression following medical, psychotherapeutic or DBS treatment (Kennedy et al. 2001, 2007; Mayberg et al. 2005). Other regions implicated in depression include those involved in reward- and decision-making pathways, such as the nucleus accumbens and dorsolateral prefrontal cortex (DLPFC) (Price and Drevets 2010). Anhedonia, or the lack of pleasure in typically pleasurable activities, is a major component of depression, and has been linked to dysfunction in the nucleus accumbens (NAcc) in patients and pre-clinical models (Bewernick et al. 2010; Price and Drevets 2010). The DLPFC participates in decision-making and has reciprocal projections with both anterior cingulate and medial prefrontal cortical regions, which participate in affect- or reward-guided decisions, both dysfunctional in MDD. The DLPFC is also a TMS target in depression, where its modulation is linked to improvements in mood (Lipsman et al. 2013a). All of these structures, and the SCC in particular, project widely in the brain, along pathways subserving many of MDD's cardinal symptoms. The SCC, for example, projects to amygdala and the insula, which participate in vegetative and homeostatic control, as well as to the medial prefrontal and anterior cingulate region, which participate in decision-making (Hamani et al. 2011). In this way, dysfunction in SCC can be linked to several key MDD symptoms. More broadly, such work can identify specific regions for DBS targeting, which can further be tailored according to the predominant clinical picture.

13.2.3 DBS Targets

Several brain targets for the management of treatment-refractory MDD with DBS are currently under investigation. These include SCC, NAcc, ventral caudate/ventral striatum (VC/VS), inferior thalamic peduncle (ITP), lateral habenula (Hab), and medial forebrain bundle (MFB) (Table 13.1). Below we review the targets that have accumulated the most experience to date.

13.2.3.1 SCC

SCC (aka subgenual cingulate gyrus, 'Area 25') is a region below the genu of the corpus callosum that sits at the confluence of at least three white matter pathways. These pathways, projecting to orbitofrontal cortex (OFC), medial prefrontal cortex (mPFC) and cingulate connect higher order, 'top-down' cortical structures with subcortical modulatory regions. As described above, the

Table 13.1 DBS studies for major depressive disorder

Study	Target	Number/type of patients	Outcome
Mayberg et al. (2005)	SCC	5 (MDD, one patient with bipolar II)	Follow-up 6 months. 4/6 responders, 2/6 remission as measured by HDRS
Jimenez et al. (2012)	ITP	1 (MDD with comorbid bulimia nervosa and borderline personality disorder)	Double-blind assessment protocol following initial period of 8 months with 'on' stimulation. No relapse of depressive symptoms with DBS turned off for 12 months. Sustained remission at 24 months with DBS on
Schlaepfer et al. (2008)	NAcc	3 (MDD)	Double-blind changes to stimulation parameters and assessment. HDRS scores decreased with stimulation and increased with stimulation off
Malone et al. (2009)	VC/VS	15 (MDD)	Follow-up from 6 to 51 months. 8/15 responders and 6/15 in remission at last follow-up measured by Montgomery-Asberg Depression Scale (MADRS)
Bewernick et al. (2010)	NAcc	10 (MDD)	At 12 months, 5/10 had achieved >50 % reduction in HDRS scores (i.e. responders). Antidepressant, antianhedonic, and antianxiety effects observed
Kennedy et al. (2011)	SCC	20 (MDD, one patients with bipolar II)	At last follow-up (3–6 years following implantation, mean = 3.5), response rate = 64.3 % and remission rate = 42.9 % (by HDRS). Considerable improvement in social functioning: 65 % of patients engaged in work-related activity at last follow-up compared to 10 % prior to DBS
Puigdemont et al. (2011)	SCC	8 (MDD)	Response and remission at 1 year, 62.5 and 50 %, respectively
Holtzheimer et al. (2012)	SCC	17 (10 MDD, 7 with bipolar II)	At 1 year follow-up, remission and response rate of 36 %. At 2 years, remission rate of 58 % and response rate of 92 %. Remission and response rates based on Hamilton Depression Rating Scale (HDRS). Efficacy similar for MDD and bipolar patients
Lozano et al. (2012)	SCC	21 (MDD)	At 6 months follow-up, response rate of 48 %; at 1-year follow-up, response rate of 29 %. Response measured by HDRS
Schlaepfer et al. (2013)	MFB	7 (MDD)	>50 % reduction in depression scores in most patients by day 7 post-op, at 12–33 weeks 6/7 responders, 4/7 in remission

SCC subcallosal cingulate, *MDD* major depressive disorder, *HDRS* Hamilton Depression Rating Scale, *ITP* inferior thalamic peduncle, *DBS* deep brain stimulation, *NAcc* nucleus accumbens, *VC/VS* ventral caudate/ventral striatum, *MFB* medial forebrain bundle

SCC has been functionally linked to a depressed state, and more broadly to the regulation of negative emotions. Currently, the most experience with MDD DBS worldwide is with the SCC target. The SCC DBS experience started in 2003 and published in 2005 in six patients with chronic, resistant disease (Mayberg et al. 2005). Four of these patients experienced a greater than 50 % reduction in depression scores (HAMD: Hamilton Depression Rating Scale), with two patients achieving a clinical remission. This patient group has since been expanded and data on 20 patients and followed for between 3 and 6 years have been presented (Kennedy et al. 2011). Response and remission rates at last follow-up were 64 and 43 %, respectively. Two other groups have reported their series with SCC DBS and found similar results. In one paper, eight patients were followed to 1 year with the authors finding response and remission rates of 63 and 50 % (Puigdemont et al. 2011). Another group followed 17 patients (10 with MDD and 7 with bipolar depression), and found that at 2 years following surgery, 92 % were responders and 58 % were in remission (Holtzheimer et al. 2012). An additional multi-centre trial of SCC DBS found response rates of 48 % at 6 months and 29 % at 12 months (Lozano et al. 2012). Such results, in the context of severe, unremitting chronic depression, are promising and have led to the design of phase III, randomized controlled trials. The results of these trials will help establish whether DBS at this target should be an accepted treatment for this specific patient population.

13.2.3.2 NAcc and VC/VS

The prominence of anhedonia in MDD motivated the investigation of targets along reward pathways with DBS. NAcc is a grey matter region comprised of an anatomic core and shell and which exists at the ventral confluence of the caudate and putamen (hence, ventral striatum). Neurophysiological studies in animal and human models have directly linked neuronal firing in the NAcc to the receipt and expectation of reward, and imaging studies using both PET and fMRI have linked NAcc striatal dysfunction to MDD (Patel et al. 2012).

Several studies have investigated NAcc and VC/VS with DBS in open-label, prospective trials. Malone et al. (2009) operated on 15 patients using the VC/VS target and at between 6 and 51 months follow-up found that eight patients were treatment responders, and six were in remission. Bewernick et al. (2010, 2012) targeted the NAcc in ten patients and at 1 year had a 50 % response rate, with further significant effects on anhedonia, as well as on comorbid anxiety. The similar results in these studies, from different centres and employing slightly different targets is encouraging, suggesting that DBS of reward pathways can have relatively stereotypic and reproducible response rates. VC/VS has also been investigated in refractory OCD (see below) and the experience with depression arose from the observation of improved mood in OCD patients. Given the established role of NAcc in reward pathways, and the preclinical and imaging literature linking NAcc activity to reward, it may be that NAcc, and its afferent/efferent projections may be the preferred target for primarily anhedonic MDD.

13.2.3.3 MFB

Rather than targeting distinct nuclei, as is the case for motor-circuit conditions such as Parkinson's disease, DBS in depression often targets axonal pathways in an effort to broadly modulate network wide activity. A recent example is MFB, an axon pathway that is part of the dopaminergic mesolimbic system connecting the ventral tegmental area (VTA) with NAcc and other key subcortical structures. Schlaepfer et al. (2013) described their experience of MFB DBS in seven patients with treatment-refractory MDD, and found that stimulation was associated with robust, and rapid, remission of depression. The rapidity of the response, which occurred within hours and days, contrast the typical time to response with SCC and NAcc DBS. In addition, the effect was seen in virtually every patient implanted, with six of seven patients classified as treatment responders at 12–33 weeks follow-up. These results, which require further investigation and validation in larger, blinded trials, are intriguing and suggest a more 'direct' route to mood change than previously observed. Coupling MFB stimulation with neuroimaging, and particularly dopamine or FDG PET, would provide additional insights into the mechanisms of the clinical response.

13.3 OCD

13.3.1 Epidemiology and Phenomenology

OCD is among the most common anxiety disorders, with a population prevalence of up to 2–3 % (Lipsman et al. 2007). The condition is marked by obtrusive, repetitive and anxiogenic thoughts (obsessions), as well as time-consuming, disproportionate, and anxiolytic behaviours (compulsions). Although obsessions and compulsions can occur in the same patient, some suffer only from obsessions or compulsions. For example, whereas some patients will have contamination obsessions and/or compulsions (i.e. 'washers') others will have compulsions to count (i.e. 'checkers'). Heterogeneity in OCD is the rule, although it appears that activation of fear and anxiety circuitry is a common thread.

OCD exists at the interface between psychiatry and neurology given the prominence of physical behaviours that patients believe are 'outside of their control'. Behaviours, or compulsions, that are meant to relieve anxiety become reinforcing, leading to a vicious cycle of thoughts and actions. Current treatment strategies include medications targeting primarily the serotonergic system, and psychotherapeutic treatments that attempt to break the cycle by altering pathological cognitions. As in depression, a substantial proportion of patients, often up to a third, remain significantly disabled, despite optimal guideline-concordant care. For these patients, novel treatment strategies, including neurosurgery, are being investigated.

13.3.2 Neurocircuitry

Similar to mood disorders, advances in neuroimaging have led to a better understanding of OCD circuitry. Such studies have implicated decision-making and fear circuitry, as well as pure motor pathways in the basal ganglia (Greenberg et al. 2010b). For example, among the most consistently activated structures is OFC that is known to participate heavily in judgement, executive functioning, impulse control and emotion-guided decision-making (Kent et al. 2003). Both fMRI and PET studies have further shown significant amygdalar activation in response to provocative, disease-relevant stimuli, as well as a failure of cortical structures, and OFC in particular, to downregulate activity within the amygdale (Saxena et al. 1999, 2004; Swedo et al. 1992). The argument for overlap between anxiety and motor circuitry is strengthened by the large number of patients with Tourette's syndrome who are diagnosed with comorbid OCD (Cummings and Frankel 1985). It is further not uncommon for patients with striatal and other basal-ganglia pathology to develop tic- and OCD-like behaviours (Cummings and Frankel 1985). Indeed, the complex regionalization of neuroanatomy, particularly within motor circuitry is now being recognized. The subthalamic nucleus, for example, a traditionally 'motor' structure is now known to have distinct associative and limbic components, with unique efferent and afferent projections. The existence of parallel, yet overlapping, circuits within the same 5-mm structure, highlights the intimate relationship between these pathways, and how dysfunction in one 'critical node' can have network wide influence, and lead to a broad constellation of symptoms.

13.3.3 DBS Targets

OCD was the first psychiatric condition to be investigated with DBS, in a report published in 1999 that described the anterior limb of the internal capsule (ALIC) as the target (Nuttin et al. 1999). Since then, several structures have been investigated, including the subthalamic nucleus (STN), VC/VS and ITP. Below we review the targets that have accumulated the most experience to date (Table 13.2).

13.3.3.1 ALIC

The ALIC is a projection pathway connecting cortical structures in the frontal and medial frontal lobe with subcortical structures and thalamus. The importance of the ALIC to disorders of mood and anxiety was recognized early, and severing this cortical–subcortical connection was the objective of initial attempts at psychiatric surgery with limbic leucotomy (Dax et al. 1948). Leucotomy has long been abandoned, replaced with stereotactic capsulotomy, a more precise and safe lesioning of the ALIC which for many years was the standard surgical approach for

Table 13.2 DBS studies for OCD

Study	Target	Patients	Outcomes
Nuttin et al. (1999)	ALIC	4	Three-quarters of patients had significant clinical benefit
Mallet et al. (2002)	STN	2	Comorbid PD and OCD; 58 and 64 % reduction in OCD scores after surgery
Anderson and Ahmed (2003)	ALIC	1	79 % reduction in YBOCS score at 3-month follow-up
Nuttin et al. (2003)	ALIC	6	Four patients had pre/post YBOCS assessments, and three-quarters showed >35 % reduction in YBOCS score
Sturm et al. (2003)	VC/VS	4	Three-quarters of patients had 'near total recovery' at 24–30 months follow-up
Aouizerate et al. (2004)	VC/VS	1	Comorbid OCD/MDD; remission of MDD at 6 months (HAM-D <7); remission of OCD after 12–15 months
Fontaine et al. (2004)	STN	1	Comorbid PD and OCD; YBOCS score reduced from 32 to 1 at 1-year follow-up
Abelson et al. (2005)	ALIC	4	Randomization to 3-week blocks of on- and off-stimulation. one patient had reduction >35 % in YBOCS score during the double-blind period
Greenberg et al. (2006)	VC/VS	10	Eight patients followed for 3 years; 50 % had >35 % reduction in YBOCS score
Mallet et al. (2008)	STN	16	Randomized, double-blind design; eight patients assigned to sham and eight to active stimulation. Twelve of 16 had >25 % reduction in YBOCS score
Plewnia et al. (2008)	VC/VS	1	YBOCS score reduced from 40 to 22 at 6-month and 1-year follow-up
Jimenez-Ponce et al. (2009)	ITP	5	49 % reduction in YBOCS at 12 months Heterogeneous patient group (schizoid, addiction, etc.)
Denys et al. (2010)	VC/VS	16	46 % reduction in YBOCS score at 8 months in open-label phase and 25 % difference in YBOCS score between active and sham stimulated patients in blinded phase; nine patients classified as clinical responders
Franzini et al. (2010)	VC/VS	2	Clinically beneficial response in 2 of 2 patients, with YBOCS score decreasing to 22 (from 38) and 20 (from 30) at 12 and 22 months, respectively
Goodman et al. (2010)	VC/VS	6	Four of 6 patients had >35 % reduction in YBOCS score at 36 months
Tsai et al. (2012)	VC/VS	4	At 15 m follow-up, 33 % reduction in mean YBOCS score, 32 % reduction in HAMD, 31 % improvement in global assessment of functioning

ALIC anterior limb of internal capsule, *OCD* obsessive–compulsive disorder, *STN* subthalamic nucleus, *YBOCS* Yale-Brown Obsessive Compulsive Scale, *VC/VS* ventral caudate/ventral striatum, *HAMD* Hamilton Depression Rating Scale, *MDD* major depressive disorder, *PD* Parkinson's disease, *ITP* inferior thalamic peduncle

treatment-refractory anxiety and mood disorders. The development of DBS permitted implantation of electrodes at the capsulotomy target without causing a lesion. Nuttin et al. (1999) described their experience with ALIC DBS in OCD in two publications, their initial experience in 1999 in four patients and a subsequent publication in 2003 in six patients (Nuttin et al. 1999). Of the patients who had pre- and post-operative assessments with the Yale-Brown Obsessive Compulsive Scale (YBOCS), 75 % saw a reduction in scores of greater than 35 %, indicating a clinically meaningful response. Abelson et al. (2005) also performed a double-blind, sham stimulation study in four patients who underwent ALIC DBS and found that one patient saw a greater than 35 % YBOCS reduction during the double-blind period.

13.3.3.2 STN

The STN is an ovoid grey matter structure that is a component of the 'indirect' motor pathway. STN receives largely inhibitory input from the globus pallidus externus (GPe) and excitatory input directly from the motor cortex, and sends excitatory output to the globus pallidus internus (GPi) and substantia nigra reticulata (SNr).

The STN is a major DBS target for patients with disabling PD, and it was in the course of PD surgery that its putative role in OCD was hypothesized. Mallet et al. (2002) reported their experience of STN DBS in two patients with comorbid PD and OCD, and found that in addition to improvements in motor scores, patients experienced significant reductions in OCD scores post-operatively. This work led to a randomized, double-blind trial of STN DBS for OCD, wherein 16 patients underwent the procedure of which 12 saw at least a 25 % reduction in YBOCS scores (Mallet et al. 2008).

13.3.3.3 VC/VS

The DBS target with the most experience to date in OCD is the VC/VS. Anatomically, the VC/VS is closely related to the NAcc which exists at the ventral interface of caudate and putamen. Sturm et al. (2003) initially reported that three out of four patients who underwent VC/VS DBS for OCD saw 'near total recovery' at 24–30 months follow-up, although no YBOCS data were provided (Greenberg et al. 2010a; Greenberg et al. 2006) operated on ten patients with severe OCD using the same target, and found that of eight patients who were followed to 3 years, 50 % had a greater than 35 % reduction in YBOCS scores, indicating a treatment response. Such results are similar to those reported by Denys et al. (2010), who found 9 of 16 patients were responders at 8 months follow-up, with a mean YBOCS reduction of 46 % in open-label follow-up. Most recently, Tsai et al. (2012) reported their experience with VC/VS stimulation in four severe OCD patients and found that at 15-month follow-up, there was a mean 31 % reduction in YBOCS scores as well as 32 % reduction in depression ratings. Such results provide further support for the role of VC/VS in both mood and anxiety pathways.

13.3.3.4 ITP

The ITP consists of a relatively small bundle of projection fibres connecting OFC with the thalamus. ITP stimulation has been proposed for both refractory OCD and MDD, and a small experience with this target is accumulating. Jimenez-Ponce et al. reported the initial experience with ITP stimulation in five patients with OCD finding a mean 49 % reduction in YBOCS scores at 12-month follow-up (Jimenez-Ponce et al. 2009). The patient group, however, was highly heterogeneous and included some with comorbid schizophrenia and addiction. Larger studies, in more homogeneous cohorts will provide additional data about this target, but such results do to confirm earlier case reports that described the safety and efficacy of ITP stimulation (Jimenez et al. 2007).

13.4 Other Emerging Indications

All psychiatric indications for DBS are currently investigational. Although a Food & Drug Administration (FDA) humanitarian device exemption (HDE) exists for the use of DBS in OCD in the United States, DBS is not yet a standard of care for any psychiatric condition. However, the early promise of DBS in psychiatry has motivated its investigation in other circuit-based disorders, such as Alzheimer's disease and anorexia nervosa.

13.4.1 Alzheimer's Disease (AD)

AD is a neurodegenerative condition marked by severe memory and cognitive impairments. Given its relationship to advancing age and associated significant disability, demographic changes in the years to come will lead to an exponential rise in cases. The societal and public health costs will be enormous, and compounded by the abject lack of any effective treatments, despite decades of intense research (Laxton et al. 2013; Laxton and Lozano 2013).

It is becoming clear that AD is a disorder of brain networks, similar to PD and other

Table 13.3 DBS studies in Alzheimer's disease and dementia

Study	Target	No. of patients	Results
Turnbull et al. (1985)	NBM	1	No significant clinical response at 8 months following surgery, but increase in temporo-parietal metabolic activity
Freund et al. (2009)	NBM	1 (PD dementia)	Improvements in neuropsychological function at 2 months. Subsequent significant decline following deactivation of device and then recovery of previous gains with activation
Laxton et al. (2010)	Fornix	6	Two of six patients saw stabilization of MMSE scores, increased metabolic activity in temporo-parietal regions
Fontaine et al. (2013)	Fornix	1	At 12 months, MMSE scores stabilized compared to baseline, increase in mesial temporal metabolism

NBM nucleus basalis of meynert, *MMSE* mini-mental status examination

neurodegenerative disorders. Focal disturbances lead to local disruption of neuronal activity, which is then propagated to synaptically connected structures within a functional network (Smith et al. 2012). By focally targeting disrupted networks, DBS has been proposed as a means of modulating activity in these circuits thereby restoring function. To date, two targets have been proposed for DBS in AD (Table 13.3), the fornix and the nucleus basalis of meynert (NBM). As part of Papez Circuit, the fornix is the principle outflow tract from the hippocampus and projects to the mammillary bodies via post-commissural fibres. A case report in 2008 described stimulation of the hypothalamic fornix in a case of severe obesity, which instead of curbing appetite led to significant improvements in verbal memory as well as spontaneous recall of autobiographical events (Hamani et al. 2008). This motivated a pilot trial of fornix DBS in six patients with mild AD, which found a significant slowing or stabilization of disease in two patients, with concomitant increases in cerebral glucose utilization in key memory circuits, including the default mode network (Laxton et al. 2010). An additional case report of fornix DBS in a patient with AD also found stabilization of memory scores at 12 months following stimulation (Fontaine et al. 2013). A large, multi-centre phase II/III trial is now being conducted to study the potential of this approach.

The NBM is a prime source of cholinergic transmission, and projects widely to key memory-related structures. Two case reports have described NBM DBS in patients with dementia, one with Alzheimer's type and the other with Parkinson's (Freund et al. 2009; Turnbull et al. 1985). The AD saw little clinical improvement but significant changes in glucose utilization on PET scan. The PD patient did see significant cognitive improvements following stimulation. The entorhinal cortex (EC) has also been explored as a stimulation target for memory enhancement. To date, however, this work has been limited to patients without preexisting memory disturbance, and exclusively tested in patients undergoing epilepsy surgery (Suthana et al. 2012, 2013). In these patients, who had hippocampal depth electrodes in place for seizure localization, researchers were able to demonstrate significant improvements in spatial memory with EC stimulation; an intriguing result that requires additional investigation.

13.4.2 Anorexia Nervosa (AN)

AN is a psychiatric condition marked by severe disturbances in weight, body- and self-perception. A common condition, with a lifetime general population prevalence of between 0.3 and 0.9 % anorexia nervosa is approximately ten times more common in females than in males (Bulik et al. 2005; Smink et al. 2012). The most obvious and striking feature of AN is a severe state of emaciation and malnourishment. As a result of chronic starvation patients are at risk for serious medical and metabolic complications that can affect virtually any body system. AN has the highest mortality rate of any psychiatric disease with mortality rates ranging from 5 to 15 % (Attia 2010; Hoek 2006; Morris and Twaddle 2007).

The imaging and anatomic literatures suggest that dysfunction in emotional circuits contribute to AN, as well as subsequent related dysfunctions in reward, perception and body-homeostatic control. Evidence is also emerging that depression, anxiety and dysregulated emotional processing impede effective therapies and lead to worse clinical outcomes (Kaye and Bailer 2011; Kaye et al. 2009). Circuit models have linked AN symptoms to interconnected regions and structures, such as the parietal lobe, insula and SCC. DBS, by intervening in a critical node in the AN circuit, may influence both core pathology and the symptoms that impede effective treatment. For these reasons, DBS for treatment-refractory AN has been proposed.

There are several published case reports and series' investigating DBS in AN. Two case reports evaluated DBS of the SCC and NAcc in patients with comorbid AN/MDD and AN/OCD, respectively (Israel et al. 2010; McLaughlin et al. 2012). In both cases, long-term follow-up was associated with improvements in weight, and in the OCD case, improvements in anxiety. One case series evaluated NAcc DBS in four adolescent females with acute AN (average illness duration 18 m), and found at mean 38 m follow-up, a mean 65 % increase in body mass index (Wu et al. 2012). A pilot trial investigating SCC DBS in six patients with chronic, refractory AN showed that at 6–9 months follow-up, four patients were at BMIs significantly higher than baseline, with five patients showing significant improvements in mood and/or anxiety (Lipsman et al. 2013c). At 6 months, DBS was also associated with significant changes in cerebral glucose metabolism on PET scans compared to baseline, most notably showing a reversal of known parietal hypometabolism. With the psychometric results preceding changes in weight, such results suggest that DBS may be influencing the most common obstacles to enduring behaviour change in these patients. Additional, larger trials, utilizing sham stimulation control, are now required to validate these results.

13.5 Future Directions

The future of DBS in psychiatry will see both technical and conceptual advances. The former will see smaller, rechargeable batteries make the procedure safer and the clinical benefits longer lasting. Improved imaging will allow more accurate targeting, as advances in tractography will permit placement of stimulating electrodes at key junctional pathways that maximize the modulatory effect. One key area of interest will be elucidating biomarkers for psychiatric conditions as well as predictors of treatment response. Recent work in MDD has shown, for example, that glucose utilization patterns in the insula, can predict response to a first-line depression treatment (McGrath et al. 2013). Similarly, work done using EEG has shown that preoperative power in specific frequency bands can predict outcomes following SCC DBS in depression (Broadway et al. 2012). Such work can help elucidate the characteristics of patients that do and do not respond to stimulation. It may also be that in the future, emerging technologies such as radiofrequency-guided nanotechnology and focused ultrasound will obviate the need for cranial access (Lipsman et al. 2013b; Stanley et al. 2012).

The number of indications for DBS in psychiatry will also continue to expand. Changes in the Diagnostic and Statistical Manual (DSM), such as a shift away from categorical labels and towards classification of broad behaviours and cognitions, will help tailor treatments to specific dysfunctional circuits. Improving our understanding of the neural circuitry maintaining these disorders will help to further define the role of DBS in their management.

References

Abelson JL, Curtis GC, Sagher O et al (2005) Deep brain stimulation for refractory obsessive-compulsive disorder. Biol Psychiatry 57(5):510–516. doi:10.1016/j.biopsych.2004.11.042

Anderson D, Ahmed A (2003) Treatment of patients with intractable obsessive-compulsive disorder with anterior capsular stimulation. Case report. J Neurosurg 98(5):1104–1108

Aouizerate B, Cuny E, Martin-Guehl C et al (2004) Deep brain stimulation of the ventral caudate nucleus in the treatment of obsessive-compulsive disorder and major depression. Case report. J Neurosurg 101(4):682–686. doi:10.3171/jns.2004.101.4.0682

Attia E (2010) Anorexia nervosa: current status and future directions. Annu Rev Med 61:425–435. doi:10.1146/annurev.med.050208.200745

Bewernick BH, Hurlemann R, Matusch A et al (2010) Nucleus accumbens deep brain stimulation decreases ratings of depression and anxiety in treatment-resistant depression. Biol Psychiatry 67(2):110–116. doi:10.1016/j.biopsych.2009.09.013

Bewernick BH, Kayser S, Sturm V et al (2012) Long-term effects of nucleus accumbens deep brain stimulation in treatment-resistant depression: evidence for sustained efficacy. Neuropsychopharmacology 37(9):1975–1985. doi:10.1038/npp.2012.44

Broadway JM, Holtzheimer PE, Hilimire MR et al (2012) Frontal theta cordance predicts 6-month antidepressant response to subcallosal cingulate deep brain stimulation for treatment-resistant depression: a pilot study. Neuropsychopharmacology 37(7):1764–1772. doi:10.1038/npp.2012.23

Bulik CM, Reba L, Siega-Riz AM et al (2005) Anorexia nervosa: definition, epidemiology, and cycle of risk. Int J Eat Disord 37(Suppl):S2–S9. doi:10.1002/eat.20107; discussion S20–S21

Cummings JL, Frankel M (1985) Gilles de la Tourette syndrome and the neurological basis of obsessions and compulsions. Biol Psychiatry 20(10):117–126

Dax EC, Freudenberg RK, Reitman F et al (1948) Prefrontal leucotomy; a review. Postgrad Med J 24(274):415–426

Denys D, Mantione M, Figee M et al (2010) Deep brain stimulation of the nucleus accumbens for treatment-refractory obsessive-compulsive disorder. Arch Gen Psychiatry 67(10):1061–1068. doi:10.1001/archgenpsychiatry.2010.122

Fontaine D, Mattei V, Borg M et al (2004) Effect of subthalamic nucleus stimulation on obsessive-compulsive disorder in a patient with Parkinson disease. Case report. J Neurosurg 100(6):1084–1086. doi:10.3171/jns.2004.100.6.1084

Fontaine D, Deudon A, Lemaire JJ et al (2013) Symptomatic treatment of memory decline in Alzheimer's disease by deep brain stimulation: a feasibility study. J Alzheimers Dis 34(1):315–323. doi:10.3233/JAD-121579

Franzini A, Messina G, Cordella R et al (2010) Deep brain stimulation of the posteromedial hypothalamus: indications, long-term results, and neurophysiological considerations. Neurosurg Focus 29(2):E13. doi:10.3171/2010.5.FOCUS1094

Freund HJ, Kuhn J, Lenartz D et al (2009) Cognitive functions in a patient with Parkinson-dementia syndrome undergoing deep brain stimulation. Arch Neurol 66(6):781–785. doi:10.1001/archneurol.2009.102

Giacobbe P, Mayberg HS, Lozano AM (2009) Treatment resistant depression as a failure of brain homeostatic mechanisms: implications for deep brain stimulation. Exp Neurol 219(1):44–52. doi:10.1016/j.expneurol.2009.04.028

Goodman WK, Foote KD, Greenberg BD et al (2010) Deep brain stimulation for intractable obsessive compulsive disorder: pilot study using a blinded, staggered-onset design. Biol Psychiatry 67(6):535–542. doi:10.1016/j.biopsych.2009.11.028

Greenberg BD, Malone DA, Friehs GM et al (2006) Three-year outcomes in deep brain stimulation for highly resistant obsessive-compulsive disorder. Neuropsychopharmacology 31(11):2384–2393. doi:10.1038/sj.npp.1301165

Greenberg BD, Gabriels LA, Malone DA Jr et al (2010a) Deep brain stimulation of the ventral internal capsule/ventral striatum for obsessive-compulsive disorder: worldwide experience. Mol Psychiatry 15(1):64–79. doi:10.1038/mp.2008.55

Greenberg BD, Rauch SL, Haber SN (2010b) Invasive circuitry-based neurotherapeutics: stereotactic ablation and deep brain stimulation for OCD. Neuropsychopharmacology 35(1):317–336. doi:10.1038/npp.2009.128

Hamani C, McAndrews MP, Cohn M et al (2008) Memory enhancement induced by hypothalamic/fornix deep brain stimulation. Ann Neurol 63(1):119–123. doi:10.1002/ana.21295

Hamani C, Mayberg H, Stone S et al (2011) The subcallosal cingulate gyrus in the context of major depression. Biol Psychiatry 69(4):301–308. doi:10.1016/j.biopsych.2010.09.034

Hoek HW (2006) Incidence, prevalence and mortality of anorexia nervosa and other eating disorders. Curr Opin Psychiatry 19(4):389–394. doi:10.1097/01.yco.0000228759.95237.78

Holtzheimer PE, Kelley ME, Gross RE et al (2012) Subcallosal cingulate deep brain stimulation for treatment-resistant unipolar and bipolar depression. Arch Gen Psychiatry 69(2):150–158. doi:10.1001/archgenpsychiatry.2011.1456

Israel M, Steiger H, Kolivakis T et al (2010) Deep brain stimulation in the subgenual cingulate cortex for an intractable eating disorder. Biol Psychiatry 67(9):e53–e54. doi:10.1016/j.biopsych.2009.11.016

Jimenez F, Velasco F, Salin-Pascual R et al (2007) Neuromodulation of the inferior thalamic peduncle for major depression and obsessive compulsive disorder. Acta Neurochir Suppl 97(Pt 2):393–398

Jimenez F, Nicolini H, Lozano AM et al (2012) Electrical stimulation of the inferior thalamic peduncle in the treatment of major depression and obsessive compulsive disorders. World Neurosurg. doi:10.1016/j.wneu.2012.07.010

Jimenez-Ponce F, Velasco-Campos F, Castro-Farfan G et al (2009) Preliminary study in patients with obsessive-compulsive disorder treated with electrical stimulation in the inferior thalamic peduncle. Neurosurgery 65(6 Suppl):203–209. doi:10.1227/01.NEU.0000345938.39199.90; discussion 209

Kaye WH, Bailer UF (2011) Understanding the neural circuitry of appetitive regulation in eating disorders. Biol Psychiatry 70(8):704–705. doi:10.1016/j.biopsych.2011.08.018

Kaye WH, Fudge JL, Paulus M (2009) New insights into symptoms and neurocircuit function of anorexia nervosa. Nat Rev Neurosci 10(8):573–584. doi:10.1038/nrn2682

Kennedy SH, Evans KR, Kruger S et al (2001) Changes in regional brain glucose metabolism measured with positron emission tomography after paroxetine treatment of major depression. Am J Psychiatry 158(6):899–905

Kennedy SH, Konarski JZ, Segal ZV et al (2007) Differences in brain glucose metabolism between responders to CBT and venlafaxine in a 16-week randomized controlled trial. Am J Psychiatry 164(5):778–788. doi:10.1176/appi.ajp.164.5.778

Kennedy SH, Milev R, Giacobbe P et al (2009) Canadian Network for Mood and Anxiety Treatments (CANMAT) clinical guidelines for the management of major depressive disorder in adults. IV Neurostimulation therapies. J Affect Disord 117(Suppl 1):S44–S53. doi:10.1016/j.jad.2009.06.039

Kennedy SH, Giacobbe P, Rizvi SJ et al (2011) Deep brain stimulation for treatment-resistant depression: follow-up after 3 to 6 years. Am J Psychiatry 168(5):502–510. doi:10.1176/appi.ajp.2010.10081187

Kent JM, Rauch SL (2003) Neurocircuitry of anxiety disorders. Curr Psychiatry Rep 5(4):266–273

Kessler RC, Berglund P, Demler O et al (2003) The epidemiology of major depressive disorder: results from the National Comorbidity Survey Replication (NCS-R). JAMA 289(23):3095–3105. doi:10.1001/jama.289.23.3095

Kessler RC, Berglund P, Demler O et al (2005) Lifetime prevalence and age-of-onset distributions of DSM-IV disorders in the National Comorbidity Survey Replication. Arch Gen Psychiatry 62(6):593–602. doi:10.1001/archpsyc.62.6.593

Lam RW, Kennedy SH, Grigoriadis S et al (2009) Canadian Network for Mood and Anxiety Treatments (CANMAT) clinical guidelines for the management of major depressive disorder in adults. III Pharmacotherapy. J Affect Disord 117(Suppl 1):S26–S43. doi:10.1016/j.jad.2009.06.041

Laxton AW, Lozano AM (2013) Deep brain stimulation for the treatment of Alzheimer disease and dementias. World Neurosurg 80(3–4):S28.e21–S28.e28. doi:10.1016/j.wneu.2012.06.028

Laxton AW, Tang-Wai DF, McAndrews MP et al (2010) A phase I trial of deep brain stimulation of memory circuits in Alzheimer's disease. Ann Neurol 68(4):521–534. doi:10.1002/ana.22089

Laxton AW, Lipsman N, Lozano AM (2013) Deep brain stimulation for cognitive disorders. Handb Clin Neurol 116:307–311. doi:10.1016/B978-0-444-53497-2.00025-5

Lipsman N, Neimat JS, Lozano AM (2007) Deep brain stimulation for treatment-refractory obsessive-compulsive disorder: the search for a valid target. Neurosurgery 61(1):1–11. doi:10.1227/01.neu.0000279719.75403.f7; discussion 11–13

Lipsman N, Sankar T, Downar J et al (2013a) Neuromodulation for treatment-refractory major depressive disorder. CMAJ 186(1):33–39. doi:10.1503/cmaj.121317

Lipsman N, Schwartz ML, Huang Y et al (2013b) MR-guided focused ultrasound thalamotomy for essential tremor: a proof-of-concept study. Lancet Neurol 12(5):462–468. doi:10.1016/S1474-4422(13)70048-6

Lipsman N, Woodside DB, Giacobbe P et al (2013c) Subcallosal cingulate deep brain stimulation for treatment-refractory anorexia nervosa: a phase 1 pilot trial. Lancet. doi:10.1016/S0140-6736(12)62188-6

Lozano AM, Lipsman N (2013) Probing and regulating dysfunctional circuits using deep brain stimulation. Neuron 77(3):406–424. doi:10.1016/j.neuron.2013.01.020

Lozano AM, Giacobbe P, Hamani C et al (2012) A multicenter pilot study of subcallosal cingulate area deep brain stimulation for treatment-resistant depression. J Neurosurg 116(2):315–322. doi:10.3171/2011.10.JNS102122

Mallet L, Mesnage V, Houeto JL et al (2002) Compulsions, Parkinson's disease, and stimulation. Lancet 360(9342):1302–1304. doi:10.1016/S0140-6736(02)11339-0

Mallet L, Polosan M, Jaafari N et al (2008) Subthalamic nucleus stimulation in severe obsessive-compulsive disorder. NEnglJMed 359(20):2121–2134. doi:10.1056/NEJMoa0708514

Malone DA Jr, Dougherty DD, Rezai AR et al (2009) Deep brain stimulation of the ventral capsule/ventral striatum for treatment-resistant depression. Biol Psychiatry 65(4):267–275. doi:10.1016/j.biopsych.2008.08.029

Mayberg HS (1997) Limbic-cortical dysregulation: a proposed model of depression. J Neuropsychiatry Clin Neurosci 9(3):471–481

Mayberg HS, Liotti M, Brannan SK et al (1999) Reciprocal limbic-cortical function and negative mood: converging PET findings in depression and normal sadness. Am J Psychiatry 156(5):675–682

Mayberg HS, Lozano AM, Voon V et al (2005) Deep brain stimulation for treatment-resistant depression. Neuron 45(5):651–660. doi:10.1016/j.neuron.2005.02.014

McGrath CL, Kelley ME, Holtzheimer PE et al (2013) Toward a neuroimaging treatment selection biomarker for major depressive disorder. JAMA Psychiatry 70:821–829. doi:10.1001/jamapsychiatry.2013.143

McLaughlin NC, Didie ER, Machado AG et al (2012) Improvements in anorexia symptoms after deep brain stimulation for intractable obsessive-compulsive disorder. Biol Psychiatry. doi:10.1016/j.biopsych.2012.09.015

Morris J, Twaddle S (2007) Anorexia nervosa. BMJ 334(7599):894–898. doi:10.1136/bmj.39171.616840.BE

Nuttin B, Cosyns P, Demeulemeester H et al (1999) Electrical stimulation in anterior limbs of internal capsules in patients with obsessive-compulsive disorder. Lancet 354(9189):1526. doi:10.1016/S0140-6736(99)02376-4

Nuttin BJ, Gabriels L, van Kuyck K et al (2003) Electrical stimulation of the anterior limbs of the internal capsules in patients with severe obsessive-compulsive disorder: anecdotal reports. Neurosurg Clin N Am 14(2):267–274

Patel SR, Sheth SA, Mian MK et al (2012) Single-neuron responses in the human nucleus accumbens during a financial decision-making task. J Neurosci 32(21):7311–7315. doi:10.1523/JNEUROSCI.0027-12.2012

Plewnia C, Schober F, Rilk A et al (2008) Sustained improvement of obsessive-compulsive disorder by deep brain stimulation in a woman with residual schizophrenia. Int J Neuropsychopharmacol 11(8):1181–1183. doi:10.1017/S1461145708009188

Price JL, Drevets WC (2010) Neurocircuitry of mood disorders. Neuropsychopharmacology 35(1):192–216. doi:10.1038/npp.2009.104

Puigdemont D, Perez-Egea R, Portella MJ et al (2011) Deep brain stimulation of the subcallosal cingulate gyrus: further evidence in treatment-resistant major depression. Int J Neuropsychopharmacol 15:1–13. doi:10.1017/S1461145711001088

Saxena S, Brody AL, Maidment KM, Dunkin JJ, Colgan M, Alborzian S, Phelps ME, Baxter LR Jr (1999) Localized orbitofrontal and subcortical metabolic changes and predictors of response to paroxetine treatment in obsessive-compulsive disorder. Neuropsychopharmacology 21(6):683–693. doi:10.1016/S0893-133X(99)00082-2

Saxena S, Brody AL, Maidment KM et al (2004) Cerebral glucose metabolism in obsessive-compulsive hoarding. Am J Psychiatry 161(6):1038–1048

Schlaepfer TE, Cohen MX, Frick C et al (2008) Deep brain stimulation to reward circuitry alleviates anhedonia in refractory major depression. Neuropsychopharmacology 33(2):368–377. doi:10.1038/sj.npp.1301408

Schlaepfer TE, Bewernick BH, Kayser S et al (2013) Rapid effects of deep brain stimulation for treatment-resistant major depression. Biol Psychiatry 73(12):1204–1212. doi:10.1016/j.biopsych.2013.01.034

Smink FR, van Hoeken D, Hoek HW (2012) Epidemiology of eating disorders: incidence, prevalence and mortality rates. Curr Psychiatry Rep 14(4):406–414. doi:10.1007/s11920-012-0282-y

Smith GS, Laxton AW, Tang-Wai DF et al (2012) Increased cerebral metabolism after 1 year of deep brain stimulation in Alzheimer disease. Arch Neurol 69(9):1141–1148. doi:10.1001/archneurol.2012.590

Stanley SA, Gagner JE, Damanpour S et al (2012) Radio-wave heating of iron oxide nanoparticles can regulate plasma glucose in mice. Science 336(6081):604–608. doi:10.1126/science.1216753

Sturm V, Lenartz D, Koulousakis A et al (2003) The nucleus accumbens: a target for deep brain stimulation in obsessive-compulsive- and anxiety-disorders. J Chem Neuroanat 26(4):293–299

Suthana N, Fried I (2013) Deep brain stimulation for enhancement of learning and memory. Neuroimage 85(3):996–1002. doi:10.1016/j.neuroimage.2013.07.066

Suthana N, Haneef Z, Stern J et al (2012) Memory enhancement and deep-brain stimulation of the entorhinal area. N Engl J Med 366(6):502–510. doi:10.1056/NEJMoa1107212

Swedo SE, Pietrini P, Leonard HL et al (1992) Cerebral glucose metabolism in childhood-onset obsessive-compulsive disorder. Revisualization during pharmacotherapy. Arch Gen Psychiatry 49(9):690–694

Tsai HC, Chang CH, Pan JI et al (2012) Pilot study of deep brain stimulation in refractory obsessive-compulsive disorder ethnic Chinese patients. Psychiatry Clin Neurosci 66(4):303–312. doi:10.1111/j.1440-1819.2012.02352.x

Turnbull IM, McGeer PL, Beattie L et al (1985) Stimulation of the basal nucleus of Meynert in senile dementia of Alzheimer's type. A preliminary report. Appl Neurophysiol 48(1–6):216–221

Wu H, Van Dyck-Lippens PJ, Santegoeds R et al (2012) Deep-brain stimulation for anorexia nervosa. World Neurosurg 98(5):1104–1108. doi:10.1016/j.wneu.2012.06.039/10.3171/jns.2003.98.5.1104

Deep Brain Stimulation for Epilepsy: Evidence for Limbic Network Disruption via Chronic Anterior Nucleus of the Thalamus and Hippocampus Stimulation

14

Paul Koch and Gordon Baltuch

14.1 Introduction

Epilepsy is a *chronic* seizure condition, classically characterized as "a continuing tendency to seizure relapse" (Shorvon and Goodridge 2013). It is estimated to affect 50 million people worldwide (Epilepsy Fact Sheet 2012). As a chronic condition epilepsy confers significant mortality, including suicide and SUDEP (Sudden Unexpected Death in Epilepsy) (Nashef and Ryvlin 2009), and morbidity, including cognitive, psychological and social impairment, risk of injury, and socioeconomic consequences (Tellez-Zenteno et al. 2007; Epilepsy Therapy Project 2013). While antiepileptic drugs have been transformative for a majority of sufferers, there remain around 20 % of patients with poor seizure control despite optimal medical therapy (Sander 2003). Some of these patients with medically refractory epilepsy are candidates for resective surgery. Up to 66 % can achieve long-term seizure freedom (Tellez-Zenteno et al. 2005). However, many are ineligible due to comorbidities, or number and location of epileptic foci. Further, the risk of permanent memory impairment is significant with resection of the dominant mesial temporal structures (Helmstaedter et al. 2003).

P. Koch, MD (✉) • G. Baltuch, MD, PhD
Department of Neurosurgery,
University of Pennsylvania,
Philadelphia, PA, USA
e-mail: paul.koch@uphs.upenn.edu

It is clear from decades of research that seizures do not simply originate from one location (e.g. temporal lobe) and spread haphazardly throughout the cortex, but rather propagate and are sustained via distinct cortical–subcortical networks (Norden and Blumenfeld 2002). Since the 1980s attempts have been made to modulate these networks in order to disrupt, or prevent seizures in medically intractable epilepsy using deep brain stimulation (DBS) with some success (Cooper et al. 1984; Kerrigan et al. 2004; Fisher et al. 2010; Tellez-Zenteno et al. 2006; Velasco et al. 2007; McLachlan et al. 2010). Although the mechanism of action of DBS is still hotly debated (Lozano and Lipsman 2013), it is clear that DBS disrupts neuronal networks (whether by activation, inhibition, or lesion) and that this is likely the source of therapeutic benefit (McIntyre and Hahn 2010).

With the recent encouraging, albeit modest, results of the SANTE trial (Fisher et al. 2010) coupled with the established success of DBS therapy for movement disorders (Rezai et al. 2008) DBS for the treatment of epilepsy is gaining ground. Furthermore, because of the favorable safety profile of DBS when compared to surgical resection (Umemura et al. 2003), the ability to adjust stimulation parameters and its reversibility, DBS for refractory epilepsy should begin to transition from a therapy of last resort to a viable treatment option.

This chapter will briefly review relevant seizure circuitry and then focus on evidence for

T. Itakura (ed.), *Deep Brain Stimulation for Neurological Disorders: Theoretical Background and Clinical Application*, DOI 10.1007/978-3-319-08476-3_14,

effective DBS of the anterior nucleus of the thalamus (ANT) and of the hippocampus for medically refractory epilepsy. Both targets are part of a wider limbic network with extensive reciprocal cortical connections and in some sense serve as "gateways" between the cortical and subcortical worlds. The ANT and the hippocampus have significant clinical evidence in their favor as DBS targets for epilepsy including a large, multi-enter, randomized controlled trial for ANT stimulation (Fisher et al. 2010). Additionally, seizures originating in the temporal lobe have been treated very successfully with resective surgery (Tellez-Zenteno et al. 2005), but for some patients surgical resection is contraindicated, making the hippocampus a natural and enticing DBS target. We will finally briefly review the safety evidence for DBS and present a representative surgical protocol for DBS implantation at our institution.

14.2 Seizure Propagation: Cortical–Subcortical Interactions

Limbic circuitry, originally proposed by Papez in 1937 as the circuit of emotional processing (Papez 1937), may be important for seizure propagation. Papez's goal was to provide an anatomic basis of the theory that emotion resulted from the interaction between the cortex and these subcortical structures (a network now thought to be involved primarily in memory encoding). Much of the cerebral cortex projects, via the cingulum, to the parahippocampal gyrus, which projects to the entorhinal cortex. The entorhinal cortex, in turn, projects into the hippocampus via the perforant pathway. The hippocampus projects outward via the fimbria and fornix to the mammillary bodies, which, in turn, project to both the hypothalamus and the ANT (via the mamillothalamic tract). From here the ANT completes the corticolimbic loop by projecting to the cingulate cortex. Thus, Papez described a network that funnels cortical fibers into the hippocampus on one end and subsequently routs pathway-connected fibers in the thalamus back to the cortex on the other.

Indeed, much animal and human evidence exists that the hippocampus and subcortical structures and their interaction with the cortex are key to seizure propagation (Norden and Blumenfeld 2002; Gale 1992). As one example, Gale describes a consistent network that is activated during limbic motor seizures in rodents (thought to be the corollary of partial complex seizures in humans) that includes (but is not limited to) the entorhinal cortex, hippocampus, amygdala and thalamus. Importantly, these regions were consistently activated *regardless of which area of the limbic region initiated seizures* (Gale 1992). If seizures propagate along predictable pathways, then interruption of those pathways via DBS could potentially prevent the generation and propagation of seizures.

There is also evidence that seizures themselves may induce cortical–subcortical network changes, possibly making epilepsy more difficult to treat and may have implications for patient selection and timing of intervention. Prolonged seizures in rats leads to progressive recruitment of subcortical structures (Gale 1992). In humans, not only does the interictal extent of cortical metabolic derangement expand as seizure frequency increases in children with intractable epilepsy (Benedek et al. 2006), but interictal thalamic and hippocampal metabolic derangements worsen with duration of epilepsy and are worse in patients with secondarily generalized seizures (Benedek et al. 2004). These results may simply reflect co-activation of nodes in a known cortical–subcortical network, but alternatively may hint at secondary epileptogenesis, a phenomenon described in animal models, whereby seizure activity from one site eventually leads to independent seizure activity from a second, remote site (Luat and Chugani 2008). Clinical outcomes data on long-term prognosis for epilepsy could be consistent with this idea: the authors of a recent comprehensive review conclude that the longer an epilepsy is active, the poorer is the long-term outcome and that further, the largest predictor of poor long-term outcome is pre-treatment seizure frequency (Shorvon and Goodridge 2013). However, the extent to which secondary epileptogenesis exists in humans is unclear and the further question of whether it is reversible is unknown. Nonetheless, it is interesting to note that several studies of

DBS for epilepsy, including the recent SANTE trial, report a seizure reduction rate of at least 50 % in some patients only after 3–6 years of stimulation (Andrade et al. 2006; Fisher et al. 2010). While these results could be explained by evolving stimulation parameters, or antiepileptic drug regimens, it is intriguing to speculate that DBS may exert a chronic, plastic effect on epileptogenic circuitry as is seen in DBS therapy for other conditions such as dystonia, or obsessive–compulsive disorder (Lozano and Lipsman 2013).

14.3 Target: Anterior Nucleus of the Thalamus (ANT)

There are several theoretical reasons to select the ANT as a target for disruption in epilepsy. First, the thalamus is a known monosynaptic gateway to the cortex. Second, thalamocortical interactions are, by themselves, responsible for certain seizure types (Avanzini et al. 2000). Third, the ANT in particular is a privileged recipient of mesial temporal lobe efferent pathways via the limbic circuit (see above). Therefore, disrupting the downstream propagation of mesial temporal epileptic firing would seem logical. An animal model of chemically induced seizures via systemic administration of pentylenetetrazol has shown that high-frequency stimulation of the ANT can attenuate the progression of cortical bursting activity to clonic seizures (Mirski et al. 1997). This high-frequency stimulation is theorized to disrupt cortical–subcortical propagation of epileptic activity. In one small clinical study of ANT stimulation for epilepsy, although there was no statistically significant reduction in overall seizures, there was a significant reduction in generalized and complex partial seizures (termed "serious seizures"), suggesting that chronic ANT stimulation may disrupt seizure propagation rather than prevent seizure onset (Kerrigan et al. 2004).

Some of the first attempts to ameliorate seizures with DBS were in the thalamus (Cooper et al. 1980) and in the ANT in particular (Cooper et al. 1984). Cooper et al. achieved control of complex partial seizures in four of six patients implanted with bilateral ANT stimulators who were refractory to medical therapy. Although these patients had seizures of non-generalized origin, the electrographic seizure foci were either indistinct, or multiple, and therefore not amenable to resection. As such, these patients were theoretically good candidates for ANT stimulation: they were not candidates for surgical resection, yet they exhibited some evidence of focality in seizure onset, which may or may not have generalized, but which required propagation through the ANT to sustain seizure activity. While all subsequent trials of ANT DBS for epilepsy have required patients to be medically refractory and to have no structural lesion amenable to resection, some have included patients with no evidence of focality either electrographically, or semiologically (i.e. primary generalized seizures) (Hodaie et al. 2002; Lim et al. 2007; Lee et al. 2006), while others required simple or complex partial seizures that then did, or did not generalize (Cooper et al. 1984; Osorio et al. 2007; Kerrigan et al. 2004; Fisher et al. 2010). All of these studies have shown positive results, although all have been small case series, with the exception of the SANTE trial (Fisher et al. 2010), reporting seizure frequency reductions compared to baseline between 49 and 75.6 % with variable follow-up periods ranging from 2 months to 7 years. Lack of controls, variable precision of ANT targeting, variable patient selection, and variations in stimulating parameters all make these data difficult to interpret. Table 14.1 provides a summary of clinical studies of ANT DBS for epilepsy.

Although the ANT is a relatively large structure, one study suggests that the internal complexity of the thalamus may make effective targeting difficult (Osorio et al. 2007). They recorded in bilateral hippocampi during bilateral ANT stimulation in four patients, with highly variable responses across patients. They also confirmed placement with post-operative MRI and found that only three of the 16 stimulating contacts (two per nucleus in four patients) were located in the ANT proper. Curiously, the patient with contacts in the ANT had the most modest reduction in seizures with stimulation.

Since ANT lesions have themselves been shown to reduce seizures (Mullan et al. 1967), the

Table 14.1 Clinical trials for anterior nucleus of the thalamus (ANT) stimulation to treat epilepsy

Study	Type	No. of patients	Seizure type	Follow up	Stimulation parameters	Results[a]
SANTE	Multi-center, double-blind, randomized controlled trial	108	Partial onset	3 months (blinded)	145 Hz, 1 min on, 5 min off (blinded)	29 % increased reduction in active vs. control groups (blinded)
Fisher et al. (2010)				25 months (unblinded)	variable (unblinded)	56 % reduction (unblinded)
Osorio et al. (2007)	Case series	4	Mesiotemporal	36 months	157 Hz (mean), 1 min on, 5 min off	75 % reduction
Lim et al. (2007)	Case series	4	Heterogeneous	33–48 months	90–110 Hz, continuous and cycling	51 % reduction
Hodaie et al. (2002)	Case series	6	Heterogeneous	11–21 months (short-term)	100 Hz, 1 min on, 5 min off	53.8 % reduction (short-term)
Andrade et al. (2006)				2–7 years (long-term)		No change long-term
Lee et al. (2006)	Case series	3	Heterogeneous	2–10 months	130 Hz, 1 min on, 5 min off	75.4 % reduction
Kerrigan et al. (2004)	Case series	5	Partial onset	12 months	100 Hz, 1 min on, 5 min off	Statistically significant reduction in 1/5 patients
Cooper et al. (1984)	Case series	6	Partial onset	3 years	60–70 Hz, continuous	Clinically significant improvement in 4/6 patients

[a]Results are given as an aggregate percentage reduction in seizure frequency compared to baseline if provided, unless otherwise noted

question of a "lesion effect" from stimulator placement is also important. Hodaie et al. (2002) reported an immediate mean reduction in seizure frequency of 56.8 % after electrode implantation compared to baseline. They found no significant change in seizure reduction out to an average of 15 months when the stimulators were turned on, nor when they were turned off for a period of 2 months in a blinded fashion. These patients were subsequently followed for 2–7 years, during which time seizure frequency reductions over baseline were maintained, but did not improve (Andrade et al. 2006). In another case series, however, some individual patients were noted to suffer an increase in seizure frequency when the stimulators were unintentionally turned off (without awareness of the patient), with return of seizure improvement with resumption of stimulation (Kerrigan et al. 2004). These results only emphasized that a randomized, controlled, blinded study was needed.

In 2010 the anticipated results of the multicenter, double-blind SANTE trial (Fisher et al. 2010) were published. To be included in this trial patients had to have partial seizures, with or without secondary generalization, in line with the logic that ANT stimulation disrupts subcortical–cortical propagation of seizures along a distinct limbic pathway. Patients had failed at least three antiepileptic drugs and had no evidence of a structural brain lesion. Patients were implanted with bilateral ANT stimulating electrodes after completing a 3-month baseline period during which their antiepileptic drug regimen remained stable. If an electrode was not within the ANT on post-operative imaging, it was replaced. Patients were randomized to stimulation on or stimulation off groups 4 weeks after implantation. The blinded phase lasted 3 months and included 108 patients. Using a model that adjusted for repeated measurements, the authors reported a 29 % greater seizure frequency reduction in the stimulation group compared to the

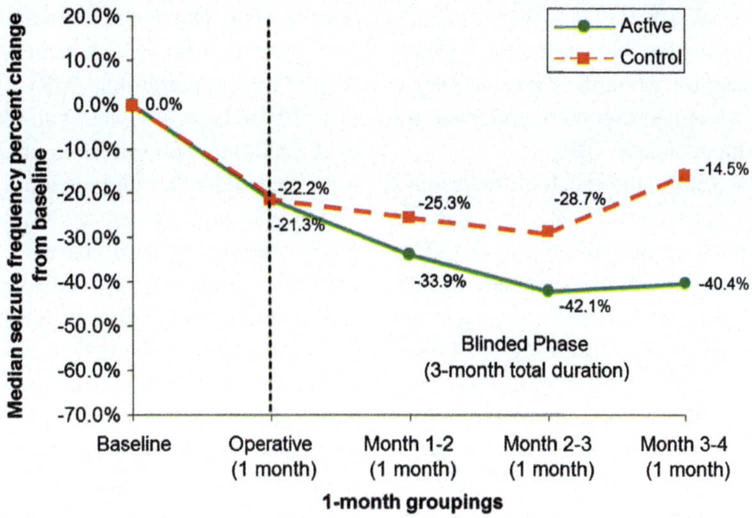

Fig. 14.1 SANTE trial: electrical stimulation of the anterior nucleus of thalamus for the treatment of refractory epilepsy. The graph shows unadjusted median total seizure frequency percent change from baseline by 1-month groupings and treatment group during the blinded phase. Patients ($n = 108$) included in this graph were those with at least 70 diary days in the blinded phase (including the outlier). The operative data point contains cumulative data from hospital discharge to 1 month post-implantation but prior to randomization (no active stimulation). Month 1–2 contains cumulative data from month 1 visit to month 2 visit. Month 2–3 contains cumulative data from month 2 visit to month 3 visit. Month 3–4 contains cumulative data from month 3 visit to month 4 visit (From Fisher et al. (2010), with permission)

control group during month 3 of the blinded phase. It is instructive to look at the (unadjusted) median seizure frequency improvement in the blinded phase over time (Fig. 14.1). Both the stimulation and the control groups saw a comparable reduction in seizures in the month after implantation, before stimulation, which may capture a conjectured "lesional effect." In the ensuing blinded months, however, the two groups progressively separate, the difference becoming significant in the third month. After the 3-month blinded phase, all patients entered an open trial of stimulation with restrictions on stimulation parameters. After month 13 stimulation parameters were allowed to vary freely. Median seizure frequency reduction at 13 months was 41 %, and increased to 56 % at 25 months. These results demonstrate a benefit of high-frequency bilateral ANT stimulation for refractory epilepsy. Further, more than having failed antiepileptic medication, 44.5 % of patients had failed vagal nerve stimulation, and 24.5 % had achieved no benefit from surgical resection, demonstrating that ANT DBS may be the therapy of choice in certain patients with partial epilepsy. Further trials need to be done in patients with primary generalized seizures, such as those with epilepsy syndromes (e.g. West syndrome, Lennox-Gastaut syndrome), who are often among the most difficult patients to treat (Sander 2003).

14.4 Target: Hippocampus

Whereas the idea behind ANT stimulation is to disrupt seizure propagation through a limbic network, hippocampal stimulation is aimed at disrupting the epileptogenic focus itself. Mesial temporal lobe epilepsy is the most common of the medically refractory chronic epilepsies. When there is a single, identifiable electrographic focus, these patients do well with removal of that focus (i.e. temporal lobectomy), 66 % of whom achieve long-term seizure freedom (Tellez-Zenteno et al. 2007). However, many of these patients have bilateral seizure foci, or develop contralateral foci after resection and thereby remain refractory. Furthermore, memory decline after resection can be substantial, particularly in those who undergo dominant temporal lobe resection, or who continue seizing postoperatively

(Helmstaedter et al. 2003). Thus, there is a subpopulation of patients with refractory mesial temporal epilepsy for whom resective surgery is not an option, who may respond to epileptogenic disruption via hippocampal DBS.

Velasco et al. (2000) did much of the original groundwork by taking advantage of ten patients undergoing hippocampal depth electrode placement for temporal lobectomy candidacy evaluation. After identifying the area of ictal onset within the hippocampus, recording electrodes were removed and chronic stimulating electrodes implanted along the hippocampal axis. They stimulated over 2–3 weeks and demonstrated a reduction in clinical seizures, reduction in interictal spiking, and temporal lobe metabolic normalization. They then examined the resected tissue after temporal lobectomy to confirm that there was no observable tissue damage from stimulation. This study was important because it demonstrated the feasibility of hippocampal stimulation for temporal epilepsy and confirmed that the ability to reduce interictal spiking on EEG correlated with seizure reduction. Indeed, another group of investigators has used the reduction of interictal spiking by at least 50 % as a necessary condition for chronic stimulation with good results (Vonck et al. 2002; Boon et al. 2007). Table 14.2 provides a summary of clinical studies of hippocampal DBS for epilepsy.

Velasco et al. (2007) again published a series of nine patients, all with significant seizure reduction after 18 months to 7 years of follow-up. Two further interesting results came of this. First, in a 1-month blinded period after implantation during which some patients remained with their stimulators off, no beneficial "lesion effect" was seen, a result confirmed by other blinded studies (Tellez-Zenteno et al. 2006; McLachlan et al. 2010) and in contrast to ANT DBS studies. This probably reflects the size and complexity of the hippocampus and suggests that in lieu of complete amygdalohippocampectomy, active disruption of local, epileptogenic circuitry may be important in reducing some temporal-origin seizures. Second, Velasco et al. (2007) found that patients with structural mesial temporal sclerosis on MRI had delayed and more modest seizure control when compared to those with a normal MRI. This is the inverse of resective surgery patients, who achieve better seizure control if they have an abnormal MRI (Tellez-Zenteno et al. 2010). Indeed, Vonck et al. (2002) and Boon et al. (2007) in their series required normal MRIs to be a candidate for chronic hippocampal DBS.

Since a primary indication for hippocampal DBS in epilepsy is the potential for substantial memory impairment following resection (Helmstaedter et al. 2003), the question of whether DBS leads to memory deficits is critical. Tellez-Zenteno et al. (2006) selected temporal lobe epilepsy patients who could not have temporal lobectomies due to risk of memory impairment and found that chronic unilateral hippocampal DBS induced no further memory impairments over baseline, although in a later study bilateral hippocampal DBS may have induced a detrimental effect on memory in two patients (McLachlan et al. 2010).

Nearly all studies of hippocampal DBS have been small, primarily open-label case series and therefore have no true controls. Tellez-Zenteno et al. (2006) attempted to address this in their study using a blinded crossover design, although only in four patients. They found a non-significant 15 % reduction in seizure frequency with stimulation, much less than the open-label studies (Table 14.2). Although these data are promising, details such as exact electrode orientation within the amygdalohippocampal complex, stimulation parameters and thresholding, long-term effects on memory and cognition and patient selection criteria can only be determined in larger prospective, randomized trials.

14.5 Side Effects and Complications

DBS has an excellent safety record in general (Rezai et al. 2008) and for epilepsy specifically (Fisher et al. 2010). Hemorrhage and infection are the two most significant potential surgical complications. In a comprehensive review of DBS for movement disorders, Rezai et al. report a hemorrhage rate of 0.2–12.5 % and an infection rate of 1–15 %. In the SANTE trial hemorrhage was reported at 4.5 %, but all were incidentally found and none were symptomatic, or clinically

Table 14.2 Clinical trial for hippocampus stimulation to treat epilepsy

Study	Type	No. of patients	Seizure type	Follow up	Stimulation parameters	Results[a]
McLachlan et al. (2010)	Blinded, cross-over design	2	Bilateral temporal onset	3 months each: stim, washout (no stim), no stim	Bilateral, 185 Hz, 90 μs, variable intensity[b], continuous	33 % reduction (stim vs. no stim)
Velasco et al. (2007)	Case series with initial blinded control period	9	Unilateral or bilateral temporal onset	1 month (stim vs. no stim), 18 months unblinded	Uni-, or bilateral, 130 Hz, 450 μs, 300 μA, 1 min on, 4 min off	All patients with significant reduction
Tellez-Zenteno et al. (2006)	Blinded, cross-over design	4	Unilateral or bilateral temporal onset	3 months stim, 3 months no stim	Unilateral, 190 Hz, 90 μs, variable intensity[b], continuous	15 % reduction (stim vs. no stim)
Boon et al. (2007) Vonck et al. (2002)	Case series	12	Unilateral[c] temporal onset	5.5–21 months	Unilateral[c], 130 Hz[d], 450 μs, variable intensity[b], continuous	30–100 % reduction in 11/12 patients
Velasco et al. (2001)	Case series	10	Unilateral or bilateral temporal onset	16 days	Unilateral, 130 Hz, 450 μs, variable intensity[b], continuous	Seizure free in all patients by day 7

[a]Results are given as an aggregate percentage reduction in seizure frequency compared to baseline if provided, unless otherwise noted

[b]Intensity of stimulation was titrated to the maximum without patient awareness

[c]One patient was noted to have bilateral temporal onset of seizures and underwent bilateral hippocampal stimulation, with 30–49 % reduction in seizure frequency during follow-up

[d]One patient was increased to 200 Hz

significant. The infection rate was 12.5 % in the SANTE trial and all were superficial with the exception of one meningeal reaction. There is also a certain rate of hardware failure and hardware erosion, usually requiring revision surgery, between 2.7 and 50 % of patients (Fisher et al. 2010; Rezai et al. 2008). No such complications were reported in the SANTE trial, although several of the case series do report such incidents (Hodaie et al. 2002; Lim et al. 2007; Velasco et al. 2007).

Regarding side effects of the stimulation itself, the SANTE trial reports one case of stimulation-induced seizures (Fisher et al. 2010) and Tellez-Zenteno observed worsening of temporal lobe seizures compared to baseline during periods when stimulation was off, suggestive of a detrimental lesioning effect, in contrast to ANT studies (Tellez-Zenteno et al. 2006). The SANTE trial found a 14.8 % rate of worsening depression and a 13 % rate of worsening memory impairment in the stimulation group, significantly greater than the controls (Fisher et al. 2010). Such psychological and cognitive effects of mesial temporal lobe stimulation have yet to be quantified in sufficient patients.

14.6 Implantation Procedure at the University of Pennsylvania

The procedure for electrode implantation begins with placement of the stereotactic frame under general or local anesthesia. The frame should be tilted so that its lateral crossbar is parallel to a line drawn from the lateral canthus of the eye to the external auditory meatus, approximating the anterior commissure (AC)–posterior commissure

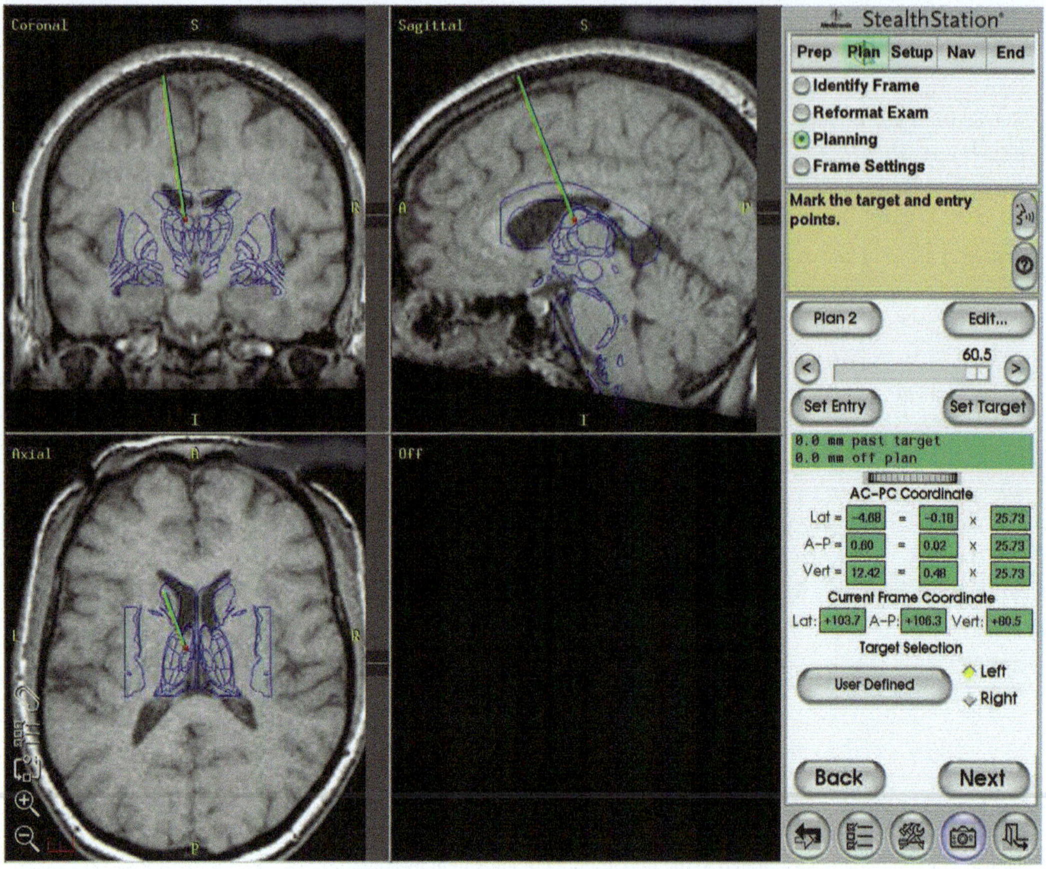

Fig. 14.2 Diagram showing the planned trajectory through the cortex to the anterior thalamic nucleus using the Medtronic surgical navigation system (Medtronic, Minneapolis, MN) with a superimposed stereotactic atlas (From Lega et al. (2010), with permission)

(PC) line. MRI fast spin echo inversion recovery and standard T2 high resolution, 1 mm slice images are obtained for targeting. Indirect localization of the desired target is obtained by identifying coordinates on a standard stereotactic atlas and referencing them to the AC–PC on an axial image. Frame position relative to the AC–PC line is also calculated. Direct radiographic visualization of the target is also possible for most potential DBS targets, including the ANT and the hippocampus. We use a surgical navigation system (Medtronic Stealth Navigator, Medtronic, Minneapolis, MN; Stryke Leibinger, Kalamazoo, MI) to plan a trajectory through the cortex that avoids sulcal vasculature (Fig. 14.2).

The patient is fixed in a Mayfield head frame supine or in a semi-sitting position. Head position is altered to optimize access to the chosen entry point and can be manipulated depending on the stereotactic target. We avoid shaving hair prior to sterile preparation. The scalp above the chosen entry point is infiltrated with local anesthetic. A burr hole is placed with assiduous attention to the angle used with the high speed drill. The dura and pia are sharply incised and cauterized with care taken to avoid surface vessels. A guide cannula is inserted and advanced into the brain to a point 10 mm from the desired target with fluoroscopic confirmation of cannula position. A monopolar single-unit recording electrode (Advanced Research Systems, Atlanta, GA or FHC, Bowdoinham, ME) can be introduced to confirm entry into thalamic or other tissue. For targeting the ANT, the lateral ventricle is invariably traversed and no unit recordings are made here. Recordings are first heard in the superficial surface of the ANT. A GS3000 (Axon Instruments, Sunnyvale, CA) or Leadpoint (Medtronic) amplifier is used to amplify signal generated by extracellular action potentials. Recordings are made using standard techniques together with a descriptive voice channel. Target neurons are identified based on the firing characteristics of the ANT, of surrounding tissue and the described firing rate of human recordings. The process is identical for other targets, with identifying electrographic features of the tissue being targeted used to confirm electrode location. For the ANT, the electrode is advanced further until recordings cease as it enters the intralaminar region, rich in white matter with a paucity of nuclei to generate signal. Recordings with a different pattern resume as the electrode enters the dorsomedial nucleus of the thalamus.

For ANT specifically, an additional step is used to confirm lead placement using characteristic EEG activity following low frequency stimulation. A stimulation lead (Radionics stimulation/lesioning probe, Integra Radionics, Burlington, MA) is inserted at the tentative stimulating location. Stimulation parameters include a frequency of five to ten cycles per second with a pulse width of 90–330 μs, a pulse amplitude of 4–5 V, and total pulse duration between 3 and 10 s. Stimulation at these frequencies in the ANT is associated with recruiting rhythms on cortical EEG (Kerrigan et al. 2004). This is called a driving response, the meaning of which is unclear. It may reflect spatiotemporal summation of individual pulses due to non-specific activation of multiple thalamocortical pathways, but is unlikely to be unique to the ANT, as it can be elicited from stimulation at other thalamic nuclei (Hodaie et al. 2002).

Following confirmation of EEG activity and removal of this lead, the final DBS stimulation lead is inserted. We use a Medtronic 3387 electrode with four platinum–iridium stimulation contacts 1.5 mm wide, with 1.5 mm edge-to-edge separation between the contacts. This configuration, with wider spacing between leads, is different than the electrode used in other, smaller DBS targets. Fluoroscopy is again used to confirm electrode placement, it is secured with a burr hole cap, and the skin incision is closed. The same sequence of steps is used for placing the contralateral electrode. With both incisions closed, the head is washed and the stereotactic frame is removed.

At our institution, the internal pulse generator (IPG) is placed on the same day as the DBS electrodes, although other neurosurgeons elect to do this at a later date. The patient is placed under general anesthesia, the scalp incision sites are re-sterilized along with the neck and upper chest. The scalp incisions are opened and the electrode wires are identified and connected to an extension wire (Medtronic 7495 lead extension). These are tunneled subcutaneously to an infraclavicular, subcutaneous pocket dissected for placement of the IPG (Medtronic model Itrel II, Soletra or Kinetra).

Postoperatively, lead placement is confirmed with MRI or CT after recovery from anesthesia. Patients are usually discharged on postoperative day 1 after a night spent in the neurosurgical intensive care unit. The procedure is generally well-tolerated, although poorly controlled epileptics require attentive postoperative monitoring following anesthesia. Several outpatient visits are necessary to optimize stimulation parameters, especially for a large, internally complex target for stimulation such as the ANT. Initial parameters are set with a frequency of 90–130 Hz, pulse width at 60–90 μs, and pulse amplitude at 4–5 V. These settings can be altered, as can which specific contacts are active to maximize clinical affect and minimize side effects. This process requires more attention in DBS for epilepsy as compared to Parkinson's or tremor because the clinical benefits do not immediately manifest with parameter alterations.

Conclusions

The limbic network is one link between the cortical and subcortical worlds and may be key to seizure propagation. The most promising DBS treatments for epilepsy may function via disruption along this pathway. With the results of the SANTE trial, deep brain stimulation has been established as a safe and effective therapy for a restricted subset of patients with medically refractory epilepsy. Future studies are needed to determine other patient populations for whom ANT DBS may be an effective option, particularly those patients with more fundamentally generalized seizures. Meanwhile, encouraging evidence is accruing for the treatment of refractory mesial temporal lobe epilepsy with hippocampal DBS, which may ultimately serve as an effective alternative for patients who cannot undergo temporal lobectomy. However, efficacy, safety, stimulating parameters, and patient selection still need to be established in large, randomized trials.

References

Andrade DM, Zumsteg D, Hamani C, Hodaie M, Sarkissian S, Lozano AM, Wennberg RA (2006) Long-term follow-up of patients with thalamic deep brain stimulation for epilepsy. Neurology 66(10): 1571–1573

Avanzini G, Panzica F, de Curtis M (2000) The role of the thalamus in vigilance and epileptogenic mechanisms. Clin Neurophysiol 111(Suppl 2):S19–S26

Benedek K, Juhász C, Muzik O, Chugani DC, Chugani HT (2004) Metabolic changes of subcortical structures in intractable focal epilepsy. Epilepsia 45(9):1100–1105

Benedek K, Juhász C, Chugani DC, Muzik O, Chugani HT (2006) Longitudinal changes in cortical glucose hypometabolism in children with intractable epilepsy. J Child Neurol 21(1):26–31

Boon P, Vonck K, De Herdt V, Van Dycke A, Goethals M, Goossens L, Van Zandijcke M, De Smedt T, Dewaele I, Achten R, Wadman W, Dewaele F, Caemaert J, Van Roost D (2007) Deep brain stimulation in patients with refractory temporal lobe epilepsy. Epilepsia 48(8):1551–1560

Cooper IS, Upton AR, Amin I (1980) Reversibility of chronic neurologic deficits. Some effects of electrical stimulation of the thalamus and internal capsule in man. Appl Neurophysiol 43(3–5):244–258

Cooper IS, Upton AR, Amin I, Garnett S, Brown GM, Springman M (1984) Evoked metabolic responses in the limbic-striate system produced by stimulation of anterior thalamic nucleus in man. Int J Neurol 18:179–187

Epilepsy Fact Sheet (2012) World Health Organization. http://www.who.int/mediacentre/factsheets/fs999/en/. Accessed 30 Sept 2013

Epilepsy Therapy Project (2013) Epilepsy Foundation. http://www.epilepsy.com/epilepsy/main_epilepsy. Accessed 30 Sept 2013

Fisher R, Salanova V, Witt T, Worth R, Henry T, Gross R, Oommen K, Osorio I, Nazzaro J, Labar D, Kaplitt M, Sperling M, Sandok E, Neal J, Handforth A, Stern J, DeSalles A, Chung S, Shetter A, Bergen D, Bakay R, Henderson J, French J, Baltuch G, Rosenfeld W, Youkilis A, Marks W, Garcia P, Barbaro N, Fountain N, Bazil C, Goodman R, McKhann G, Babu Krishnamurthy K, Papavassiliou S, Epstein C, Pollard J, Tonder L, Grebin J, Coffey R, Graves N, Group tSS (2010) Electrical stimulation of the anterior nucleus of thalamus for treatment of refractory epilepsy. Epilepsia 51(5):899–908

Gale K (1992) Subcortical structures and pathways involved in convulsive seizure generation. J Clin Neurophysiol 9(2):264–277

Helmstaedter C, Kurthen M, Lux S, Reuber M, Elger CE (2003) Chronic epilepsy and cognition: a longitudinal study in temporal lobe epilepsy. Ann Neurol 54(4):425–432. doi:10.1002/ana.10692

Hodaie M, Wennberg RA, Dostrovsky JO, Lozano AM (2002) Chronic anterior thalamus stimulation for intractable epilepsy. Epilepsia 43(6):603–608

Kerrigan JF, Litt B, Fisher RS, Cranstoun S, French JA, Blum DE, Dichter M, Shetter A, Baltuch GH, Jaggi JL, Krone S, Brodie M, Rise M, Graves N (2004) Electrical stimulation of the anterior nucleus of the thalamus for the treatment of intractable epilepsy. Epilepsia 45(4):346–354

Lee KJ, Jang KS, Shon YM (2006) Chronic deep brain stimulation of subthalamic and anterior thalamic nuclei for controlling refractory partial epilepsy. Acta Neurochir Suppl 99:87–91

Lega BC, Halpern CH, Jaggi JL, Baltuch GH (2010) Deep brain stimulation in the treatment of refractory epilepsy: update on current data and future directions. Neurobiol Dis 38:354–360

Lim S-N, Lee S-T, Tsai Y-T, Chen I-A, Tu P-H, Chen J-L, Chang H-W, Su Y-C, Wu T (2007) Electrical stimulation of the anterior nucleus of the thalamus for intractable epilepsy: a long-term follow-up study. Epilepsia 48(2):342–347

Lozano AM, Lipsman N (2013) Probing and regulating dysfunctional circuits using deep brain stimulation. Neuron 77(3):406–424. doi:10.1016/j.neuron.2013.01.020

Luat AF, Chugani HT (2008) Molecular and diffusion tensor imaging of epileptic networks. Epilepsia 49(Suppl 3):15–22

McIntyre CC, Hahn PJ (2010) Network perspectives on the mechanisms of deep brain stimulation. Neurobiol Dis 38(3):329–337

McLachlan RS, Pigott S, Tellez-Zenteno JF, Wiebe S, Parrent A (2010) Bilateral hippocampal stimulation for intractable temporal lobe epilepsy: impact on seizures and memory. Epilepsia 51(2):304–307. doi:10.1111/j.1528-1167.2009.02332.x

Mirski MA, Rossell LA, Terry JB, Fisher RS (1997) Anticonvulsant effect of anterior thalamic high frequency electrical stimulation in the rat. Epilepsy Res 28(2):89–100

Mullan S, Vailati G, Karasick J, Mailis M (1967) Thalamic lesions for the control of epilepsy. A study of nine cases. Arch Neurol 16:277–285

Nashef L, Ryvlin P (2009) Sudden unexpected death in epilepsy (SUDEP): update and reflections. Neurol Clin 27(4):1063–1074. doi:10.1016/j.ncl.2009.08.003

Norden AD, Blumenfeld H (2002) The role of subcortical structures in human epilepsy. Epilepsy Behav 3(3): 219–231

Osorio I, Overman J, Giftakis J, Wilkinson SB (2007) High frequency thalamic stimulation for inoperable mesial temporal epilepsy. Epilepsia 48(8):1561–1571

Papez JW (1937) A proposed mechanism of emotion. Arch Neurol Psychiatry 38(4):725–743

Rezai AR, Machado AG, Deogaonkar M, Azmi H, Kubu C, Boulis NM (2008) Surgery for movement disorders. Neurosurgery 62(Suppl 2):809–838. doi:10.1227/01.neu.0000316285.52865.53; discussion 838–809

Sander JW (2003) The natural history of epilepsy in the era of new antiepileptic drugs and surgical treatment. Epilepsia 44(Suppl 1):17–20

Shorvon SD, Goodridge DM (2013) Longitudinal cohort studies of the prognosis of epilepsy: contribution of the National General Practice Study of Epilepsy and other studies. Brain 136(Pt 11):3497–3510. doi:10.1093/brain/awt223

Tellez-Zenteno JF, Dhar R, Wiebe S (2005) Long-term seizure outcomes following epilepsy surgery: a systematic review and meta-analysis. Brain 128(Pt 5):1188–1198. doi:10.1093/brain/awh449

Tellez-Zenteno JF, McLachlan RS, Parrent A, Kubu CS, Wiebe S (2006) Hippocampal electrical stimulation in mesial temporal lobe epilepsy. Neurology 66(10):1490–1494. doi:10.1212/01.wnl.0000209300.49308.8f

Tellez-Zenteno JF, Dhar R, Hernandez-Ronquillo L, Wiebe S (2007) Long-term outcomes in epilepsy surgery: antiepileptic drugs, mortality, cognitive and psychosocial aspects. Brain 130(Pt 2):334–345. doi:10.1093/brain/awl316

Tellez-Zenteno JF, Hernandez Ronquillo L, Moien-Afshari F, Wiebe S (2010) Surgical outcomes in lesional and non-lesional epilepsy: a systematic review and meta-analysis. Epilepsy Res 89(2–3):310–318. doi:10.1016/j.eplepsyres.2010.02.007

Umemura A, Jaggi JL, Hurtig HI, Siderowf AD, Colcher A, Stern MB, Baltuch GH (2003) Deep brain stimulation for movement disorders: morbidity and mortality in 109 patients. J Neurosurg 98(4):779–784. doi:10.3171/jns.2003.98.4.0779

Velasco AL, Velasco M, Velasco F, Menes D, Gordon F, Rocha L, Briones M, Marquez I (2000) Subacute and chronic electrical stimulation of the hippocampus on intractable temporal lobe seizures: preliminary report. Arch Med Res 31(3):316–328

Velasco F, Velasco M, Velasco AL, Menez D, Rocha L (2001) Electrical stimulation for epilepsy: stimulation of hippocampal foci. Stereotact Funct Neurosurg 77(1–4):223–227, 64610

Velasco AL, Velasco F, Velasco M, Trejo D, Castro G, Carrillo-Ruiz JD (2007) Electrical stimulation of the hippocampal epileptic foci for seizure control: a double-blind, long-term follow-up study. Epilepsia 48(10):1895–1903. doi:10.1111/j.1528-1167.2007.01181.x

Vonck K, Boon P, Achten E, De Reuck J, Caemaert J (2002) Long-term amygdalohippocampal stimulation for refractory temporal lobe epilepsy. Ann Neurol 52(5):556–565. doi:10.1002/ana.10323

15 Complications of Deep Brain Stimulation

Kenji Sugiyama

15.1 Introduction

Two recent double-blinded multicenter studies have compared the effects of deep brain stimulation (DBS) and the best medication therapy. Deuschl et al. have conducted a multicenter study (ten centers) involving 156 patients with advanced Parkinson's disease and have shown statistically significant superior improvements in the DBS group, both on the United Parkinson's Disease Rating Scale (UPDRS) motor scores (55 % improvement in the DBS group vs. 21 % in the medication group) and Activities of Daily Living (ADL) scores (58 % in the DBS group vs. 28 % in the medication group) (Deuschl et al. 2006). Weaver et al. (2009) have reported that in their Veterans Affairs Cooperative Studies Program (VACSP), which is a multicenter double-blinded study involving 255 patients with advanced Parkinson's disease, the patients in the DBS group showed superior improvements compared to those in the best medication group on UPDRS motor scores (71 % improvement in the DBS group vs. 32 % in the medication group) and ADL scores (+14 points in the DBS group vs. −1.5 points in the medication group) (Weaver et al. 2009). In both studies, DBS has shown better effects than the best medication, but these studies have also shown higher incidence rate of complications in the DBS group (Deuschl et al.: 13 % in the DBS group vs. 4 % in the medication group, Weaver et al.: 40 % in the DBS group vs. 15 % in the medication group). These findings have suggested that methods that result in the avoidance of these complications need to be determined.

15.2 Types of Complications

Complications that are related to DBS have been divided into the following three different categories: (1) those related to the surgical procedure, (2) those related to problems with the DBS machinery or the wiring, and (3) those related to the DBS-stimulated neuronal structures or networks.

Category (1) includes intracranial hemorrhages, infections, epilepsy, and air embolisms. Category (2) includes machinery breakdown, electrode breakage, skin erosion over the implantable pulse generator (IPG) or electric wires, and related infections. This category also includes complications related to electromagnetic fields surrounding patients. Category (3) includes psychiatric or cognitive malfunctions and the increased risks for suicide after DBS.

K. Sugiyama, MD, PhD
Department of Neurosurgery,
Hamamatsu University School of Medicine,
Hamamatsu, Shizuoka, Japan
e-mail: kesugi@hama-med.ac.jp

T. Itakura (ed.), *Deep Brain Stimulation for Neurological Disorders: Theoretical Background and Clinical Application*, DOI 10.1007/978-3-319-08476-3_15,

15.3 Intracranial Hemorrhage

15.3.1 Incidence Rate

Among all of the complications, intracranial hemorrhage is the one that should be given meticulous attention to try to avoid, because it directly affects to the patient's morbidity and mortality after DBS surgery. The incidence rates reported by studies with a large number of patients, and published after 2006, range from 0 to 5 % for any hemorrhage and from 0 to 2 % for symptomatic hemorrhages. Follet et al. have reported intracranial hemorrhage in three cases (1 %) and in one death, among 299 DBS patients in their VACSP study (Follett et al. 2010). Deuschl et al. (2006) have also reported intracranial hemorrhage in three cases (3.8 %) and in one death, among 78 DBS patients. A meta-analysis study of subthalamic nucleus (STN)-DBS by Kleiner-Fisman et al. (2006) have shown 3.9 % hemorrhagic rate among 921 cases in 34 studies. Pahwa et al. (2006) have also reported 2.9 % hemorrhagic rate in an American Academy of Neurology (AAN) review of 360 DBS cases, which included 288 patients with Parkinson's disease (Table 15.1).

Table 15.1 Incidence rate for complications related to surgical procedure

	Complications related to surgical procedure		
	Intracranial hemorrhage	Epilepsy	Air embolism
Follett KA $n=299$	2	–	–
Deuschl G $n=78$	3.8	–	–
Kleiner-Fisman G $n=921$	3.9	1.5	–
PahwaR $n=360$	2.9	2.9	–

Each number indicates the reported incidence rate (%) for each complication. Blanks indicate that there was no description in each report

15.3.2 Risk Factors for Intracranial Hemorrhage

The risk factors for intracranial hemorrhage have been reported to include a previous history of hypertension and older age (Sansur et al 2007; Elias et al. 2009; Ben-Haim et al. 2009). Xiaowu et al. (2011) have indicated that the incidence rate of intracranial hemorrhages increased 2.5 times in patients with hypertension than in other patients.

With respect to surgical methods, patients undergoing stereotactic coagulation had 5.4 times higher incidence rate of hemorrhage than those undergoing DBS (Xiaowu et al. 2011; Terao et al. 2003; Blomstedt and Hariz 2006). When the electrodes penetrate the ventricular wall or pass through a gyrus, the rate of hemorrhagic complications increases (Elias et al. 2009; Ben-Haim et al. 2009; Zrinzo et al. 2011). The usage of microelectrode recording techniques has been shown to increase the hemorrhagic rate (Zrinzo et al. 2011). Limiting the electrode penetration frequency has been shown to decrease the rate (Gorgulho et al. 2005). There have been two different reports on hemorrhagic risks with the use of the simultaneous multi-microelectrode technique (so called Ben-Gun method): one has shown an increase (Park et al. 2011), while the other has reported the same risk of hemorrhage as the single microelectrode technique (Temel et al. 2007).

15.3.3 How to Avoid Hemorrhages

While deciding between treatment with coagulation or DBS, the patient's risk factors for hemorrhage should be considered. DBS surgery is more beneficial for the patients with risk factors, such as elderly patients or patients with a previous history of hypertension.

The use of gadolinium-enhanced magnetic resonance imaging (MRI) is recommended for surgical navigation and for determining the electrode trajectory from the surface of the cortex to the target sites to prevent injuring any enhanced vessels. Electrode trajectory penetrating ventricular wall

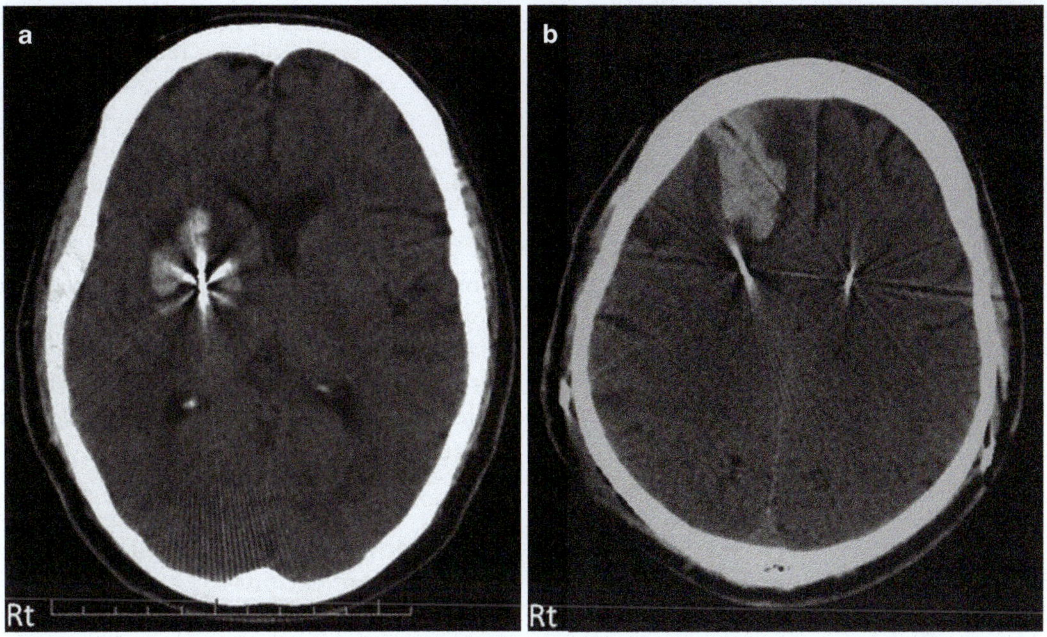

Fig. 15.1 Two different types of intracranial hemorrhagic complications. (**a**) Deep-seated hemorrhage that occurred in the basal ganglia around the electrode track and that was thought to be due to damage to the vessels by the electrodes, especially the microelectrodes. (**b**) Shallow subcortical hemorrhage, which sometimes occurred in the outer area of the electrode track. This type of hemorrhage was thought to be due to venous congestion caused by coagulation of the surface veins of the cerebral cortex

should be avoided. It is also recommended that attention is given to maintaining the patient's blood pressure in the normal range during the operation. The frequency of the use of microelectrode technique in DBS surgery should be minimized.

We experienced six cases of nonsymptomatic intracranial hemorrhages among 308 patients undergoing stereotactic procedures. The sites of the hemorrhages in our cases were divided into two types. One involved deep-seated hemorrhages that occurred in the basal ganglia around the electrode track, and the other involved shallow subcortical hemorrhages, which sometimes occurred around the outer area of the electrode track (Fig. 15.1). The former type of hemorrhage seemed to be caused by damage to the vessels by the electrodes, especially microelectrodes (Fig. 15.1a). The latter type of hemorrhage seemed to be due to venous congestion caused by coagulation of the surface vein of cerebral cortex (Fig. 15.1b). After we recognized that one case of subcortical hemorrhage was caused by the thoughtless coagulation of seemingly minor thin veins, we stopped performing coagulations of any cortical veins in the stereotactic operative procedure.

We ordinarily use semi microelectrodes for unit recording as their tips are not as sharply pointed as the tips of microelectrodes. For these procedures, we first use a dull-point catheter to make an electrode root to 10 mm above the target, which is considered the essential area for unit recording. We think that this procedure also reduces the hemorrhagic risk.

15.4 Mechanical Complications

15.4.1 Incidence Rate of Mechanical Complications

The incidence rates that are reported in studies with a large number of and published after 2006

Table 15.2 Incidence rate for complications related to DBS machinery trouble or related to wiring

	Complications related to DBS machinery trouble or related to wiring		
	Infection	Erosion or ulcer of the skin	Malfunction of DBS systems
Follett KA $n=299$	7.7	–	2
Deuschl G $n=78$	2.6	3.8	1.3
Kleiner-Fisman G $n=921$	–	–	–
PahwaR $n=360$	2.9	1	4.9

Each number indicates the reported incidence rate (%) for each complication. Blanks indicate that there was no description in each report

and are related to DBS systems range from 4 to 9.7 %, and these incidences include the mechanical failure of the IPG, pull out or migration of the intracranial electrode, and breakage of the electrodes or extension cords (Seijo et al. 2007; Tabbal et al. 2007; Voges et al. 2007. Boviatsis et al. 2011; Dashti et al. 2008; Fernandez et al. 2011; Hu et al. 2011).

Deuschl et al. (2006) have reported one case (1.3 %) of abnormal DBS stoppage among 78 DBS patients. Follet et al. (2010) have reported an incidence rate of 2 % for malfunctions among 299 DBS patients in their VACSP study, but the reasons for these malfunctions were not reported. Kleiner-Fisman et al. (2006) have reported that 4.4 % of patients underwent reoperations because of malfunctions of the DBS system, infections, or migration of the intracranial electrodes among 921 patients in their meta-analysis study of STN-DBS. Pahwa et al. (2006) have also reported a rate of 2.9 % for electrode migration cases and a rate of 2.0 % for the inappropriate positioning of the electrodes in an AAN review (Table 15.2). That review has also reported that 5 % of 360 cases (18 cases) underwent replacement surgery for the intracranial electrode due to breakage, migration, or inadequate positioning of electrodes, 4.4 % of cases (16 cases) underwent replacement surgery of extension cord, 4.2 % of cases (15 cases) underwent replacement surgery of IPG due to malfunction of IPG, and 0.6 % of cases (2 cases) developed allergic reactions to DBS systems.

15.4.2 Risk Factors of Mechanical Complications

Fernandez et al. (2011) have indicated that the most frequent place for breakage of the electrode or extension cord is the connection area of the intracranial electrode and the extension cord, and there is a tendency for breakage when this part is subjected to a twisting force.

15.4.3 How to Avoid Mechanical Complications

In order to avoid mechanical complications, the wiring, the angles and positions of the intracranial electrodes, the extension cords, and especially the connection of these two cords have to be taken into account. Wiring with sharp angle should be avoided particularly for intracranial electrodes around burr holes or for extension cords around the IPG implantation site. In ordinary patients with involuntary movement, such as Parkinson's disease, sub-pectoral muscle implantation of the IPG as well as subcutaneous implantation is a preferable method from a cosmetic point of view, and it has an advantage in the prevention of skin erosion or infection of the skin above the IPG. However, sub-pectoral muscle implantation is not preferable for the patients who have a well-developed pectoral major muscle, such as male patients with generalized dystonia. In these patients, strong involuntary contractions of the pectoral muscle can cause stress to the extension wire and subsequently lead to breakage of the wires at the entrance under the pectoral muscle.

15.4.4 Effects of Electromagnetic Fields on DBS Systems

It is required that patients be informed to pay attention to electromagnetic fields in their surroundings or to machines that generate electromagnetic waves in their daily life. According to the Medtronic, Inc. manual of DBS system, it is recommended that cellular phones or radios be kept at least 10 cm away from IPGs. In addition, it is possible that IPGs can be shut off by passing through security gates at the airport or stores and, thus, it is recommended that patients pass through the middle of the gate. It is also recommended that doctors turn down the stimulation voltage of Soletra IPGs to 0 volt and then switch off the Soletra IPGs when they use monopolar electrodes or when computed tomographic scans are performed (Medtronic 2010a).

15.4.5 MRI Measurements After DBS System Implantation

After two MRI-related accident reports, in which one patient developed permanent (Henderson et al. 2005) and the other developed transient neurological deficits (Spiegel et al. 2003), there has been debate about the MRI sequences permissible after DBS implantation. A product company has proposed guidelines for performing MRI on patients with implanted DBS systems, and they have adopted a specific absorption rate (SAR) of less than 0.1 W/kg (Medtronic 2010b). However, several clinical and experimental reports have cast doubts on the adequacy of this SAR value. Baker et al. have reported in their phantom experiments that the linearity between the SAR and temperature increases with MRI measurements differed between MRI machines, and they concluded that the SAR value is an unreliable guideline of MRI safety (Baker et al. 2004). A subcommittee of the Society of Japanese Stereotactic and Functional Neurosurgery conducted a survey on the performance of MRI on patients with DBS implantation in 49 facilities in 2010 in Japan. This survey has revealed that a total of 2,136 MRI procedures that used SAR values above 0.1 W/kg have been performed on patients who had undergone DBS surgeries in these institutions, and no accidents have been reported. Similar to the Japanese survey, Larson et al. (2008) have reported the performance of 1,071 MRI scans on 405 cases with SAR values of 3 W/kg with no accidents. Nazzaro et al. (2010) have reported 1,092 MRI scans that used SAR values above 0.1 W/kg on 249 patients with DBS systems without any accidents. Tagliati et al. (2009) have surveyed 40 institutions comprising 3,304 patients with implanted DBS systems. In their report, all 3,304 patients had undergone at least one MRI, and only one IPG stoppage in one patient was reported. When considering the disadvantages of not conducting MRIs on elderly patients with diseases such as Parkinson's disease, we strongly hope that these SAR guidelines will be reconsidered and the MRI-tolerable IPG will be developed as soon as possible.

15.5 Infections, Skin Erosions

15.5.1 Incidence Rate of Infection and Skin Erosion

The incidence rate of skin erosion above the DBS system or infection of the DBS system has been reported to range from 2.9 to 7.7 % (Bhatia et al. 2008; Bhatia et al. 2011a; Sillay et al. 2008). Deuschl et al. (2006) have reported two cases (2.6 %) of infection and three cases (3.8 %) of skin erosion around the DBS system among 78 DBS patients. Follet et al. (2010) have reported a rate of 7.7 % of infection around implanted DBS systems among 299 DBS patients in their VACSP study. Pahwa et al. (2006) have reported a rate of infection of 2.9 % (ten cases) after DBS implantation in their AAN review (Table 15.2). Bhatia et al. (2011b) have conducted a meta-analysis of 35 studies published from 1997 to 2009 comprising 3,550 patients and reported an average infection rate of 4.7 %. The most commonly identified pathogen was *Staphylococcus aureus*, which was found in 62 % (8/13 infected patients among 139 DBS patients) of the cases reported by Gorgulho et al. (2009) and in more than 50 % of the cases reported in the meta-analysis by Bhatia et al (2011a).

15.5.2 Risk Factors for Infections Related to DBS Implantation

Bhatia et al. (2011a) have stated the following specific risk factors in their meta-analysis: (1)

frontal subcutaneous connector bulk, (2) straight frontal skin incision, (4) age under 58 years, and (5) age over 65 years. There are two reports on the externalization of electrodes, with one indicating that it is a risk factor of infection (Constantoyannis et al. 2005) and the other reporting that there is no relation to DBS infection (Bhatia et al. 2011a).

15.5.3 How to Avoid the Side Effects of Infections or Skin Erosions

A strategy that avoids infections and skin problems is a matter to consider during all of DBS surgeries, however, it requires much attention to avoid these problems for the patients with ages that fit into the risk factors (age under 58 and over 65), for the patients who have a thin scalp or who have an increased susceptibility to infection, such as patients with diabetes mellitus. Patient management and precautions on handling the DBS device should be made as they are for ventriculo-peritoneal shunt surgery, such as bathing the patients and washing their head and body thoroughly before the operation, not opening the package containing the DBS system until immediately before its use, and avoiding grasping the DBS system with the surgeons' hand instead of with a surgical instrument. Hockey-stick or crescent incisions, are recommended, instead of linear incisions, which cross over the burr hole, or intracranial electrodes. In addition, placing the stimulating electrodes, extension wires, and connectors under or around the skin incision should be avoided. For patients with very thin scalp, there are several ways worth considering for the placement of the connector. One is to drill out skull to make a space for connector placement, which is actually not easy to do because of the limited exposed area by skin incision for burr-hole surgery. We otherwise recommend that the connectors be placed at patient's neck area under his jaw where it will be surrounded by loose soft tissue without any underlying bone. It is also recommended that the electrodes and connecting wires be placed as deep as possible, especially under the scalp area.

15.6 Epilepsy and Air Embolisms

15.6.1 Incidence Rate of Epilepsy and Air Embolisms

Epilepsy has also been reported as a complication related to DBS therapy. Its incidence reported in the literature has widely varied from 0 to 13 %. Kleiner-Fisman et al. (2006) have reported that 1.5 % of the patients in their meta-analysis study of STB-DBS developed epilepsy. Pahwa et al. (2006) have also reported that 2.9 % of the patients in their AAN review developed epilepsy (Table 15.1). In their meta-analysis of DBS complications described in 32 reports from 1991 to 2008, Coley et al. (2009) have reported that 2.4 % of patients developed epilepsy among 1,445 patients in 14 out of 16 reports (two of the reports were omitted because of data duplication, and no descriptions of seizures as a complication). A total of 74 % of these seizures occurred around the time of electrode implantation, and many of these patients suffered intracranial hemorrhages. Coley et al. (2009) have also indicated that the risk of seizures associated with the chronic stimulation period is 0.5 %. Chang et al. (2011) have reported that air embolisms occurred in 1.3 % (6 out of 467 cases) of DBS surgeries, but there have been no reports of air embolism complications in the large number case studies (Table 15.1).

15.6.2 Risk Factors of Epilepsy and Air Embolisms

Pouratian et al. (2011) have chosen the following three possible risk factors of seizure complications in an univariate analysis: 1) abnormal postoperative imaging, such as hemorrhages, edema, or ischemia; 2) age over 60; and 3) transventricular electrode trajectories, but only abnormal postoperative imaging was identified as a significant factor in a multivariate analysis. Chang et al. (2011) have reported no statistically significant relationships of air embolisms during surgery with patients' ages, diagnoses, or DBS targets.

15.6.3 How to Avoid Epilepsy and Air Embolism Complications

As for the risk factors for seizure complications, these causes are merely related to subcortical damage during DBS procedure. It is recommended that procedures be followed that avoid hemorrhagic risks and that the penetrations by electrodes be limited to prevent brain injury and edema.

Air embolism complications are often due to the adoption of a sitting position during DBS surgery. The surgeons who use a sitting position or semi-sitting position for DBS surgery have to pay attention to prevent air embolisms, or they need to consider avoiding the sitting or semi-sitting positions in DBS surgeries.

15.7 Complications Related to the Stimulation of Neuronal Networks and Structures

15.7.1 Outline of the Complications

This complication is not only related to electrical stimulation of targeted neuronal structures or the neuronal circuits themselves but also to stimulation of the surrounding structures of targeted area by spreading current. Because the activation threshold of neuronal fibers is generally 40–50 times less than that of neuronal soma (Nowak and Bullier 1998), these complications are easy to provoke when stimulating electrodes placed near untargeted neural fiber pathways. Electrodes in the ventral intermediate (Vim) thalamic nucleus can cause paresthesia of patients' extremities when the current spreads to the ventral caudal (Vc) thalamic nucleus, which is posterior to the (Vim) nucleus, and these can cause rigidity or dysarthria by current sprea to the internal capsule. In addition, electrodes in the internal globus pallidus (GPi) can cause scintillation when current spreads to the optic tract underlying the GPi. However, recent concerns for these complications have arisen with respect to cognitive and psychiatric symptoms and the suicide risks accompanying STN-DBS surgery. Saint-Cyr et al. have proposed cognitive and psychiatric status should be included in the surgical indications for STN-DBS. This is because they observed that verbal fluency declined, 9 % developed some psychiatric symptoms, and only half of the patients were able to return to their original work after STN-DBS surgery (Saint-Cyr and Albanese 2006).

15.7.2 Cognitive Status

Although there have been reports of a decline in verbal fluency after STN-DBS, some reports have shown improvements on the Mini-Mental State Examination (Daniele et al. 2003). Weaver et al. (2012) have compared STN-DBS and GPi-DBS studies (the VACSP study) and have found that patients in both groups showed decreased verbal fluency and cognitive function, but the STN-DBS group showed greater cognitive decline as compared to the GPi-DBS group according to the Mattis Dementia Rating Scale conducted 3 years after the surgery. These declines were statistically significant, but the extent of the decline was not very large (2.6/144 points in the GPi group and 6.2/144 points in the STN group). There have been no comparison studies conducted between DBS and non-DBS groups about cognitive decline in double-blinded manner. Parsons et al. (2006) have reported in their meta-analysis of 28 studies of STN-DBS comprising 612 patients that no changes were observed on the Mini-Mental Status Examination or on attention after STN-DBS surgeries, and only a moderate decline in verbal fluency was observed. They concluded that STN-DBS is a rather safe procedure with respect to cognitive functions (Parsons et al. 2006).

15.7.3 Psychiatric Symptoms

There are several case reports on psychiatric symptoms, but no typical trends have been

Table 15.3 Incidence rate for complications related to DBS neuronal structures or networks, especially related to psychiatric, cognitive symptoms, and suicidal risks

	Complications related to DBS neuronal structures or networks				
	Depression (minor depression)	Mania	Suicide (suicide attempt)	Cognitive decline	Other psychiatric symptoms
Follett KA $n=299$	1.6 (31.4 %)	–	0.3 (1)	–	–
Deuschl G $n=78$	5.1	–	1.3	3.8	5.1
Kleiner-Fisman G $n=921$	6.8	1.9	–	–	3.5
PahwaR $n=360$	–	–	0.1 (0.74)	–	–

Each number indicates the reported incidence rate (%) for each complication. Blanks indicate that there was no description in each report

observed with respect to the development of some psychiatric symptoms such as mood changes, depression, and apathy after DBS, especially STN-DBS surgeries. From patient management point of view, the most important psychiatric symptom in patients with Parkinson's disease is the emergence of depression, which is closely related to suicide risks. Follet et al. (2010) have reported incidence rates of major depression and minor depression after DBS as 1.6 % and 31.4 %, respectively in the VAC study. Kleiner-Fisman et al. (2006) have reported a 6.8 % of depression, a 1.9 % of mania, and a 3.5 % of other psychiatric symptoms, while Deuschl et al. (2006) have reported a 5.1 % of depression, a 1.2 % of apathy, and a 5.1 % rate of other psychiatric symptoms (Table 15.3).

There are two different reports on depression or mood, with one reporting a decline (Berney et al. 2002) and the other reporting an improvement of mood (Daniele et al. 2003). Bejjani et al. (1999) have reported the acute development of depression after electrical stimulation of a lower electrode placed in the STN, possibly due to stimulation of the substantia nigra pars reticulata (SNr). However, there is also a report that showed the development of a manic state after stimulation of a lower electrode placed in the STN (Kulisevsky et al. 2002). In addition, symptoms that suggest dopamine dysregulation symptoms, such as excessive gambling or shopping, have been reported (Saint-Cyr and Albanese 2006). We have reported our experience with the acute development of hallucinations and delusions after STN-DBS surgery in 2002 (Sugiyama 2002). We assumed that these hallucinations and delusions occurred because the microlesioning of the outer part of the SNr in the STN-DBS surgery caused disinhibition of the ventral anterior thalamic nucleus, resulting in a mismatch between what is happening in reality and their memory (Fig. 15.2).

15.7.4 Suicide Risks

Suicide risks are closely related to major depression. Follet et al. (2010) have reported three cases (among 299 cases, 1 %) of depression who attempted suicide in the VAC study. Deuschl et al. (2006) have reported one case of suicide among the 78 patients who underwent DBS. Large incidence rate of suicide after STN-DBS has been reported by Burkhard et al. (2004) (6 out of 140 cases, 4.3 %), by Soulas et al. (2008) (two suicide (1.5 %) and 4 attempted suicide (3 %) out of 200 patients). Voon et al. (2008) have reported in their multicenter study comprising 5,311 patients that 24 of them committed suicide (0.45 %) and 48 attempted suicide (0.90 %) and 0.26 % suicide rate 1 year after STN-DBS surgery. In addition, they have

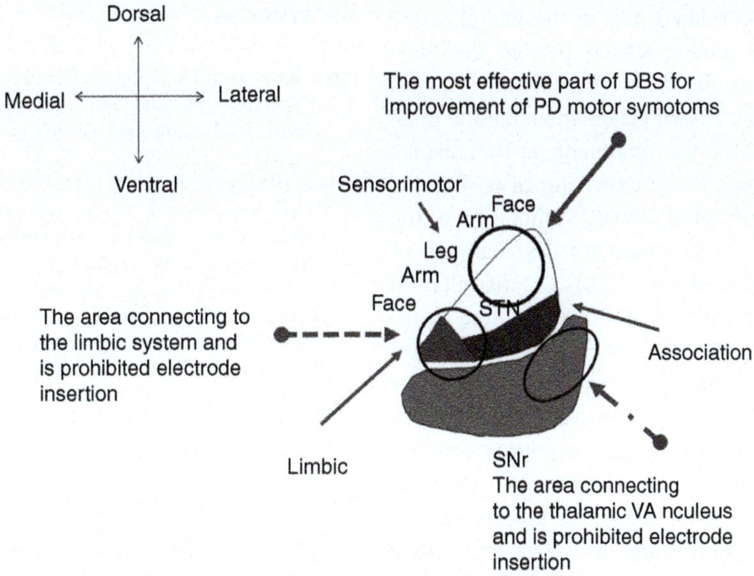

Fig. 15.2 Functional topography related to deep brain stimulation (*DBS*) surgery in and around the subthalamic nucleus (*STN*). The schema indicates a coronal section of the STN and substantia nigra pars reticulata (*SNr*). The STN was separated into three different functional topographic areas: the sensorimotor part of the dorsolateral STN, the association part of the ventro-lateral STN, and the limbic part of the most medial STN. The most effective part for the treatment of the motor symptoms of Parkinson's disease is at the most dorso-lateral part of the STN, and electrical stimulation of the limbic part (the most medial part of the STN) has been used for the treatment of patients with intractable obsessive–compulsive disorder by some groups. There are fiber connections from the lateral part of the SNr to the thalamic ventral anterior nucleus, the injury of which can cause disinhibition of the temporal lobe, and hallucinations and delusions. Electrical stimulation or injury by electrodes is prohibited in these two areas because they are thought to cause inhibition of the orbito-frontal lobe or excitation of the temporal lobe

described the three following risk factors for suicide: (1) relatively younger age, (2) early onset of Parkinson's disease, and (3) a preoperative suicide attempt. The World Health Organization has reported that the incidence rate of suicide in the world population is 16 per 100,000 persons, while it is 25 per 100,000 persons in Japan. Myslobodsky et al. (2001) have reported a suicide rate for patients with Parkinson's disease of 122 out of 144,364 patients (0.085 %). Therefore, if these numbers are simply compared, the suicide rate after STN-DBS has been reported by Voon et al. to be 5.3 times higher than that in the population of patients with Parkinson's disease, 17.7 times higher than that in the Japanese population, and 28 times higher than that in the world population. However, these data cannot be directly compared because of the selection biases of the patient populations. Patients who undergo STN-DBS are patients with advanced refractory Parkinson's disease. No studies published so far have compared suicide risks among patients with advanced refractory Parkinson's disease who have had DBS surgery and those who have not had DBS surgery.

15.7.5 How to Avoid Cognitive or Psychiatric Complications

Because the mechanisms underlying the development of psychiatric symptoms after DBS surgery are unclear, methods to avoid these complications also remain under investigation. However, the topography within the STN is well known to divide into the following three parts: the motor-related part in the lateral upper STN, the association-related part in the lateral lower STN, and the limbic-related part in the most medial part of the STN (Parent and Hazrati 1995). It has been well established that the most effective part for the treatment of Parkinson's motor symptoms is the upper dorsal part of the STN (Yokoyama et al. 2006). Stimulation of the medial STN has been used for the treatment of intractable obsessive–compulsive disorder in some groups (Mallet et al. 2008), and the therapeutic effect is thought to occur due to inhibition of the orbitofrontal lobe. It is unclear whether similar inhibition occurs on the normal orbitofrontal lobe without hyper-excitation, but the possibility cannot be denied. In addition, Middleton and Strick (1996) have proposed the idea that microlesioning the SNr can cause disinhibition of the magnocellular division of the ventral anterior thalamic nucleus and hyperexcitability of the temporal lobe, which results in hallucination and delusion symptoms that are the same as L-dopa-induced hallucination and delusion symptoms. This topography was summarized in Fig. 15.2. Based on this hypothesis, we now use the following guidelines for STN-DBS: (1) Determine the exact location of the motor area, which is the dorsolateral part of the STN, to avoid electrical stimulation to the medial limbic part of the STN; and (2) Avoid micro-lesioning of the SNr. For this purpose, we use a unit recording technique to search for the precise ventral border of the STN, and when the background noises reduce, we stop advancing the electrode to prevent the micro-lesioning of the SNr. For the same reason, we do not advance the chronic stimulating electrodes into the SNr. We think that the precise identification of the ventral border of the STN is not essential for the STN-DBS procedure because the dorsolateral part of the STN is the most important part for the improvement of the motor symptoms of Parkinson's disease.

Attention should be constantly paid to the suicide risks in patients who undergo DBS surgery. This requires multidisciplinary management by not only neurosurgeons or neurologists but also by psychiatrists and psychologists for the patients who underwent DBS surgery.

References

Baker KB, Tkach JA, Nyenhuis JA et al (2004) Evaluation of specific absorption rate as a dosimeter of MRI-related implant heating. J Magn Reson Imaging 20(2):315–320

Bejjani BP, Damier P, Arnulf I et al (1999) Transient acute depression induced by high-frequency deep-brain stimulation. N Engl J Med 340(19):1476–1480

Ben-Haim S, Asaad WF, Gale JT et al (2009) Risk factors for hemorrhage during microelectrode-guided deep brain stimulation and the introduction of an improved microelectrode design. Neurosurgery 64(4):754–762; discussion 762–753

Berney A, Vingerhoets F, Perrin A et al (2002) Effect on mood of subthalamic DBS for Parkinson's disease: a consecutive series of 24 patients. Neurology 59(9): 1427–1429

Bhatia S, Oh M, Whiting T et al (2008) Surgical complications of deep brain stimulation. A longitudinal single surgeon, single institution study. Stereotact Funct Neurosurg 86(6):367–372

Bhatia R, Dalton A, Richards M et al (2011a) The incidence of deep brain stimulator hardware infection: the effect of change in antibiotic prophylaxis regimen and review of the literature. Br J Neurosurg 25(5): 625–631

Bhatia S, Zhang K, Oh M, Whiting D et al (2011b) Infections and hardware salvage after deep brain stimulation surgery: a single-center study and review of the literature. Stereotact Funct Neurosurg 88(3):147–155

Blomstedt P, Hariz MI (2006) Are complications less common in deep brain stimulation than in ablative procedures for movement disorders? Stereotact Funct Neurosurg 84(2–3):72–81

Boviatsis EJ, Stavrinou LC, Themistocleous M et al (2011) Surgical and hardware complications of deep brain stimulation. A seven-year experience and review of the literature. Acta Neurochir (Wien) 152(12): 2053–2062

Burkhard PR, Vingerhoets FJ, Berney A et al (2004) Suicide after successful deep brain stimulation for movement disorders. Neurology 63(11):2170–2172

Chang EF, Cheng JS, Richardson RM et al (2011) Incidence and management of venous air embolisms during awake deep brain stimulation surgery in a large clinical series. Stereotact Funct Neurosurg 89(2): 76–82

Coley E, Farhadi R, Lewis S et al (2009) The incidence of seizures following Deep Brain Stimulating electrode implantation for movement disorders, pain and psychiatric conditions. Br J Neurosurg 23(2):179–183

Constantoyannis C, Berk C, Honey CR et al (2005) Reducing hardware-related complications of deep brain stimulation. Can J Neurol Sci 32(2):194–200

Daniele A, Albanese A, Contarino MF et al (2003) Cognitive and behavioural effects of chronic stimulation of the subthalamic nucleus in patients with Parkinson's disease. J Neurol Neurosurg Psychiatry 74(2):175–182

Dashti SR, Baharvahdat H, Spetzler RF et al (2008) Operative intracranial infection following craniotomy. Neurosurg Focus 24(6):E10

Deuschl G, Schade-Brittinger C, Krack P et al (2006) A randomized trial of deep-brain stimulation for Parkinson's disease. N Engl J Med 355(9):896–908

Elias WJ, Sansur CA, Frysinger RC (2009) Sulcal and ventricular trajectories in stereotactic surgery. J Neurosurg 110(2):201–207

Fernandez FS, Alvarez Vega MA, Antuna Ramos A et al (2011) Lead fractures in deep brain stimulation during long-term follow-up. Parkinsons Dis 2010:409356

Follett KA, Weaver FM, Stern M et al (2010) Pallidal versus subthalamic deep-brain stimulation for Parkinson's disease. N Engl J Med 362(22):2077–2091

Gorgulho A, De Salles AA, Frighetto L et al (2005) Incidence of hemorrhage associated with electrophysiological studies performed using macroelectrodes and microelectrodes in functional neurosurgery. J Neurosurg 102(5):888–896

Gorgulho A, Juillard C, Uslan DZ et al (2009) Infection following deep brain stimulator implantation performed in the conventional versus magnetic resonance imaging-equipped operating room. J Neurosurg 110(2):239–246

Henderson JM, Tkach J, Phillips M et al (2005) Permanent neurological deficit related to magnetic resonance imaging in a patient with implanted deep brain stimulation electrodes for Parkinson's disease: case report. Neurosurgery 57(5):E1063; discussion E1063

Hu X, Jiang X, Zhou X et al (2011) Avoidance and management of surgical and hardware-related complications of deep brain stimulation. Stereotact Funct Neurosurg 88(5):296–303

Kleiner-Fisman G, Herzog J, Fisman DN et al (2006) Subthalamic nucleus deep brain stimulation: summary and meta-analysis of outcomes. Mov Disord 21(Suppl 14):S290–S304

Kulisevsky J, Berthier ML, Gironell A et al (2002) Mania following deep brain stimulation for Parkinson's disease. Neurology 59(9):1421–1424

Larson PS, Richardson RM, Starr PA et al (2008) Magnetic resonance imaging of implanted deep brain stimulators: experience in a large series. Stereotact Funct Neurosurg 86(2):92–100

Mallet L, Polosan M, Jaafari N et al (2008) Subthalamic nucleus stimulation in severe obsessive-compulsive disorder. N Engl J Med 359(20):2121–2134

Medtronic (2010a) Medtronic DBS therapy. Implanted neurostimulators. Medtronic Inc., Mineapolis

Medtronic (2010b) MRI guidelines for Medtronic deep brain stimulation systems. Medtronic Inc., Mineapolis

Middleton FA, Strick PL (1996) The temporal lobe is a target of output from the basal ganglia. Proc Natl Acad Sci U S A 93(16):8683–8687

Myslobodsky M, Lalonde FM, Hicks L (2001) Are patients with Parkinson's disease suicidal? J Geriatr Psychiatry Neurol 14(3):120–124

Nazzaro JM, Lyons KE, Wetzel LH et al (2010) Use of brain MRI after deep brain stimulation hardware implantation. Int J Neurosci 120(3):176–183

Nowak LG, Bullier J (1998) Axons, but not cell bodies, are activated by electrical stimulation in cortical gray matter. I. Evidence from chronaxie measurements. Exp Brain Res 118(4):477–488

Pahwa R, Factor SA, Lyons KE et al (2006) Practice Parameter: treatment of Parkinson disease with motor fluctuations and dyskinesia (an evidence-based review): report of the Quality Standards Subcommittee of the American Academy of Neurology. Neurology 66(7):983–995

Parent A, Hazrati LN (1995) Functional anatomy of the basal ganglia. II. The place of subthalamic nucleus and external pallidum in basal ganglia circuitry. Brain Res Brain Res Rev 20(1):128–154

Park JH, Chung SJ, Lee CS et al (2011) Analysis of hemorrhagic risk factors during deep brain stimulation surgery for movement disorders: comparison of the circumferential paired and multiple electrode insertion methods. Acta Neurochir (Wien) 153(8):1573–1578

Parsons TD, Rogers SA, Braaten AJ et al (2006) Cognitive sequelae of subthalamic nucleus deep brain stimulation in Parkinson's disease: a meta-analysis. Lancet Neurol 5(7):578–588

Pouratian N, Reames DL, Frysinger R et al (2011) Comprehensive analysis of risk factors for seizures after deep brain stimulation surgery. Clinical article. J Neurosurg 115(2):310–315

Saint-Cyr JA, Albanese A (2006) STN DBS in PD: selection criteria for surgery should include cognitive and psychiatric factors. Neurology 66(12):1799–1800

Sansur CA, Frysinger RC, Pouratian N et al (2007) Incidence of symptomatic hemorrhage after stereotactic electrode placement. J Neurosurg 107(5):998–1003

Seijo FJ, Alvarez-Vega MA, Gutierrez JC et al (2007) Complications in subthalamic nucleus stimulation surgery for treatment of Parkinson's disease. Review of 272 procedures. Acta Neurochir (Wien) 149(9):867–875; discussion 876

Sillay KA, Larson PS, Starr PA (2008) Deep brain stimulator hardware-related infections: incidence and management in a large series. Neurosurgery 62(2):360–366; discussion 366–367

Soulas T, Gurruchaga JM, Palfi S et al (2008) Attempted and completed suicides after subthalamic nucleus stimulation for Parkinson's disease. J Neurol Neurosurg Psychiatry 79(8):952–954

Spiegel J, Fuss G, Backens M et al (2003) Transient dystonia following magnetic resonance imaging in a patient with deep brain stimulation electrodes for the treatment of Parkinson disease. Case report. J Neurosurg 99(4):772–774

Sugiyama K, Yokoyama T et al (2002) Hallucination and delusion associated with electrode implantation into the subthalamic nucleus. Brain Science (Japan) 24:475–480

Tabbal SD, Revilla FJ, Mink JW et al (2007) Safety and efficacy of subthalamic nucleus deep brain stimulation

performed with limited intraoperative mapping for treatment of Parkinson's disease. Neurosurgery 61(3 Suppl):119–127; discussion 127–119
Tagliati M, Jankovic J, Pagan F et al (2009) Safety of MRI in patients with implanted deep brain stimulation devices. Neuroimage 47(Suppl 2):T53–T57
Temel Y, Wilbrink P, Duits A et al (2007) Single electrode and multiple electrode guided electrical stimulation of the subthalamic nucleus in advanced Parkinson's disease. Neurosurgery 61(5 Suppl 2):346–355; discussion 355–347
Terao T, Takahashi H, Yokochi F et al (2003) Hemorrhagic complication of stereotactic surgery in patients with movement disorders. J Neurosurg 98(6):1241–1246
Voges J, Hilker R, Botzel K et al (2007) Thirty days complication rate following surgery performed for deep-brain-stimulation. Mov Disord 22(10):1486–1489
Voon V, Krack P, Lang AE et al (2008) A multicentre study on suicide outcomes following subthalamic stimulation for Parkinson's disease. Brain 131(Pt 10):2720–2728
Weaver FM, Follett K, Stern M et al (2009) Bilateral deep brain stimulation vs best medical therapy for patients with advanced Parkinson disease: a randomized controlled trial. JAMA 301(1):63–73
Weaver FM, Follett KA, Stern M et al (2012) Randomized trial of deep brain stimulation for Parkinson disease: thirty-six-month outcomes. Neurology 79(1):55–65
Xiaowu H, Xiufeng J, Xiaoping Z et al (2011) Risks of intracranial hemorrhage in patients with Parkinson's disease receiving deep brain stimulation and ablation. Parkinsonism Relat Disord 16(2):96–100
Yokoyama T, Ando N, Sugiyama K et al (2006) Relationship of stimulation site location within the subthalamic nucleus region to clinical effects on parkinsonian symptoms. Stereotact Funct Neurosurg 84(4):170–175
Zrinzo L, Foltynie T, Limousin P et al (2011) Reducing hemorrhagic complications in functional neurosurgery: a large case series and systematic literature review. J Neurosurg 116(1):84–94

Index

T. Itakura (ed.), *Deep Brain Stimulation for Neurological Disorders: Theoretical Background and Clinical Application*, DOI 10.1007/978-3-319-08476-3,

The manufacturer's authorised representative in the EU is Springer Nature Customer Service Centre GmbH, Europaplatz 3, 69115 Heidelberg, Germany. If you have any concerns regarding our products, please contact ProductSafety@springernature.com

Printed and bound by CPI Group (UK) Ltd, Croydon, CR0 4YY
22/09/2026
02221056-0004